YOUR HOME, YOUR HEALTH, AND WELL-BEING

What you can do to design or renovate your house or apartment to be free of outdoor AND indoor pollution

YOUR HOME, YOUR HEALTH, AND WELL-BEING

by David Rousseau
W. J. Rea, M.D.
Jean Enwright

A Cloudburst Press Book
Hartley & Marks, Publishers

Published by
Hartley & Marks, Ltd.
3663 West Broadway
Vancouver, B.C.
V6R 2B8

Third Printing, 1989

ISBN 0-88179-017-6 paperback

Cover photo courtesy of Richard MacMath,
Sunstructures, Inc., Ann Arbor, Michigan.

CONTENTS

INTRODUCTION

DON'T BE ALARMED, BUT BE PREPARED

The most significant physical feature of civilization has been our move away from the natural environment and into a built environment. Our homes and cities have changed dramatically through time, but never so rapidly as in the brief period since WW II. Our buildings of only two generations ago were loose and forgiving, because they were built from natural materials and relied largely upon natural lighting and ventilation. Increasingly, however, today's built environments are closed systems filled with synthetic materials, often with conditions that are beyond the control of the people who use them. In the last fifty years, drafty, daylit buildings of wood or masonry relatively free from noxious chemicals have been replaced by tightly sealed, deep core buildings filled with a vast variety of synthetic products, and jammed with mechanical and electrical equipment. The result is a growing body of evidence suggesting that today's man-made environments are a major cause of irritation, stress, and disease.

The California Department of Consumer Affairs, in a 1982 report on air quality, concluded: "There is increasing evidence that many modern buildings are damaging the health of the people who live and work in them. Building design changes intended to conserve energy, new materials used in construction, and the presence indoors of numerous hazardous substances, are combining to make this indoor environment where most Americans spend 90 percent of their time, an unhealthy place." Home building technology has been advancing rapidly in the past two decades, and widespread new building codes for ALL homes now specify airtightness and insulation levels unheard of a decade ago. While the capability for improved comfort, energy efficiency, and control of indoor air quality are part of this new technology, indoor air quality remains entirely dependent on reduction of the contaminants in the home AND the provision of effective ventilation.

Along with our new knowledge about environmental hazards, new advances in home ventilation systems are appearing rapidly, and we must keep pace with these changes in order to prevent environmental disasters in our homes.

"Environmental disease" is a recently coined term for a range of ailments affecting a growing number of people who suffer allergic reactions to the chemical and biological conditions around them. It is now becoming clear that environmental disease can be acquired with repeated exposure to chemical irritants, and that it may be aggravated by unwanted physical and psychological stress. Continued exposure to toxic conditions, even at low levels, may also be responsible for a large number of the chronic problems that we have come to accept as part of the aging process. The increase in minor skin problems that often accompanies aging is an example of this. The proliferation of new chemical products and their introduction into building materials, furnishings, finishes, and maintenance products, is continuing at an alarming rate and often without the consumer's knowledge.

When these chemically treated materials are brought into airtight, poorly ventilated buildings, the resulting stress conditions press the limits of human adaptability.

Both in the workplace and in public places our experience with these new conditions has been very limited; our control over them is equally limited. In contrast, our home is the one place where we *can* have a large degree of control. For those concerned about preventive health measures and for those who are already sensitive or hypersensitive to environmental conditions, the home can be made a sanctuary, as free as possible from the assaults on health and peace of mind suffered elsewhere.

This book will be about the home as a place to promote well-being, and will delineate the steps necessary to make it so. It is based on the concept of using design to reduce environmental stress—good design which incorporates a firm understanding of human needs. For design to be health promoting, more than the traditional attention to spatial planning and esthetics is required; it must also include planning for total environmental quality, including air quality and freedom from toxic chemicals. Our traditional view of architectural design as an esthetic, practical process must be expanded to include a more complete and holistic understanding of the links between people and the built environment. Though many of the pieces in this complex linkage are not yet understood, we already have a large body of knowledge and a number of clues that can be integrated into health directed home design and renovation.

This book will serve as a guide to healthy home design by discussing the environmental factors in the home and how to assess them; design principles and practical details for preventing environmental problems; materials by generic type and their health-related properties; and specific features designed for the chemically hypersensitive. Included is an introduction to the medical problem of hypersensitivity (environmental illness) by a well-known expert in the field, and a personal account by someone who suffers from this condition.

The continually growing number of hypersensitive people can be seen as a warning that certain environmental conditions will promote illness. Freedom from sensitivity may be considered a valuable and, perhaps, temporary condition for many of us who now enjoy good health. The best ways to perpetuate good health are through positive environmental conditions and a health promoting lifestyle.

A Note on the Organization of this Book

Because of the interconnected nature of environmental information, and to avoid repetition, it has been necessary to include many cross references. (To understand radon, for example, one must read the sections on: indoor hazards, ventilation, construction notes, and testing for contamination, all of which are treated separately.)

ACKNOWLEDGEMENTS

The author expresses grateful thanks to co-author Dr. William J. Rea for his valuable manuscript suggestions. He also wishes to thank Mary Oetzel, and Dona Shrier, environmental housing consultants, and Dr. Ronald Greenberg, clinical ecologist, for their assistance.

Acknowledgement is also due to the Human Ecology Research Foundation of the Southwest, and the Human Ecology Action League, and to the published work of Bruce Small, Dr. Mike Samuels and Hal Zina Bennett, Dr. Iris Bell, Karl Raab, The Canada Mortgage and Housing Corporation, The U.S. Environmental Protection Agency, and the U.S. Department of Energy.

A special thanks goes to Susanne Tauber, editorial director of Hartley and Marks, Publishers, whose continuing inspiration and endless patience made it all possible.

This book is dedicated to all who believe that environmental awareness begins at home, and whose concerned, informed actions are helping restore our planet to health.

Health and Comfort Factors for Each Room

BASEMENT
Chapter 15

AIR QUALITY & VENTILATION	Flue gases: p. 52–53, 56, 65–67; Ventilation: fig. 18-8; Chimney Safety: p. 144–45
LIGHTING	Stairs: fig. 2-2
THERMAL COMFORT	Humidity: p. 22–25, 137
SOUND CONTROL	fig. 29-68, 29-70, 29-72, 29-75
OTHERS	Radon: p. 50, 68–71, fig. 29.3; Fungus: p. 61, 75–76, 151; Dampness: fig. 29-3 to 29-7

BATHROOM
Chapter 14

AIR QUALITY & VENTILATION	Ventilation: p. 121, fig. 18-10, 18-13; Radon: fig. 7-7
LIGHTING	Color: p. 10
THERMAL COMFORT	Humidity: p. 22, 137, fig. 18-15, 18-20; Separate Heating: p. 138–39
SOUND CONTROL	p. 33
OTHER	Fungus Control: p. 153; Dampness: p. 129–30; Water Quality: p. 157, 167, Table 21-1, 21-2

BEDROOM/RETREAT Chapter 13		
	AIR QUALITY & VENTILATION	Cross Ventilation: fig. 18-6; Air Purification: p. 131–35
	LIGHTING	Daylight: p. 18–20, fig. 2–4, 29–1; Color: p. 18
	THERMAL COMFORT	Separate Heating: p. 138–39
	SOUND CONTROL	p. 33, fig. 29-68 to 29-74
	OTHER	Bedding: p. 192; Furniture: p. 190

ENTRY Chapter 9		
	AIR QUALITY & VENTILATION	Weatherseal: p. 183
	LIGHTING	Daylight: fig. 2-4, 2-5
	THERMAL COMFORT	Separate Heating: p. 138–39
	SOUND CONTROL	p. 30-32
	OTHER	Exhaust gases: fig. 8-1, 18-16

- GARAGE Chapter 17
  - AIR QUALITY & VENTILATION — Exhaust Gases: p. 52–53, fig. 17-1, 18-16
  - OTHER — Storage: p. 74, Ch. 16

- KITCHEN Chapter 11
  - AIR QUALITY & VENTILATION — Range Exhaust: fig. 11-1; Electric Cooking: p. 66
  - LIGHTING — Daylight: fig. 29-1; Electric Lighting: fig. 2-3, 11-7, 29-80 to 29-83
  - THERMAL COMFORT — Humidity: fig. 18-15, 18-20
  - SOUND CONTROL — p. 29–30, Table 4-1
  - OTHER — Appliances: p. 199–200; Food Storage: p. 59–60; Water Quality: Ch. 21, Table 21-3

- LIVING ROOM Chapter 10
  - AIR QUALITY & VENTILATION — Cross Ventilation: fig. 18-2, 18-3, 18-5, 18-6; Chimney Safety: p. 144–45
  - LIGHTING — Daylight: p. 18–20, fig. 2-4 to 2-6, 29-1
  - THERMAL COMFORT — Heating/Cooling: Ch. 19
  - SOUND CONTROL — p. 30–32, fig. 29-69 to 29-75
  - OTHER — Furniture: p. 190; Floor Cover: p. 187

- SANCTUARY Chapter 25
  - AIR QUALITY & VENTILATION
    - Air Purification: p. 131–35, fig. 18-21
  - LIGHTING
    - Daylight: p. 18–20, fig. 29-1
  - THERMAL COMFORT
    - Separate Heating: p. 138–39; Humidity: p. 25, fig. 3-2
  - SOUND CONTROL
    - p. 33, fig. 29-68 to 29-74
  - OTHER
    - Materials Selection: Ch. 22

- STORAGE Chapter 16
  - AIR QUALITY & VENTILATION
    - Separate Ventilation: p. 74

- SUNSPACE/ GREENHOUSE Chapter 12
  - AIR QUALITY & VENTILATION
    - Extra Ventilation Capacity: fig. 18-6
  - LIGHTING
    - Ultraviolet Exposure: p. 16, 19; Sunlight: fig. 29-1
  - THERMAL COMFORT
    - Humidity: p. 22–25; Radiant Comfort: fig. 3-1
  - OTHER
    - Fungus: p. 61, 75–76; Pest Control: p. 47, 73

MAJOR CONTAMINANTS IN THE HOME, AND THEIR SOURCES

Contaminant	Sources	References
AMMONIA	Household ammonia, window cleaners, cleaners, glue, paint.	Chapter 20
ASBESTOS	Street dust, old plaster, ceiling tile, wallboard, floor tile, heating ducts, insulation.	Chapters 6, 28
CARBON DIOXIDE	Poor ventilation, fuel burning stoves and heaters, faulty chimneys, respiration.	Chapters 5, 6, 7, 18
CARBON MONOXIDE	Auto exhaust, open flame, fuel burning stoves and heaters, faulty chimneys, natural oxidation of household chemicals.	Chapters 5, 6, 7, 8, 11, 17, 19, 27
CHLORINE AND ORGANOCHLORINES	Bleach, scouring powder, pesticides, chlorinated water, plastics and rubber.	Chapters 5, 6, 7, 20, 21
DUST	Pollens, soil, auto exhaust, industrial emissions, pets, construction, smoking, cooking, fires, carpets, fabrics, building materials	Chapters 6, 7, 18, 20, 29
FORMALDEHYDE	Incinerators, auto exhaust, industrial emissions, insulation, glue, carpet, fabric treatments, paints, waxes, polishes, insecticides, paper treatments, plastics, wood treatments, concrete and plaster additives, wallboard, toothpaste, mouthwash, germicides, cosmetics.	Chapters 5, 6, 7, 18, 20, 22, 27
FUNGUS	Yard and garden, dampness in bathrooms and basements, walls, ceilings and floors, mildew in bedding, carpets, fabrics and clothing, refrigerators, spoiled food, humidifiers.	Chapters 3, 6, 7, 8, 11, 12, 14, 15, 19
GAS (Natural Gas, Propane, Butane)	Heating and cooking fuel, campstoves, lanterns,lighters, hairspray.	Chapters, 7, 11, 19, 22

Contaminant	Sources	References
LEAD	Auto exhaust, industrial emission, water pipes, old paint.	Chapters 6, 21
MERCURY	Industrial emissions, paints, contaminated water	Chapters 6, 22
PHENOLS	Disinfectants, cleaners, glues, mildew cleaner, plastics, wood preservatives, waxes and polishes, air fresheners.	Chapters 6, 20
NITROGEN OXIDES	Auto exhaust, industrial emissions, fuel burning stoves and heaters, faulty chimneys, cooking.	Chapters 6, 11, 18, 19
OTHER VOLATILE ORGANIC COMPOUNDS		
Alcohols	shellac, inks, cleaners, disinfectants, rubber and plastics, cosmetics, medications, food flavorings, liquor	Chapters 16, 20
Fuels and lubricants	gasoline, diesel, motor oils, household oils	Chapters 16, 17
Propellants and refrigerants	aerosol sprays, air conditioners, refrigerators, heat pumps	Chapters 11, 19, 20
Solvents	paints, varnishes, cleaners, glues, waxes, polishes, dry cleaning fluid	Chapters 6, 20
Wood resins	plant terpenes from softwoods (pine, fir, spruce, cedar, cypress, hemlock), cones, needles or pitch, turpentine	Chapter 22
Scents	perfumed soaps and cleaners, plants and flowers, artificial flavorings	Chapters 18, 20
OZONE	Urban air pollution, electronic air cleaners and ionizers, electric motors, photocopiers.	Chapters 5, 6, 7, 18
RADON	Soil, rock, deep well water, concrete, stone, brick, gypsum board.	Chapters 6, 7, 27, 29
SULFUR DIOXIDE	Industrial emissions, fuel oil and coal burning.	Chapters 6, 7, 18

HOMEBUYER'S/RENTER'S CHECKLIST

When looking for a home to rent or buy, the usual concerns are for the suitability of the floor plan, the home's appearance its location, condition, and price. The health conscious buyer or tenant will also check the home for a number of the health and comfort concerns covered in this book. This is absolutely essential if there is a chemically sensitive individual in the household.

This list includes the most important of the home's possible environmental problems. Using it when evaluating or comparing homes will require a lot of careful observation. You might find it helpful to apply a scoring system, giving a 4 for example to indicate an excellent or preferred condition, a 2 for an average or acceptable one, and a 0 for an unacceptable one.

Your observations will be the most important part of the evaluation, so spend plenty of time looking at details, crawling in attics, and sniffing around basements. Go prepared with a flashlight, screwdriver, clipboard, and plenty of note paper.

This list starts with the outdoor items, and proceeds from the largest to the smallest. If you do not feel competent to judge a prospective home in this way, there are professionals who survey homes, looking particularly for maintenance, structural, electrical, and plumbing problems. If you make inquiries, you may be able to find a health conscious home survey professional. (Eg., Under Building Inspection Services, in the Yellow Pages of the Telephone book.)

The Home's Site

Air Pollution: Check for agriculture, industry, urban or automotive pollution.

Light and Sun: Are there obstructions, such as tall buildings or trees?

Noise: Check for sources, such as highway, street, rail, airport, industry, or business.

Wind: Check for exposure to storm winds.

Electromagnetic Fields: Are there high power lines, radio, T.V., or microwave installations nearby which may cause hazardous fields.

The Yard

Drainage: Check for low spots and poorly drained clay soil.

Allergenic and Poisonous Plants: Are there plants which are known allergens to family members. Check for plants which are poisonous to children and pets.

The Building Materials

Insulation: Check for Urea Formaldehyde Foam Insulation (U.F.F.I.), or residues if it has been removed. It appears as a light brown, foamy mass, or as a residual crust or powder. Check attic and basement perimeters, especially where wires or pipes enter walls. Remove electrical cover plates on outside walls and look for foam or residue. **Any U.F.F.I. is unacceptable.**

Inside finish: Look for the preferred materials of lath and plaster, cement, ceramics, and hardwood where possible. Check for interior plywood, simulated wood wall board, or vinyl finished wall board (like that used in mobile homes) which are sources of indoor pollution.

Frame materials: Check for wood assemblies joined with glue, or types of wood whicha re allergenic to family members.

Exterior Finish: Check for preservative treated wood, particularly creosote (black and tarry), or pentachlorophenol treatments (usually light green). These are hazardous.

Condition: Is there rot, mildew, and moisture damage, such as blistering paint? Use a small penknife to probe wood for soft, rotting areas.

The Foundation

Soundness: Check for cracks, or signs or excessive settling, like gaps between foundation and framing, lifted chimney flashing.

Drainage: Check for downpipes discharging onto the ground, water stains, or other signs of poor drainage.

Rot: Check for wood exposed to earth or to excessive moisture.

Insect Attack: Check for termite tubes or cells, wood parts less than 1 ft. above ground, or lack of proper metal guards and flashings. Beetle, worm, or ant infestation is usually apparent from bore holes in wood, with powdery or granular castings below.

The Basement/Crawlspace

Drainage: Check floor drains or sumps by running a hose in them for 5 minutes to see if they back up. Check carefully for water marks or damage from flooding.

Dampness: Are there cracks in walls or slab, leaking or sweating pipes, and damp insulation?

Fungus: Are there musty odors, mildew stains, and wood in contact with damp concrete?

Ventilation: Check for inadequate or blocked ventilation openings or windows.

The Roof

Attic Ventilation: Check for inadequate or blocked gable vents, soffit vents, and ridge vents.

Insulation: Check for inadequate or uneven coverage. Check if loosefill insulation is blocking vents and recessed lights, or sifting into living space.

Roofing Materials: Check for asphalt materials close to doors or opening windows if there are chemically sensitive people in the household.

Condition: Check for leaks, damaged shingles, and corroded flashings which may lead to dampness in the attic.

The Kitchen

Range: Gas ranges, whether new or old, are serious sources of indoor pollution.

Ventilation: Are there unvented ranges or vent hoods without outside ducts? Preferred ventilators are rated for 200 cfm. or more. (Check the identification plate.) There should be at least one opening window.

Cabinets: Are there particle board (pressed board) cabinet frames which release formaldehyde?

Floor covering: Check for soft vinyl or cushion vinyl flooring, and particle board floor underlayment. These contribute to air pollution. Kitchen carpet is unacceptable, because it traps moisture and spills.

Moisture damage: Check for dampness or rot under cabinet tops, around sinks, at baseboards, or at splash boards.

The Bathroom

Ventilation: Look for a vent fan rated for 100 cfm. or more (check the identification plate), or at least one opening window.

Moisture Damage: Check around tub and shower, behind and under toilet, and behind sink for mildew, dampness, or rot.

Floor Covering: Is there carpet or particle board underlayment? These are prone to moisture damage, and are also sources or indoor pollution.

Heat: Look for a heater or heat lamp adequate for quick drying of bathroom moisture.

The Living Room

Cross Ventilation: Look for at least two opening windows, preferably on opposite sides.

Floor coverings: Is there permanently fastened carpeting or underlayment. These contribute to air pollution and cannot be safely cleaned.

The Bedrooms

Ventilation: Look for at least one opening window.

Soundproofing: Check for windows facing noise sources or unsoundproofed walls or ceiling adjoining noisy rooms.

Storage: Look for adequate storage for clothing and possessions, preferably separated from the bedroom.

The Garage

Common Wall: Are there openings or connections between garage and living space? Detached garages are best.

The Windows

Type: Check for inadequate single glass in cold regions or in noisy locations. Metal frames are best where there is someone who is chemically sensitive in the household.

Weatherseal: Are there poor fitting or stuck windows? Look for weatherstrips (and thermal breaks on metal frames to prevent condensation).

Adequate Ventilation: Are there enough opening units to provide whole house ventilation in warm weather?

Condition: Check for rot in frames and sash. Check condition of putty or gaskets.

Heating/Cooling/Water Heating Systems

Fuel: Look for electric systems, where possible. Fuel burning appliances, particularly gas and oil, are sources of indoor pollution.

Type: Look for liquid type radiators, where possible. Warm air systems and electric baseboard heaters aggravate dust problems.

Chimneys: Where fuel burning appliances are necessary, check for sound chimneys, free of cracks. There must be a combustion air supply to each unit, and a draft control on oil burner chimneys.

Condition: Are there signs of fuel leaks or aging equipment?

The Electrical System

Type of Wiring: Look for the preferred conduit or metallic sheathed cable systems, where possible. Is there knob and tube wiring (in older homes) that may have to be replaced due to fire hazards? (This is made up from single wires passing through porcelain "knobs and tubes.")

Circuit Adequacy: Look for a minimum of 24 circuits in the supply panel for a full sized home, and at least one three pin grounded outlet per wall in every room. If fuses are in use. are they the "safety type" which cannot be tampered with? Check for old or inadequate kitchen wiring which may be a hazard.

Condition: Is there brittle, cracked wire insulation, particularly in ceiling boxes. Check for careless or dangerous looking connections or additions.

The Water System

Water Quality: Check municipal water quality if on a city system. This information is available from the water works or health department. If a well or spring is in use, ask for recent water test results or take one yourself.

Plumbing Type: Look for the preferred all copper water supply piping. Are there iron or plastic segments which will have to be replaced?

Condition: Check any iron drain pipes for leakage or corrosion.

Miscellaneous

Asbestos: In older homes is there crumbling plaster or ceiling tile in which may contain asbestos? In broken pieces the fibers can be seen as irregular white strands.

Mildew problems: In cold or damp climates check all indoor surfaces carefully for stains or odors from fungus.

Paint types: There may be lead based paints in older houses. Any room that has not been painted for more than 20 years may have lead based paint, and may need to be repainted.

Radon: Check with local health authorities, or the United States Environmental Protection Agency's regional office (the Environment Ministry in Canada), to find out if radon is a problem in the area. If it is, get radon test results for the home before buying or moving in.

Septic Tank: Ask for a plan of the septic tank and leach field. Check carefully for signs of surface seepage over the field. Flush toilets repeatedly to see that the tank does not "back up" causing drains to overflow.

SECTION I

Health Related Factors in the Home

1 INDOOR AIR QUALITY

Indoor air quality is the best, most accessible indicator for evaluating the health aspects of an interior environment. Though interiors influence us via a range of physical and psychological factors (discussed in later chapters), the air breathed within a building has a major effect, containing as it does chemical components and traces from both the building itself, and its surrounding air, as well as from its occupants and their activities. Sampling this air with our senses or with sophisticated instruments can provide us with a great deal of information relevant to our health.

Basically, air is a mixture of gases essential to life. It is made up of nitrogen, oxygen, carbon dioxide, and a large number of trace gases, as well as varying amounts of water vapor. What we call "natural" air is found out of doors in settings relatively free from industrial, urban, or automotive pollution. It carries a host of "dust" particles containing soil, microorganisms, pollens, and other plant and animal byproducts. It also contains a large number of other components, such as minerals and ash, and various gases from natural processes. This dust will vary greatly from region to region, as well as with season and weather conditions. Its components are not essential to us, and can be serious irritants to the ten percent of us suffering from pollen and dust related allergies. It also contains toxic man-made substances which are hazardous to everyone.

"Natural" air would, of course, be ideal for human life, but it is no longer readily available except in remote, unsettled regions. The air most of us breathe carries industrial pollution, and particles and gases from human settlement, including automotive exhaust, agricultural chemicals, smoke and gases from heating fuels and incinerators, and a large number of other toxic products. These components are concentrated in urban areas, where they interact with sunlight, moisture, and heat, to create what we all recognize as smog. This man-made atmosphere has been recognized as a serious hazard to health for more than a century. However, some of the hazardous factors in polluted air cannot even be seen or sensed, and have only been recently identified. Yet this is the condition of the air available to most of us, and this is the air we bring into our buildings to breathe, recirculate, and then expel.

Because the air we breathe has such a direct influence on us, air quality often becomes the central issue when evaluating the healthfulness of an interior. An air sample's chemical composition can be measured with tremendous accuracy by complex equipment that can detect some components in concentrations as small as a few parts per million (ppm), or even parts per billion (ppb). Whether such levels are hazardous to our health is a subject for lively debate among a variety of professionals, government regulatory agencies, and environmental advocates. While the debate continues, legal battles are also being waged over responsibility for injuries suffered due to exposure to hazardous substances in the workplace and in the home.

The term "air quality" actually describes very complex assessments based on assumptions, as well as established facts about what makes an air supply good or even acceptable from a health standpoint. Maximum concentration standards have been set for many components of air, and in some places these have become a part of regulations or recommendations for public buildings and workplaces. But there are other components, even those recognized as hazardous, for which maximum levels have not been established. *In any case, the existence of recommendations or regulations does not mean that these standards will be applied and monitored, or that so-called "acceptable" levels are safe for everyone.*

Not only is our home the one environment over which we can exert a large measure of control, it is also the place in which most of us spend more than half of our lives. The qualities of this place are very important to our health, safety, and comfort. When we consider the quality of this home environment there will be little need to refer to technical standards, or for costly measurement techniques. Though we can learn from the public debate about air standards, our goal will be to avoid or eliminate all objectionable conditions in our homes, and to design them so that they will be well suited to the people living there. To do this, some knowledge will be useful, and for the most part our senses will be the only sophisticated "instruments" required for measurement. However, for some things, such as radioactive radon, testing will be needed.

The Recent History of Air Quality in the Home

Only two generations ago the home was a much simpler environment. A few basic building materials and a small range of finishes and fabric types made up the list of components that might be included. Concrete, masonry, softwoods, and asphalt products were the basic structural materials, and oil base paints, varnishes and sealants, paper products, ceramics, hardwoods, and fibers such as cotton, wool, and jute, made up the finishes and furnishings. Plastics and modern adhesives were just being introduced to the building industry, and most of the surfacing and finishing, such as plaster and woodwork, was still being done on site by craftsmen who selected and mixed their own materials. During this period, the major man-made hazards to health were combustion byproducts, such as carbon monoxide and carbon dioxide (which could be produced by poorly vented or unvented stoves or heaters), lead from paints and plumbing, a few household pesticides and cleaning chemicals (sometimes used indiscriminately), asbestos, and a few other items.

The building was usually not insulated or weather-sealed to any extent, and vapor barriers for moisture control were virtually unknown. *Natural infiltration of fresh air, at rates that provided one and a half complete air changes or more each hour, were the* norm, and it was safe to assume that any pollution buildup would be safely diluted. But with the advent of automatic heating and air conditioning systems, there was a new need for tighter buildings which would allow indoor climate control with a minimum of outside influences. At the same time, the available outdoor air in many urban regions was deteriorating rapidly as automobile traffic increased.

As the heating and cooling of large commercial buildings required heavy investments, and as operating costs grew, the tendency toward more tightly sealed and climate controlled buildings increased dramatically. At the same time, the popularity of large glass areas in modern building design, and the settlement of regions with extreme climates, such as the southwest desert, led to the present situation, in which the operation of many buildings relies heavily on cheap energy to run cooling/heating plants. These plants, in order to maintain a reasonable level of comfort against the assault of harsh climates on glass buildings, and to overcome excess interior heat, must recirculate most of the air they handle, since incoming air must be expensively cooled or heated before it can be introduced. These same concerns have now become felt by apartment dwellers, and in family homes, though homes and home designs have changed more slowly.

With the energy crisis of the mid 1970's and the increased cost of all forms of energy came both the development of the energy efficient house, and reduced air quality standards for commercial buildings (especially allowable carbon dioxide levels and air

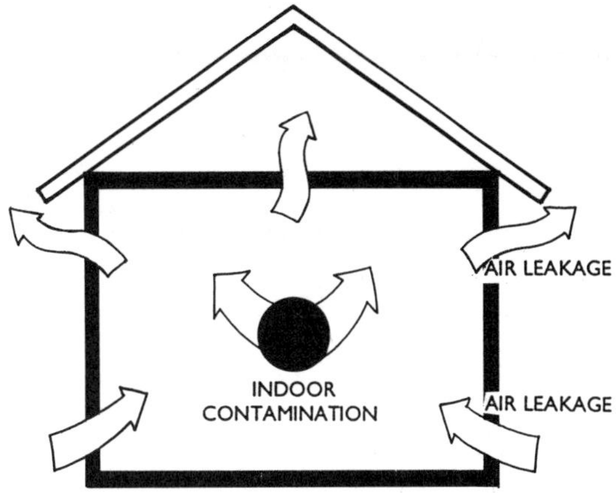

Fig. 1-1 Older Leaky House. *Indoor air contamination is readily diluted by random air change. Safer building materials also contribute to a lower contamination load.*

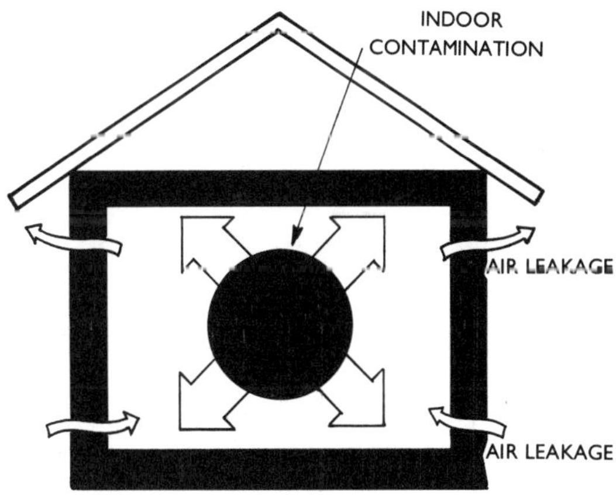

Fig. 1-2 Newer Tight House. *Indoor air contaminants can build up in a tight house unless air change is intentionally provided. The total contamination load is high, due to the prevalence of new synthetic building materials.*

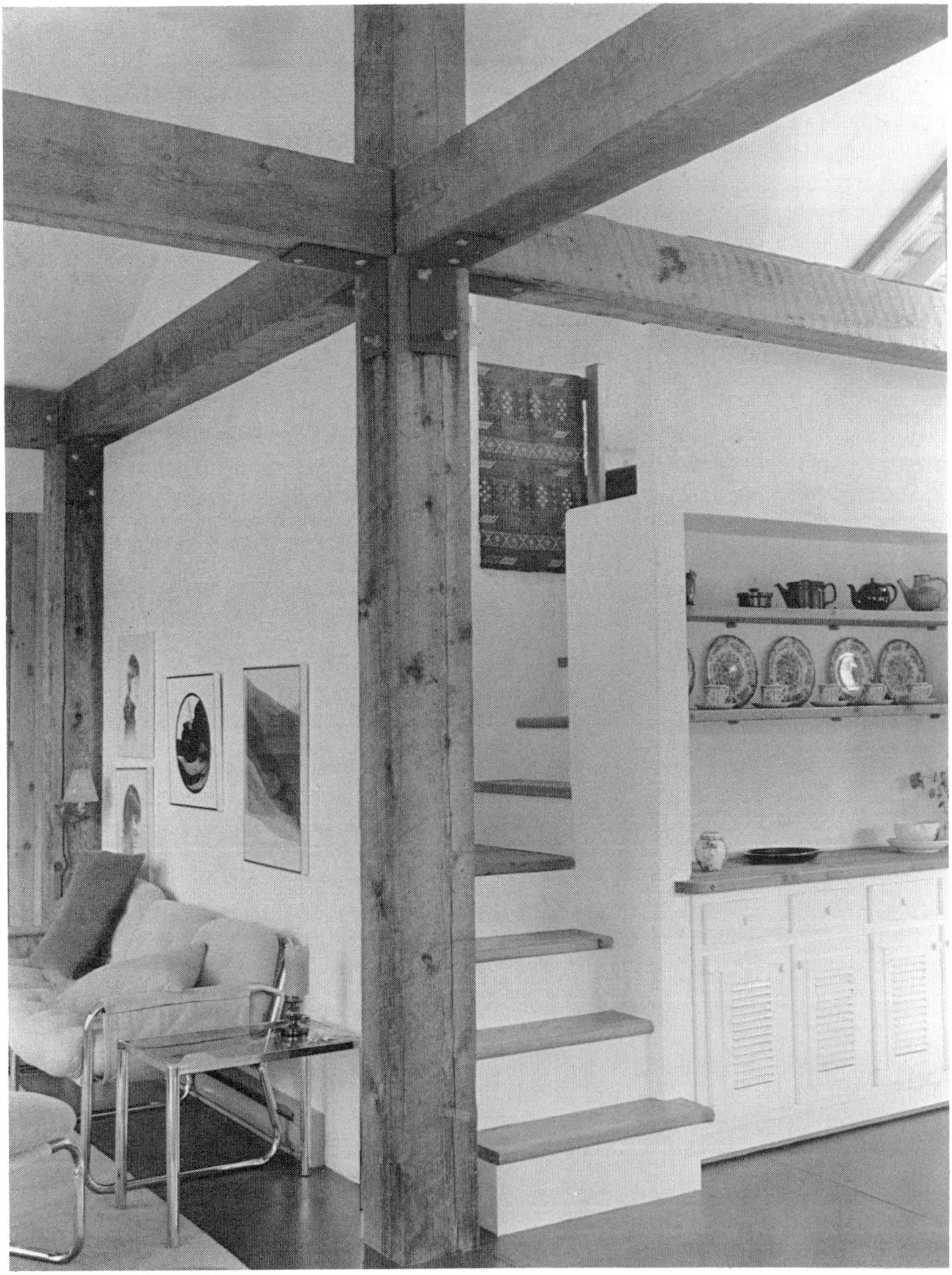

A contemporary interior with traditional, non-contaminating walls and ceilings, and furnishings of steel, glass, and natural fibres. Photo: G. Czember

change rates). The result for home design has been a dramatic increase in energy consciousness leading to new residential building standards. The drafty, uninsulated house of an earlier era has been replaced with a heavily insulated, well sealed building with small windows and controlled ventilation rates. *Today an energy efficient home's fresh air supply during the cooling or heating season may be less than one half an air change per hour, or one third of what it was a generation ago.* And the fresh air needed to dilute the hazardous products of combustion, cooking, respiration, electrical equipment, and the ever-present release of toxic chemicals from building materials, finishes, cleaners, household and garden chemicals, fabrics, and other products is still more necessary.

Over the last twenty years the use of chemicals in the production of building materials and fabrics has increased more than five fold (particularly with the plastics and polymers used in finishes and adhesives). At the same time the number of household products available for cleaning, sanitizing, deodorizing, polishing, and "protecting" has increased from a few hundred to many thousand. In fact, it is very difficult to find any manufactured item today which does not contain chemicals to which many people are uncomfortably sensitive, and which will be clearly irritating or dangerous to some. Their long term effects on human health remain largely unknown, because manufacturers have not been required to investigate them, and are often not required to divulge a full list of contents for their products. In evolutionary terms, our entire experience with these conditions covers only two generations, a very brief moment in human history.

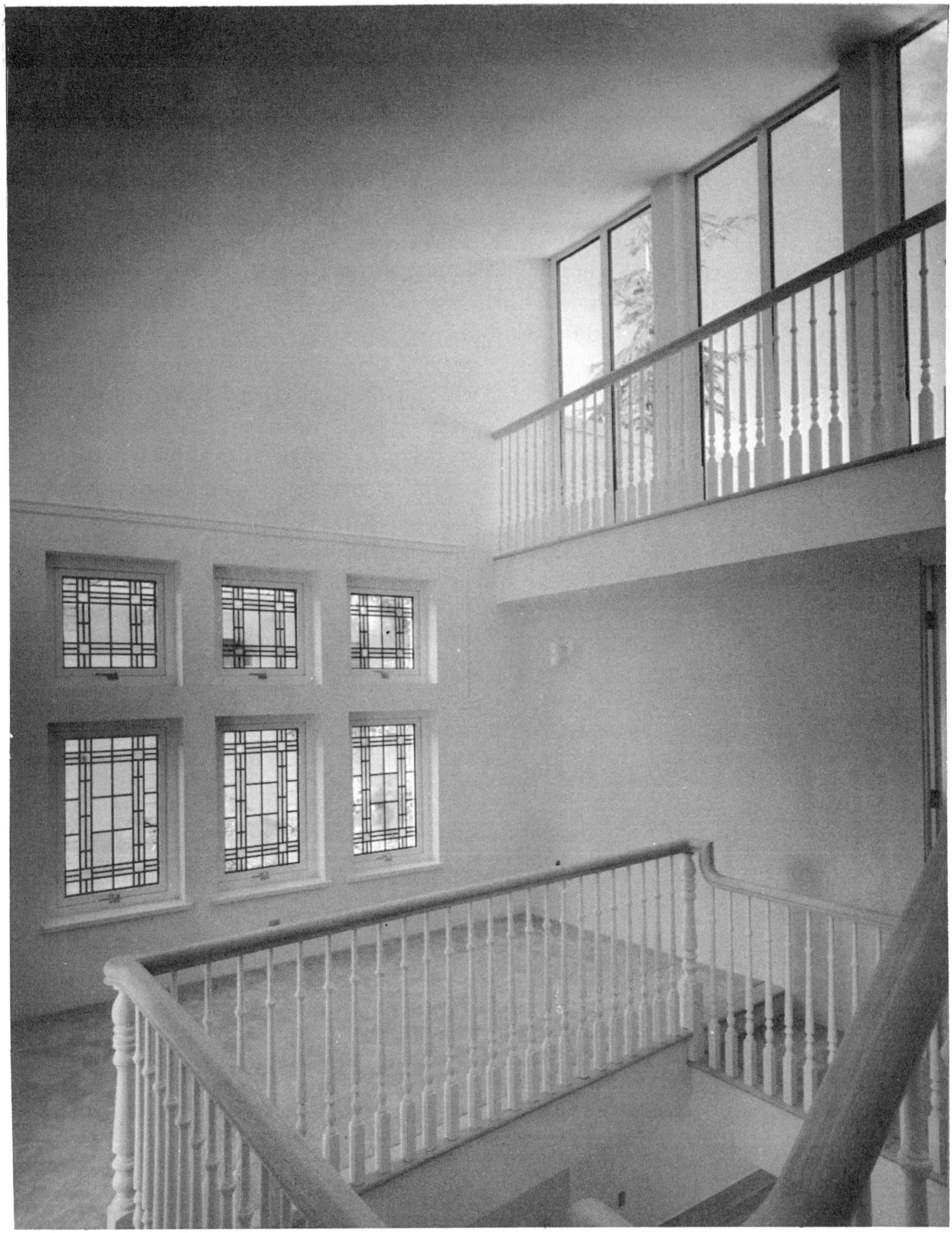

Dramatically placed abundant natural light is a special feature in this clean air house. Design by D. McIntyre and E. M. Sterling. Photo: Anthony Fulker Photography

2 LIGHT AND COLOR

Like all living creatures we are influenced by the rhythm of day and night, sun and moon, and the change of seasons. Light is also the most potent force through which most of us experience our surroundings. Psychologists tell us that vision dominates 70% of our senses, and light is one of the strongest poetic metaphors that we know in literature and religion. It has been described as emanating from the gods, as an earthly force, and as an illusion. The light in our homes is also important for good physical and emotional health. Though the importance of light for physical health has been recognized for centuries, the role of light in treating depression is only now being discovered.

Light is essential to most living things. *Our daily and seasonal rhythms are determined by inner biological clocks which are set by changes in light.* It's the bright morning light which stimulates us to make a start each day, while the soft light of evening invites rest. The bright summer sun energizes us to prepare for winter and survival. Sunlight also acts on the skin to produce essential vitamin D, increases calcium absorption and bone growth, and through the eyes it stimulates the pituitary, which regulates gland and brain function. *Of course, excessive sunlight (or exposure to strong lamps, such as sunlamps) can also be dangerous to our health and can cause skin cancer.*

How We are Affected by Light

The eye receives light reflected from an object and, after focusing for distance and adapting for brightness conditions, forms an image on the retina. This image is interpreted by the brain, where it is associated with memories of other images. Our perceptions are influenced by many things, such as the objects' qualities, the lighting on it, the background, patterns, and intensities of light, and the condition of the person observing. Our vision is most acute over a very small area (about 2°) at the center of our field of view. Beyond that, color and detail are only perceived throughout a wider central zone, about 45° wide. This makes the position of the observer very important when considering the impact of any visual information.

Our visual *attention* is strongly influenced by the brightness of the objects we see, the brightest being most noticed. Our eyes can adapt to a wide range of overall brightness, but are quite sensitive to variations between lighter and darker areas of the same visual field. This is called contrast, and we experience excessive contrast as glare. When limits of acceptable contrast are exceeded, we become uncomfortable, and experience eyestrain and headaches. In some situations it can even be hazardous, as where glare from a poorly placed window or lamp makes it difficult to judge stairs, or where eyestrain caused by poor lighting leads to fatigue, errors, and accidents. Good lighting is especially necessary for older people. Our vision deteriorates with age, so that higher light levels and better contrast become necessary for detailed tasks, such as reading. This becomes significant for most people after the age of 50.

COLOR AND PERCEPTION

Color influences our perceptions and emotions, and the colors of the light we absorb may affect our well-being. Every source of light is made up of colors that affect the way we see the color of things. A perfectly white surface will faithfully reflect all colors of the light that falls on it, while a colored surface will selectively reflect only those colors in the light that are related to it. A blue surface will appear blue and bright under some light, such as midday natural light containing blue, yellow, and green, but will appear very dark and muddy under evening light which is mostly red. This phenomenon is very important when selecting electric lamps to suit a certain mood, or to give our skin an appealing appearance. Lighting designers use "warm" lamps in homes and clothing stores, for example, where their yellow and red colors flatter us, but will use "cool" lamps, such as daylight or cool white fluorescents, in a doctor's examining room, where observing slight changes in skin color may be an important part of diagnosing disease.

The colors we see influence our mood and psychological condition in subtle ways, and while studies are difficult to interpret and not very conclusive, a few things can be said with certainty. Though our responses to color are generally very individual, and a product of our personality and experience, warm colors, such as red and yellow, are generally associated with feelings of warmth and with emotional stimulation. These are termed the "active" colors. Bright light has a similar "activating" effect on us, up to the point where it becomes irritating. Cool colors, such as green and blue, are generally associated with feelings of coolness and more "passive," relaxing, and thoughtful states. Under suitable circumstances, dim light has a similar relaxing effect for many people. Color can also influence children's performance in school, and their comfort at home. Psychologists have experimented with color schemes for schools and found that many children will perform better in rooms with "active, stimulating" color schemes, and feel more relaxed in other areas with more "passive" color schemes. This suggests that a room's color scheme can be matched to its intended use with some success. A child's play or study area, for example, can be decorated with bright, warm active colors, and a sleeping area with cool, subdued colors.

There are also therapeutic uses of color, particularly for children, but there is a curious paradox in color response among children who are extremely active or very passive. The very active seem to find bright, warm colors *relaxing,* rather than stimulating, while passive children seem to be *activated* by cool colors, rather than relaxed.

Color is also useful in altering the perception of rooms and objects. Rooms finished in white, or very light colors, appear larger, while rooms with darker walls appear smaller. On the other hand, objects such as furnishings appear smaller when they are colored white or finished in light colors, while furniture that is dark appears heavy and massive.

NATURAL AND ELECTRIC LIGHT

We evolved over millions of years under the light of the sun, with our daily and seasonal activities determined by the available daylight. For thousands of years, firelight and torches were our only artificial lights. It is less than two hundred years since more effective lights, such as gas and petroleum lamps, began to appear. After this our activity and productivity expanded dramatically.

Electric lights have been with us for only a century, and fluorescent tube lamps have been in common use for a mere forty years, yet they have profoundly changed our whole civilization. In our homes and workplaces—even in our city streets—we can function at any time of the night almost as if it were daytime. *For most of us the influence of natural daily variations in light has been almost entirely erased by electric lighting, and yet the length of time we have had to help us adapt to these new conditions is, in evolutionary terms, almost none.*

Natural light varies with region, season, weather conditions, and time of day. In southern regions there is usually stronger light, more sunshine, and less variation of day length with the change of seasons. In the zone south of the 38th parallel (roughly a line connecting San Francisco and Washington D.C.) our adaptations to natural light have been distinctly different from those in the North. Southern homes, particularly those in the deep south, have thicker walls, smaller windows, and more shade to protect the living areas from excess sunlight and heat. Homes in the north, and particularly the Pacific Northwest region, are far more likely to have large glass areas and little shading to allow full admission of weak winter light.

LIGHT AND STRESS

Winter, in the Northeast and Northwest, is often described as "depressing". *For many of us this depression actually becomes a physical condition, resulting in part from a lack of stimulating light.* A vacation in the tropics, or a visit to a tanning studio, may be the answer for some, but more exposure to daylight may be all that is necessary. Recent research with new lamp types suggests that some people can reduce winter depression by changing the lamps in their homes and workplaces. Advocates of the new "full spectrum" lamps believe that their light is good for health because it closely resembles daylight. (However, this is not scientifically established.) (Careful choice of color in the decor of these places can also make a difference.) *When we attempt to maintain a busy schedule during periods when much of the natural stimulation of daylight is absent, we undoubtedly leave ourselves open to fatigue and unwanted stress.*

At the same time that we are understimulated by natural light, we may be overstimulated at inappropriate times by electric light. During the natural daily cycle we are first stimulated by the growing morning light. In many areas it is a light rich in the cool green and blue colors which tend to stimulate mental focus, and which reach their peak at noon. By mid afternoon the light is growing weaker and warmer in color with more orange and red, culminating at sunset. These colors emphasize emotion, and they signal the day's end. For many of us this natural daily variation has been eradicated, because we spend our days in workplaces or schools lit by cool, bright, and forceful fluorescent lamps. Not only is this constant, unvaried stimulation stressful, failing to provide the necessary relaxation and relief, but it is quite different from the *quality* of stimulation provided by daylight. Then, at the end of the workday, we may ride a brightly lit bus or train home, to spend the evening in a brightly lit room, or watching a television. When the time comes for rest, sometimes in a bedroom with a harsh streetlamp outside the window, insomnia may be waiting instead.

DAYLIGHT AND SUNLIGHT

Natural light has two components, sunlight and skylight (often referred to as daylight). *Sunlight* is the light coming either directly from, or reflected from the sun. It is usually strong and harsh, and though most of us consider it essential to atmosphere in the home, it can be problematic. *Daylight* is indirect light from the sun that has been scattered by clouds, or else is coming from a part of the clear sky where there is no sun. This type of light is characteristic of overcast days or of the northern sky.

Sunlight—as long as it is not overwhelming—has its place in our homes where it can provide cheer, free heat, and pleasant variations. It is less acceptable in a work area, where glare control is essential for good concentration. For this reason it is usually inappropriate to arrange a reading area where strong sunlight can reach. Sunlight produces strong contrast and sharp shadows, while daylight has soft, pleasing qualities that are appropriate in most activity areas.

Light Pollution

The idea that light can pollute has grown out of recent experience with commercial lighting, where, over the last forty years, higher and higher levels of electric light have been utilized. The use of new, highly efficient fluorescent tubes, together with the experience of extremely productive wartime industry in intensely lit, windowless (for blackout purposes) buildings, led to a great change in lighting standards for the workplace. Before 1945 a common background lighting level for the workplace was 200 Lux or 20 candlepower (a unit of light intensity), but now the common range is between 500 and 1500 Lux (150 candlepower), or even more. Electric lighting at such levels, particularly in poor or monotonous arrangements, is very disturbing to many people. There are too many public buildings, schools, and workplaces where rows of fluorescent strips or luminous ceiling panels overwhelm the senses, and destroy the shadow, color, and relief necessary to pleasant seeing. For those who spend their working life in these stressful environments the home can be a place of relief, with more subtle, controlled lighting to encourage rest and emotional release. Electrical and magnetic fields produced by lighting are also considered to be a source of pollution affecting us, though these are not well understood.

On Shadow

One of the important properties that is often misunderstood in lighting design is the value of the shadow that is cast by an object when it is lit by direct light. This shadow is the absence of light adjacent to something that helps to describe its presence. Indirect lighting and continuous lighting (such as strip lights or luminous ceilings) are intended to erase shadow. This type of lighting, when used alone, lacks an entire level of interest and natural subtlety. It is inappropriate to most situations, particularly the home. Shadow reveals light, depth, texture, and form. A room without shadow is more like the inside of an empty refrigerator than a dwelling place.

Lamp Types

INCANDESCENTS

The first electric lamps were made from glass globes enclosing a carbon filament which glowed when heated. This is fundamentally the same "incandescent" lamp that we use in our homes today. Though materials and manufacturing techniques have improved, the incandescent lamp still produces the familiar "bright spot" of light so rich in the warm (red and orange) colors of the spectrum. This sort of light is closest to late afternoon sunlight or the light from a bright fire in nature. It is a directional light which casts shadows, and its colors enhance our features.

FLUORESCENTS

The gas tube fluorescent lamp is based on an entirely different principle. In this lamp a gas, usually mercury vapor, is heated and energized with an electric current. When current passes through the gas, it glows with intense ultraviolet, violet, blue, and green light. Once the gas is energized the glow can be maintained with a very small electric current. This mercury vapor light, if used by itself, would be very harsh to the eye, and a health hazard, but it is mostly contained within the tube, where it causes a chemical phosphor coating inside the glass to glow with a more uniform light. This light is usually rich in green and yellow, and is the greater part of the light we see from a fluorescent fixture. The selection of the phosphor lining of the tube broadly determines the color of light that the tube will produce. The available common types include cool white, warm white, daylight, and full spectrum.

The fundamental differences between incandescent and fluorescent lamps is in their colors, light qualities, and operating costs. Most incandescent lamps are warm in color, compared to the cool colors of fluorescents. The light from an incandescent lamp is steady and soft, while the light from a fluorescent lamp is vibrating and sharp. Incandescent lamps cast shadows while fluorescent lamps light uniformly, erasing shadow. Incandescent lamps are very hot while operating and consume large amounts of electricity for the light they produce, while fluorescents are cool and consume far less electricity. Fluorescent lamps also produce more high energy electromagnetic fields than the incandescent ones.

It has been found that where fluorescent lighting dominates a space, many people will describe the light as "annoying, vibrating, or glaring". Some also find the lack of shadow disorienting. Eye stimulation from fluorescent sources is quite different from that of natural light or other lamp types. Most fluorescents produce very specific colors which do not stimulate the eye evenly as do other lights. Their light also vibrates on and off rapidly sixty times per second. Though we do not consciously perceive this as flicker, worn lamps and poor installations do flicker, and there is evidence that this causes eye strain, confusion, and may even impair one's judgment. These lamps also lack certain colors present in daylight, which are important to the eyes' ability to adapt for brightness. If unscreened these lamps also produce electromagnetic radiation, which may be a hazard.

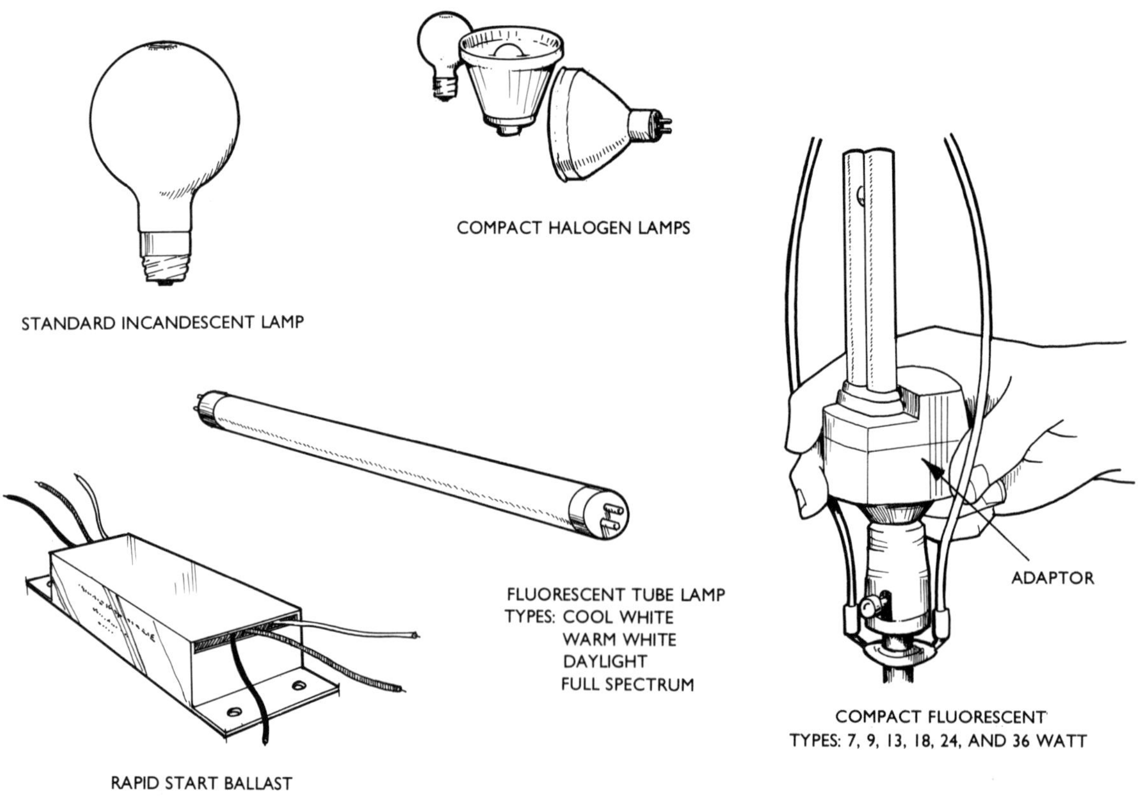

Fig. 2-1 Common Lamp Types For Home Use

QUARTZ, HALOGEN, AND COMPACT FLUORESCENTS

Recently, new families of both types of lamps have become available for the home. There are new incandescent lamps (the quartz types) which are compact and much more intense than conventional bulbs. Halogen or metal halide lamps are another family of new lamp types that are very bright, consume less electricity, and have different color values from conventional lamps. Both these types are expensive, but well suited to small reading lamps and fixtures for dramatic interest, such as display lighting. However, they can only be used in specially designed fixtures. They may produce a peculiar odor, irritating to the hypersensitive. A new, compact fluorescent lamp type is also appearing on the market that is about five to eight inches long. It produces a much softer and warmer light than other fluorescents and is efficient and cool running. It is also very adaptable and can easily replace incandescent lamps in most types of fixtures. This lamp is much more appropriate, particularly for home use, than previous fluorescents. The full spectrum lamps which are being sold as a "natural" replacement for conventional lamps are of doubtful value in improving conditions in the home. Though the debate over this continues, the U.S. government recently ruled that they could not be advertised as aids to health.

Healthful Home Lighting

Natural light, with all of its variety and subtlety, is fundamental to health, and well designed electric lighting is essential for comfort and mood. In most home situations natural light is the major daytime light source, supplemented by electric light, as needed. The task of designing home lighting for the evening hours is an entire design problem in itself.

A well designed lighting scheme will provide: safe light levels for traffic areas; good light to minimize eyestrain for task areas, such as kitchens and reading places; and clues for orientation, such as the position of the horizon, floor, thresholds, stairs, and doorways. It will also focus attention on such things as paintings or plants, reveal objects by casting shadows, and provide much needed visual variety and rest. Lighting can also be planned to help define personal territories in the home, increase or reduce the apparent size of a room, and reveal or moderate interior colors.

In northern regions, large amounts of daylight exposure are very desirable, with some sunlight exposure as well. Here skylights are also very popular. Curtains or blinds for daylight control may only be needed to darken bedrooms for rest and for living spaces in midsummer. In the South and Southwest deep porches, awnings, blinds, and tinted glass are commonly used for year round control.

LIGHT AND LIGHTING HAZARDS

Ultraviolet Radiation There are some potential health hazards in home lighting from light exposure, or from dangerous equipment. Both sunlight and the light from some electric lamps contains ultraviolet (u.v.) radiation. This is an invisible, high energy light that causes sunburn, and can cause eye damage and skin cancer. There is a good deal of debate about how much u.v. exposure is safe for us, and general disagreement about whether small amounts of u.v. indoors from sunlight or electric light can be beneficial. However, there are some hazards that can be clearly identified.

Excessive exposure to sunlight will cause sunburn, while prolonged exposure to sun increases the risk of skin cancer. Skin cancer is more common in people who live in sunny climates, and more pronounced among those who work outdoors. U.V. exposure is an emerging area of concern as new evidence collects which suggests that global levels of u.v. light from the sun may be rising. This is due to the damage being done to the protective ozone layer of the upper atmosphere by industrial emissions, the use of fluorocarbons in aerosol cans and refrigerators, and auto exhaust. Fortunately, nearly all of the u.v. in sunlight is blocked from entering our homes by the glass in our windows, but plastics, such as acrylic and polycarbonate, do not stop u.v. unless treated to do so. *Many skylights and greenhouse systems, as well as some unbreakable windows, such as those found in trailers, are made from transparent plastics and can produce sunburn indoors.* This u.v. light will also cause the rapid decay of fabrics and furnishings indoors, and can contribute to chemicals and gases in indoor air. This is also true of materials that are exposed to heat near windows or heaters.

If you have plastic windows or skylights, take care to limit your exposure to sun just as you would outdoors, and keep fabrics, *especially synthetic carpets and drapes,* which outgas (see the chapter, The Indoor Hazards), away from direct light. Enamelled metal blinds are the safest type of sun shades, and will last longest.

Eye injury can also occur with excessive u.v. exposure. Headaches, dizziness, and temporary blindness, similar to that experienced by welders who have not protected their eyes properly, can result from too much sun.

Fluorescent tube lamps also produce small amounts of u.v., though this varies with lamp types. The very small amounts of indoor u.v. produced by daylight, or "natural" fluorescent lamps, appear to be safe and should not be a cause for concern. The full spectrum fluorescent lamps have been engineered to closely simulate natural light, and can sometimes be useful in the home where natural light is poor. Like the daylight fluorescent lamp, they also give the most "natural" color appearance. Warm white and compact fluorescent lamps have the least u.v. and give the most flattering skin color, while the cool white lamps have modest amounts of u.v. and the poorest color qualities for most things.

Any fluorescent lamp should be located at least four feet away from you and the plastic covers designed for the lamp should always be in place. To reduce electromagnetic radiation, a 1 mm mesh metal screen can be placed over the lamp.

Toxic Polychlorinated Bi-Phenyls Old fluorescent "rapid start" type lamps may introduce another hazard. The ballasts (an electronic device which starts the lamp) may contain very toxic PCB's, which can leak and contaminate your home. To check if you have a rapid start fixture with a potentially leaky ballast, remove the cover from the lamp and look for a metal box about 2" x 8", usually mounted between the tubes. The ballast has six or more colored wires leading from it. If there are any signs of oily or black deposits leaking from the ballast, discard it immediately and *do not let it touch your skin.* It is difficult to be certain if it has PCB's in it, but even those that do not are filled with asphalt products which can be polluting if they leak. Lamps made in the last 7 years are more likely to be safe, but it is safest to discard rapid start lamps more than 10 years old.

Irritating Gases Conventional incandescent household lamps operate at high temperatures, which can cause problems for people suffering from asthma or environmental sensitivity. House dust is stirred up by the heat from the lamp, and this dust, as well as airborne contaminants, and even heated parts of the light fixture, can generate irritating particles and gases when close to the hot bulb. Compact fluorescents are good replacements for standard bulbs because they do not get hot during operation, do not have oil filled ballasts, give a pleasant light, and outlast ten or more common bulbs while using one quarter the electricity.

Other lighting hazards include fire danger from old or damaged fixtures, and using lamps too large for a particular device. Always follow the recommended lamp size ratings printed on the fixture.

LOCATING LIGHT FOR SAFETY

Good light levels are most important near stairs, doors, and work areas such as kitchen counters and workbenches. Reading areas and desks must also have good light to reduce eyestrain. The light on stairs should be direct and located as high above the steps as possible. In this way the stair treads will cast a small shadow to help make the edges of each step more apparent, the person on the stair will not cast a large, confusing shadow, and the lamp will be well above eye level where it cannot cause glare.

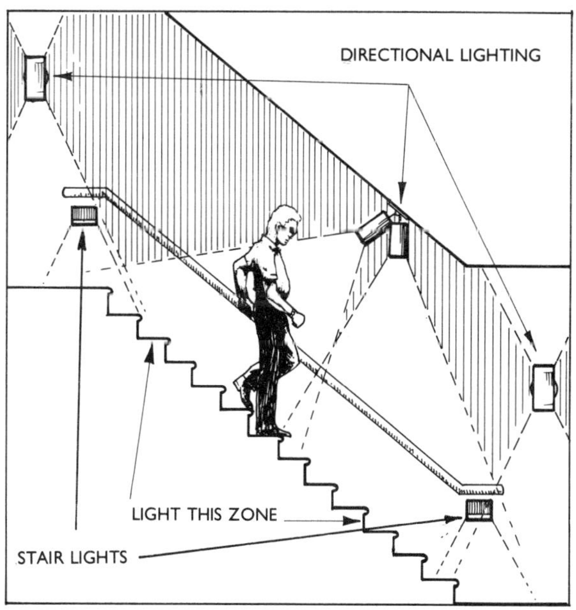

Fig. 2-2 Stair Lighting. *Use* Directional Lighting *on stairs to ensure the visibility of treads. Place lights so that they do not cause glare, particularly when descending. Consider special wall mounted* Stair Lights *for the elderly or visually handicapped.*

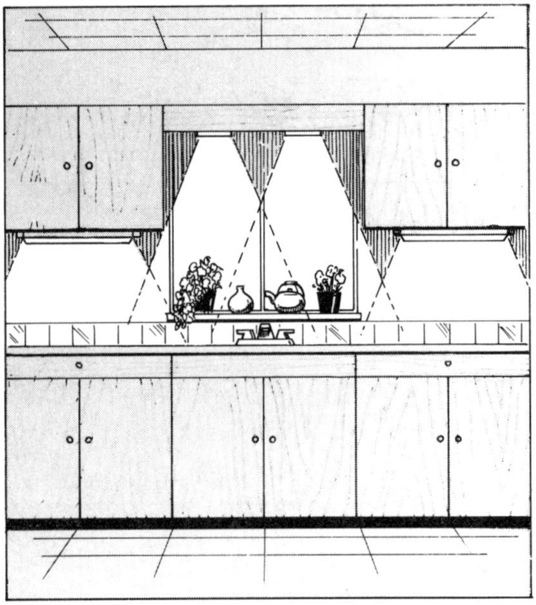

Fig. 2-3 Kitchen Lighting. *Use directional lighting in the kitchen to illuminate work areas without glare.*

The best direction for lighting work surfaces in kitchens and at desks is from above eye level, and in front of the usual working position. Two overlapping sources from both right and left sides is a good arrangement. Small lamps mounted under upper kitchen cabinets can be very good if they are properly shielded for glare. The shields should be made from safe and fireproof metal or enamelled metal.

DESIGNING LIGHTING FOR PLEASURE AND RELAXATION

Good lighting is a powerful tool for making your home a pleasant place to be. As you walk through your home, think of the places and features which are most important to you, and use light to emphasize them. There may be a painting or plant shelf which really lends appeal to the room. Locating it to receive good daylight, and lighting it for the evening with a suitable lamp, will be most effective. A quiet corner may be more subtly lit or left in partial shadow for rest and relief. Color is also an effective device for improving the appearance of our homes and changing the way we feel in them. Adding light and color are the most direct and least expensive renovations we can make, and should be a fundamental part of planning a new home. Bright color is particularly important to children under five, who learn a great deal about their environment from color.

Windows And Other Daylight Features

Generally, east, south, and west windows will require some form of external shade or awning if you live in a region with very strong light. This may be a roof overhang, a porch roof, or an awning. Controlling excess sunlight from inside with blinds is not very effective for reducing summer heat problems.

If you live in an area with more moderate sunshine, you may only need some shading on south windows. This shading can be carefully arranged to admit sun in winter and to exclude it in the mid summer. Remember that draperies and floor coverings should be kept away from direct sun to prevent their giving off fumes. Where sun enters the home, metal blinds and ceramic tile floor coverings are best.

If you live where the sunny season is short, you may wish to use some special daylight

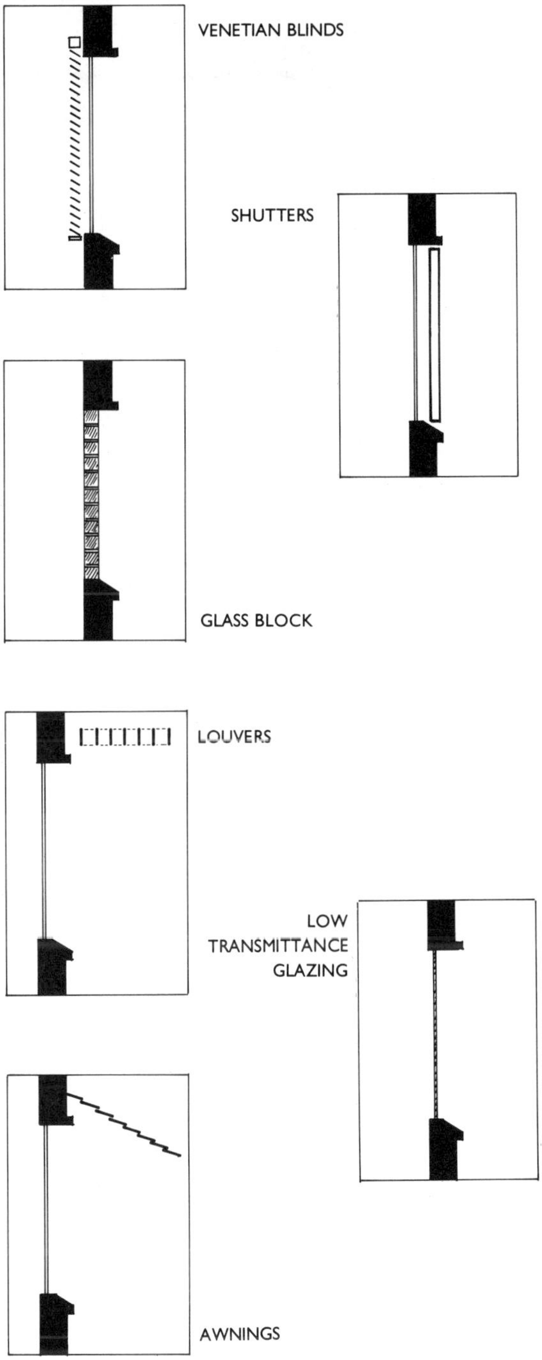

Fig. 2-4 Daylight Control Devices

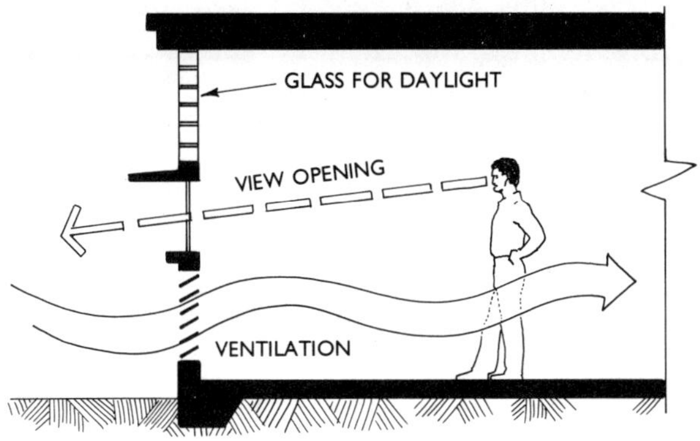

Fig. 2-5 Daylighting. *For optimum control, the three functions of wall openings are best handled separately:* Glass For Daylight *is located where it will not promote glare; the* View Opening *is located for the best view angle; the* Ventilation *opening is placed for optimum air flow.*

techniques together with windows or skylights. Windows in these regions, particularly those facing the steady north light, can be enhanced by the use of glass block walls, or by adding a pond or light colored paving outside to help reflect light into the room. Replacing the glass in a sunlit window or greenhouse with a rigid plastic sheet, such as polycarbonate, will allow entry of full spectrum sunlight, which can be beneficial to plants but must also be treated with caution. These materials can outgas when heated, and the u.v. light admitted can increase indoor pollution. (See the chapter The Sunspace/Greenhouse.) Greenhouse windows can also be very effective aids to daylight, as well as allowing indoor gardening. Windows framed with metals without any rubber or soft plastic parts are the best choices for people with chemical sensitivities.

Skylights are a very effective device for brightening an interior naturally. These should usually not be located facing south, due to excessive summer sun, and care must be taken to locate them where they can be reached for occasional cleaning. It is essential that skylights have double or triple plastic or glass to minimize winter condensation which can lead to moisture damage and mold growth. Remember that any glass used in a skylight must be treated safety glass, or wire reinforced glass. If they admit excess sun, skylights in some circumstances must be protected with shading devices. These shades can be arranged to block most of the direct sun while reflecting indirect light inside. (See the chapter The Sunspace/Greenhouse.)

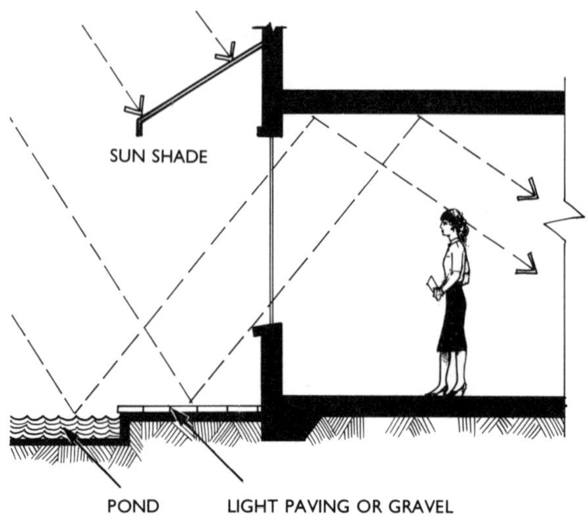

Fig. 2-6 Bouncing Daylight. *Daylight can be bounced into the home with a reflective* Pond, *or* Light-colored Paving or Gravel. *A* Sun Shade *prevents excess glare and overheating.*

3 THERMAL COMFORT

The air temperature and humidity in our homes are major factors for maintaining comfort and good health. Extreme conditions of temperature and humidity cause discomfort, promote the spread of microorganisms which cause disease, and can seriously irritate the respiratory system. High temperatures and humidity also increase the outgassing of such air pollutants as formaldehyde from building materials, which are linked with lowered resistance to bacterial and viral infection. This is particularly critical in the homes of people suffering from respiratory illness, or those with hypersensitivity to airborne allergens and contaminants. It is also important for cases of common colds, flu, and coughs.

Temperature

The air in our homes is usually maintained between about 65°F and 75°F by heating or cooling. This air, circulating throughout the home, will also lose or gain heat as it contacts the people, furnishings, appliances, and parts of the building. This is called *convective heat,* and is easily measured and controlled. The other form of heat that is particularly important for comfort is *radiant* heat. This is the heat we feel when standing in the sun, or near a fire, even when the air is very cold, and is independent of air temperature. Radiant heat can dramatically affect comfort in the home, even when air temperature is maintained at comfortable levels. Sitting indoors in sunlight we may easily become overheated, even though the air around us is at a pleasant temperature. Conversely, a fully heated room with large windows or skylights will feel cold in the winter, especially at night, due to radiant heat loss from our bodies.

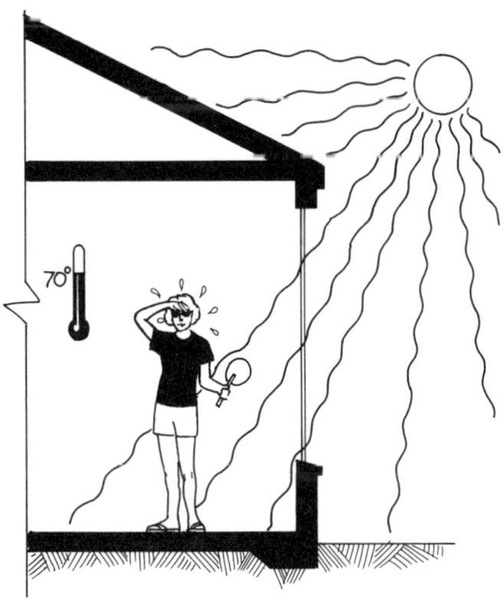

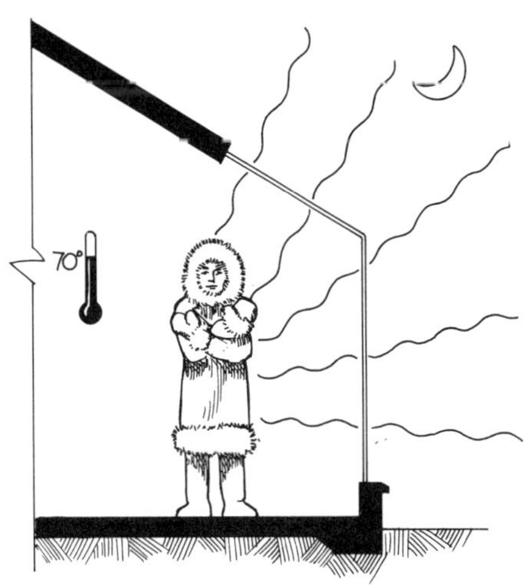

Fig. 3-1 Radiant Temperature

Radiant heat can make us uncomfortably warm, even when the air temperature is comfortable.

Radiant loss can make us uncomfortably cool, even when the air temperature is comfortable.

Humidity

All air contains water vapor in varying quantities due to weather conditions, evaporation of water from our bodies, and from cooking, bathing, and laundry. The capacity of air to carry water is based on its temperature, with cold air having the least capacity, and warm air the greatest. The amount of water vapor present in air is measured by a unit of Relative Humidity (R.H.%), which is a percentage of the maximum capacity of air to carry water at any given temperature. Thus 100% R.H. is called "saturated" air, and 50% R.H. air is carrying half its potential water vapor.

Humidity and temperature cannot be separated when considering their effect on comfort and health. 85°F air is comfortable to most people if the humidity is very low, but 70°F feels hot if the air is humid. For this reason a graph of temperature and relative humidity has been developed showing a comfort zone. This zone indicates the recommended relationship between temperature and humidity for best comfort and health. Simple measurements made in the home can be easily compared to this graph to determine where corrections might be needed. (See Fig. 3-3.)

Air inside your home will contain more or less humidity than outside air based on the following conditions:

- The amount of heating or cooling of air taking place within the house, and the kind of heating system used.
- The amount of moisture being produced in the house by cooking, washing, and breathing.
- The amount of ventilation, particularly in kitchens and bathrooms.
- The amount of insulation, vapor sealing, and weatherstripping in the structure.

Generally, a poorly sealed home being heated by a warm air furnace in a cold, dry climate such as the American Mid-West is the most likely to have a dry air problem. The reason for this is that outdoor air contains very little moisture when well below freezing. The heating of this air increases its capacity to carry moisture, thus decreasing its relative humidity. Heated air within the house then acts as a "vapor pump," forcing precious moisture through the leaky walls and ceiling, and further drying the house. The effect of the moving air coming from the heat ducts is to further aggravate the drying effect on our bodies. Under these conditions the relative humidity may drop to 10% R.H. or even less, a level which not only is irritating and unhealthful, but also harmful to household goods and plants. A home in the Great Lakes region or in the southeastern U.S. or Gulf Coast, may have a problem with *high* humidity during the late summer months, particularly where ventilation and fresh air supply are inadequate. In these regions during the hot season, the relative humidity of outdoor air may hover around 90% R.H.. This air, trapped inside a poorly ventilated house, may quickly reach 100% R.H. due to breathing and cooking. Such saturated air feels very oppressive, will contribute to the growth of fungus, and can damage the home and its contents. Air conditioning during humid summer months will generally reduce the humidity inside the home, particularly where air conditioning units are equipped to remove the water condensing from chilled humid air. This effect, or the effect of an electric de-humidifier, may be negated, however, where poor vapor sealing allows outdoor humidity to seep back through the walls. (See the Construction Notes chapter.) Evaporative type air conditioners are not effective in humid climates.

Air movement can reduce the discomforts of overheated and humid air. There is a pleasant, cooling feeling as moving air passes our skin, though this effect decreases as relative humidity increases. In winter months, however, this effect can make even comfortably heated air feel too cool, if it is moving too quickly.

The best range of relative humidity for health and comfort is between 40% and 60%. In this range, our respiratory system can function normally without excessive drying, perspiration will not readily collect, and fungus growth and the spread of bacteria will not be encouraged. Building materials, fabrics and furnishings, and paper goods are also least affected by humidity in this range. At 50% relative humidity, 80% of people surveyed tend to feel comfortable with a 70° room temperature, if they are at rest and lightly clothed, and if air movement is moderate. Many house plants can also be easily maintained at this level, though they may prefer more moisture.

MEASURING RELATIVE HUMIDITY

Most homes have some way of measuring indoor temperature, even if it is only a thermometer on a wall thermostat, but few have the means to measure relative humid-

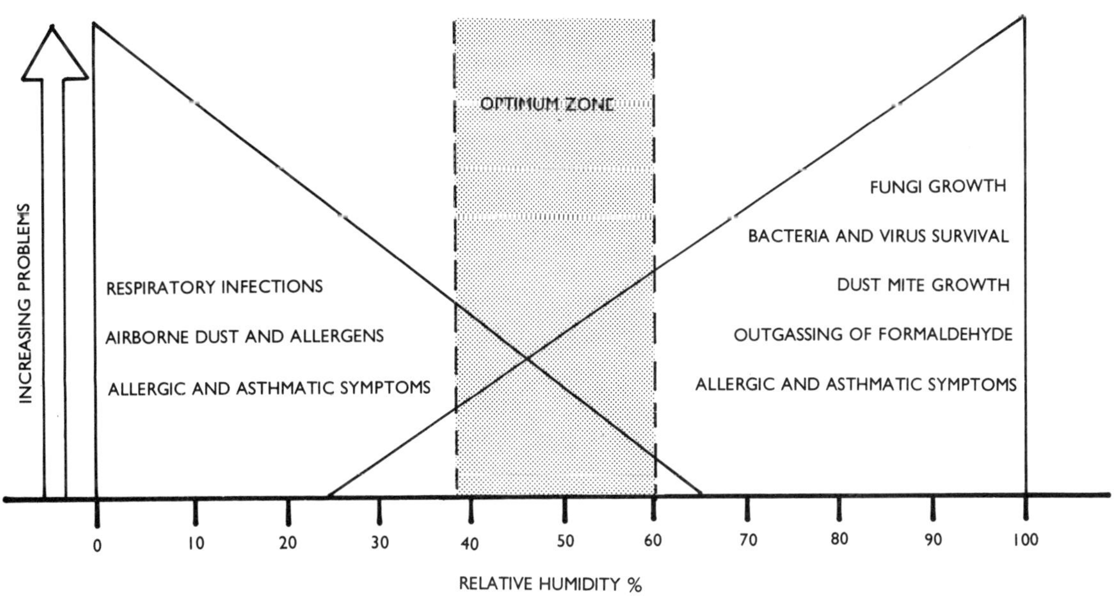

Fig. 3-2 The Effects of Relative Humidity on Health. *(Adapted from Arundel, Sterling, et.al.* Environmental Health Perspective, *V. 65, pp. 361-361, 1986.)*

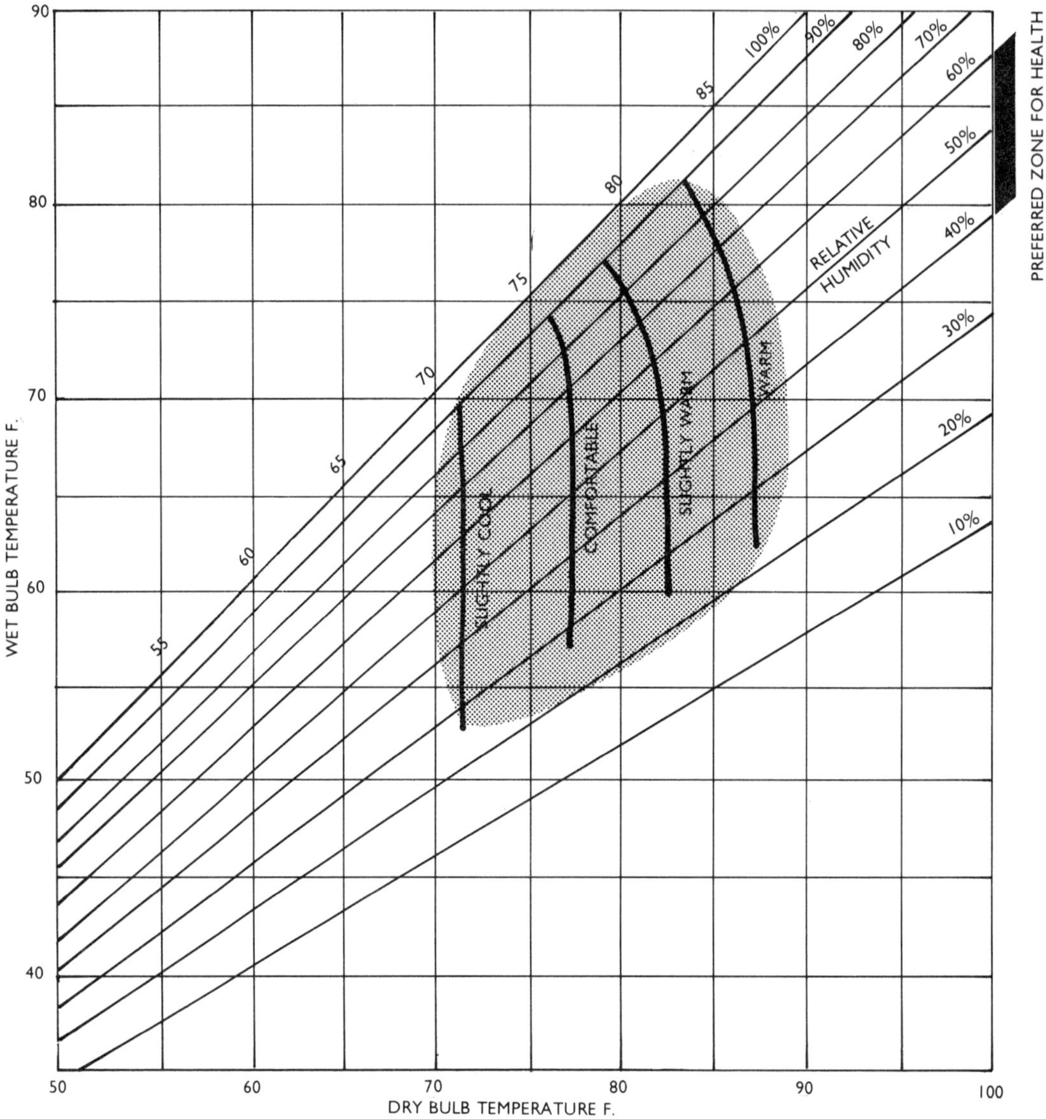

Fig. 3-3 Relative Humidity and Comfort. *Comfort is dependent on both* Temperature *and* Relative Humidity. *The shaded zone indicates the usual range of comfortable temperature and humidity for people at rest when the air movement is moderate. Read room temperature on the bottom scale and humidity on the diagonal scale. Note that the* Preferred Humidity Zone *for health is between 40% and 60%. (Adapted from American Society of Heating, Refrigeration, and Air Engineers Fundamentals Handbook.)*

Note: *To determine relative humidity from temperature measurements, locate dry bulb temperature on the bottom scale and wet bulb temperature on the left hand scale. Trace the vertical and horizontal lines to their meeting point and read the humidity from the diagonal scale. (See the chapter Home Heating for details.)*

ity. Simple, inexpensive devices are widely available for this purpose, and are very useful where extreme humidity may be a problem. The simplest ones are the "wet bulb" type, though other "direct reading" units are also available. The wet bulb system uses a pair of thermometers, one of which has a gauze sleeve over the bulb end. The gauze sleeve is moistened with water, which evaporates, cooling the thermometer. The difference in readings between the two thermometers is the relative humidity, the smallest difference indicating the highest humidity. (See Fig. 3-3.)

This chart indicates relative humidity for the usual range of household temperatures. The dry thermometer reading is read on the bottom scale, and the wet thermometer on the side. Where the lines extended from these points meet is the diagonal line of relative humidity for those values. A good rule of thumb for household health and comfort is that the wet bulb thermometer should read about 10° to 12° F. below the dry bulb for common household temperatures. This is equivalent to about 50% humidity.

Where a wet bulb thermometer is not available, a simple yet useful test can be performed with a single utility thermometer of the type commonly used for measuring indoor or outdoor temperature. (For instructions, see the Home Heating/Cooling chapter.)

REMEDIES

If possible, try to solve your humidity problems without the aid of humidifiers or dehumidifiers. Though helpful in extreme climates, such as the American South-West and South-East, these devices can be a nuisance to maintain and operate, and can add a health risk to the home. This is especially true of humidifiers with a water filled pan or reservoir connected to a wick designed to add moisture to the air by evaporation. These parts easily become a breeding place for airborne microorganisms which will promote illness. The "legionnaires disease" which struck a convention at a hotel, killing several people, was traced to organisms growing in the air conditioning system. In the home, local moisture can be safely provided with a pan of water placed on a heater, or a small vaporizer.

Low humidity caused by winter heating in dry climates is best controlled by improved air vapor barriers and sealing of the building, so as to keep in more of the water vapor generated inside the home. Better insulation and weatherstripping will also reduce the demand for heating, and the resulting dryness. Radiant heating systems are significantly better than forced air for minimizing dryness problems. (See the Construction Notes and Home Heating chapters.)

Excess humidity is best managed by good ventilation. Where possible, use natural air flow to improve comfort and reduce the need for air conditioning. House fans and specific ventilation of kitchens and bathrooms are also helpful. (See the Home Ventilation chapter.) Where necessary, dehumidifiers can be installed, either in individual rooms, or for the whole house. ***They must be drained and cleaned daily, to prevent mold and other organisms growing in the drip pans.*** Wherever air conditioning is used for cooling and humidity control, proper insulation of roofs and walls, and complete air and vapor sealing of all areas, including crawl spaces under floors, is essential. Just as moisture will be driven out by heating in dry climates, moisture will seep in when cooling in humid climates.

It is not necessary for the climate in our homes to be controlled uniformly, despite the design intent of central heating and cooling systems. Just as light, color, sound, and other environmental factors may vary widely from one room to the next, and even within the same room, varied temperature and air movement are also desirable features. A cool draft, or a sun warmed corner, can contribute a delightful sense of variety in our homes. Many people find, for example, that cooler and better ventilated bedrooms help them to sleep well, though the same conditions would be too cool for a sitting area. In many regions, kitchens will not need heating, due to the heat generated by appliances, as well as people's heightened activity in the kitchen. Ventilating kitchens is at least as important as air conditioning them for the hot season.

Energy costs are closely linked to heating and cooling efficiency. A properly sealed, insulated, and ventilated (both naturally and mechanically) home, with a well planned heating and cooling system, will deliver comfort, health, *and* financial benefits.

HUMIDITY HAZARDS

Two common humidity problems occur in houses which can contribute both to building damage and to health problems.

Surface Condensation Cold indoor surfaces such as windows or poorly insulated walls and ceilings will collect condensation during cold weather. Condensation occurs when warm, moisture-laden indoor air meets a surface cold enough to draw the moisture from the air. Moisture damage to window frames and wall and ceiling materials can result in serious rot problems as well as growth of highly allergenic fungi.

Exhausting humid air from bathrooms and kitchens will help to reduce buildup of indoor moisture, but in cold climates it will also be necessary to insulate walls, ceilings and windows well to prevent cold surface condensation. Careful insulation and double or triple glass or insulated shutters are good remedies.

Hidden Condensation Air leakage through gaps in outside walls and ceilings will allow warm, moisture-laden air to escape into cold building cavities. In these cavities condensation can occur, resulting in rot and fungus growth.

Tight air sealing of all inside surfaces is essential in cold climates to prevent hidden condensation problems. Though both are necessary, the effect of sealing cracks is far greater than what is achieved by using vapor retarding materials such as plastic or foil to protect insulated cavities. (See the Construction Notes chapter.)

4 SOUND

Sound and Noise

Sound is physical energy causing rapid vibration of the air around us. When we hear a sound our brains interpret it and give it meaning based on our learning and experience. Some sounds provide essential information, others are for social communication, or for pleasure, such as music. *Noise,* on the other hand, is any unwanted sound. The sounds we call noise are usually too loud, too meaningless (such as a rattling refrigerator), too meaningful (such as an overheard conversation), or too monotonous (such as the rumble of street noise). *Noise, according to many psychologists and doctors, is one of the most significant pollutants of modern life.* Noise contributes to tension, and to psychological and physical deterioration, increasing the incidence of heart disease, ulcers, and high blood pressure. Noise affects children in the womb, and affects their development at home and in school. Studies of schools in noisy locations show significant deficiencies in attention span and learning skills among children compared to those in quieter locations.

HOW SOUND TRAVELS

Sound travels in waves radiating outward from its source. Sound is easily reflected by hard surfaces and readily absorbed by soft surfaces. Sound will travel great distances over paved areas or water because it is reflected upward and outward from their surfaces. This is why, in a typical house, street noise may be higher on the upper floor than it is at street level.

Indoors, sound is reflected back and forth by walls, ceilings, and floors, until finally it diminishes and disappears. This may go on for only a tiny fraction of a second in some rooms with soft surfaces, but it may be prolonged for one or two seconds in rooms with hard surfaces. The nature of sound in a room is changed by this process of reflection and absorption, with certain pitches being absorbed first and others lasting longer. The kind and amount of sound reflection will affect how we perceive any indoor space. A highly reflective room will seem "bare" and larger than it actually is. In extreme cases this can be very disturbing, and will interfere with the sound of speech and music.

Rugs, draperies, and upholstery will reduce the movement of sound and change our perception of a room. A highly absorptive room will seem crowded and small; it may even be unpleasant in extreme cases.

A city street lined with buildings acts much like an outdoor room. The reflected sound will travel upward and affect apartments on the lower floors quite significantly. The noise levels in second and third floor apartments on busy streets have been found equal to those in light industries or in the cab of a heavy truck. Balconies over the street can be so noisy that normal conversation is impossible, and hearing damage will result if too much time is spent there.

Sound travels through surfaces in two ways. "Leakage" occurs when sound passes through cracks or openings in solid surfaces. This effect will spoil the soundproofing of a carefully engineered soundproof wall, for example, if an opening is made for plumbing or wiring, or if a window is poorly installed. "Transmission" occurs when sound makes a surface vibrate and itself becomes a source of sound. Single paned windows and lightweight walls act this way, and will allow annoying noise to enter the home.

HOW SOUND AFFECTS US

Sound affects us profoundly. Very quiet places may be relaxing, or they may be troubling, depending on the individual and his or her activity. Noisy places are very irritating to most people. However, a certain amount of background sound, such as is found in a comfortable office environment, is often considered "activating" and beneficial to alertness and productivity. Sound of any type can be very aggravating to most of us when we are tired or ill.

Loud or very irritating noise is always detrimental to everyone, and will cause physiological damage and psychological stress. Noise will interrupt needed deep sleep, it will promote fatigue, increase tension, leading to disease, and cause non-reversible hearing loss. Hearing loss with age has been found to be largely due to noise exposure. Studies of old people living in quiet places show that most have perfect hearing well into their eighties and nineties.

Hearing damage begins with the loss of ability to hear the higher pitches, and is caused by damage to the microscopic sensory hairs within the ear. It can be measured after only a few years of heavy noise exposure, such as in industry. When this happens there is loss of some ability to appreciate music and other subtleties of sound. If noise exposure continues, hearing damage will progress, leading to a loss of hearing for the middle pitches. At this point the ability to understand speech will become impaired. The final stages of hearing loss may involve total loss of hearing, and possibly tinnitus, a very serious condition where there is an uncontrollable ringing sensation in the ears.

The sound levels we encounter when operating power tools, home appliances (such as blenders and vacuums), and listening to loud music are high enough to cause progressive hearing damage over an extended time.

SOUND LEVELS

Sound energy is measured in decibels (dB). The decibel scale is logarithmic, which means that an increase of 10 decibels indicates that a sound has increased tenfold in intensity. The reference point for the scale of sound intensity is 0 decibels. This is defined as the smallest sound which can be heard by a person with unimpaired hearing. In practice, this means that a loud sound, such as an electric saw at 100 dB, is ten billion times more intense than the smallest sound which can be heard.

Sound intensities up to about 60 dB are considered comfortable background levels. Sound intensities between 60 and 80 dB are considered noisy but will not cause hearing damage. Sounds between 80 and 100 dB are considered loud and, with lengthy exposure, will cause hearing damage. Occupational health standards in the United States and Canada typically allow only 2 hours of exposure per day to 100 dB noise without ear protection, yet this is only one hundredth of the intensity of loud music played through earphones. Noise in excess of 110 dB is very painful and will cause rapid hearing damage.

Table 4-1

How Common Sounds Affect Hearing

	Decibels (dB)	Source
PAINFUL (Rapid hearing damage.)	140	*Jet aircraft takeoff 100 ft. away*
	130	*Jet aircraft taxiing 100 ft. away*
	125	*Propeller airplane takeoff 100 ft. away*
VERY LOUD (Hearing loss.)	120	*Very loud music with earphones*
	110	*Rock concert 50 ft. away*
LOUD (Hearing loss over time.)	100	*Operating an electric circular saw, jackhammer* 10 ft. away
	90	*Operating a very loud blender, vacuum cleaner*
NOISY	80	*Street noise entering a city apartment*
	70	*Typical office background noise*
		Street noise entering a suburban home.
COMFORTABLE	60	*Comfortable conversation*
	50	*Quiet suburban area, no traffic*
	40	*Rural area, no traffic*
	30	*Whisper*
	20	*Very quiet rural home*
	10	*Very light breeze in a field*
	0	*Threshold of hearing*

Measurement of sound levels is complex and is not necessary in the home. Use this table to discover the sources of intense, damaging sounds to which you may be exposed, and which you must protect yourself against to prevent hearing loss.

SOUND EXPOSURE IN THE HOME

For the average city dweller today only about one half of his or her hearing loss comes from exposure in the workplace. The other half happens at home, in city streets, on public transportation, or in leisure activities. The most *damaging* exposure in homes comes from listening to loud music, operating noisy power tools and appliances, and, in very busy locations, from urban or industrial noise. *Irritating* noise in homes comes from many sources, including streets, construction, neighbors, televisions and radios, furnaces, refrigerators, fans, and noisy pipes.

You can avoid damaging noise exposure at home by changing your personal habits, such as turning down the music, and wearing ear protection when operating tools. For household work, good ear protectors are the snug fitting earmuff types available at hardware or safety supply stores. Though not widely known, hearing protection is important even if you are only hammering nails. Irritating noise is more difficult to control and will require careful attention to some features in the home and yard.

The most insidious effect of chronic noise exposure is that we are able to eventually accept and adapt to very damaging conditions. Prolonged exposure to irritating or even painful noise will eventually lead to apathy or torpor, and the loss of our ability to react in our own defense.

CONTROLLING SOUND

Controlling noise at its source is the most effective way to reduce irritation. Four methods of sound control can be used in the home.

Exclusion Reflective or absorptive devices such as solid walls, double windows, trees, hedges, and fences can all be used to exclude outside noise.

Absorption Soft surfaces can be used to absorb noise that enters a room or is generated there, before it becomes a problem.

Isolation Noise from one part of the home can be prevented from spreading to another by the use of massive walls and floors, or special resilient wall and ceiling treatments.

Masking Unavoidable noise can be masked by more pleasant sounds, such as the sound of falling water.

Street Noise Vegetation and fencing will substantially reduce the entry of street noise into the home. Because noise tends to rise from street level, the most effective controls are dense hedges or solid fences close to the street. (See the chapter The House and Its Site.) Though tall, mature trees also effectivly absorb noise, they must be planted in a dense row, and this is often often not acceptable because it will interfere with light and with air circulation. A lawn or mulched ground cover is also somewhat more effective than a hard surface for reducing noise. Falling water, such as a fountain in the garden, can provide a pleasant masking sound to make outdoor living more enjoyable.

Outside Walls There are two types of outside walls or shared walls between apartments which can be used for sound control. A *massive* wall of concrete or masonry is

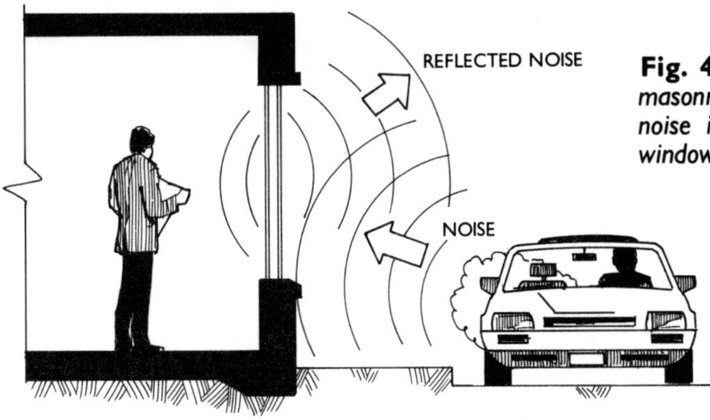

Fig. 4-1 Reflected Street Noise. *With massive masonry or concrete walls and double windows, street noise is reflected by the walls and absorbed by the windows.*

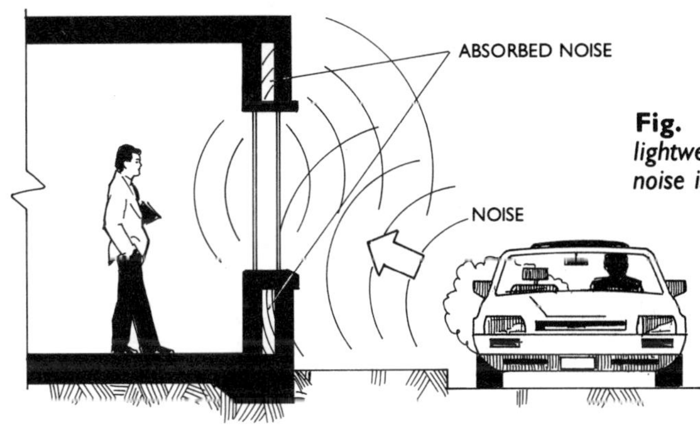

Fig. 4-2 Absorbed Street Noise. *With lightweight double walls and double windows, street noise is absorbed by both the walls and windows.*

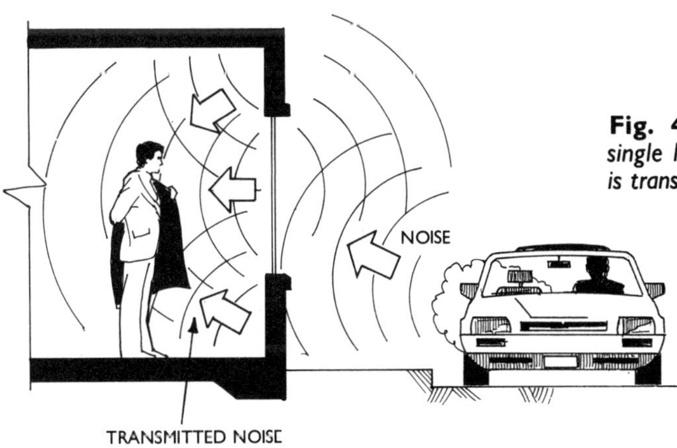

Fig. 4-3 Transmitted Street Noise. *With a single lightweight wall and single windows, street noise is transmitted by both the wall and windows.*

highly effective in reducing sound penetration. This type of wall will simply reflect and absorb sound. It will not transmit it because it is too heavy to be easily vibrated. A *resilient* double wall of lightweight construction is also effective. While each side of this wall does absorb sound and then vibrate, it will not transmit sound to the other side because the two walls are independent. Single walls of lightweight construction, such as those of common frame buildings and mobile homes, will not be effective for reducing sound transmission, because they easily vibrate, transmitting the sound to the other side. Small cracks in walls will also reduce their effectiveness at preventing the entry of sound. (See the Construction Notes chapter for details.)

Windows Single glass is not effective for reducing noise. Double or triple glass, in sealed insulating units or storm shutters, will dramatically reduce the transmission of noise. ***Often changing to sealed double windows is all that is necessary to control objectionable street noise in a busy city location.*** These units should be tightly fitted and sealed, so that they can be securely closed when necessary. Remember that if it is necessary to open windows facing a busy street for ventilation, the noiseproofing effect of the entire wall will be lost. Here alternative ways to ventilate the room should be found. (See the Home Ventilation chapter.)

Home Planning You can plan your home carefully to reduce the irritation from noise generated inside. Kitchens, televisions, childrens' play areas, and workshop areas are the worst sources of noise indoors. Where possible do not locate them adjacent to quiet areas, such as bedrooms or studies. Where necessary, shared walls between these zones can be soundproofed. (See the chapter Construction Notes.) Bedrooms on the quiet side of the home, away from the street, will also be more restful than those on the street side.

Interior Features Thick rugs and heavy drapes are effective absorption surfaces for controlling sound indoors. Soft furniture and fabric wall hangings will also help. To test a room for sound absorption stand in the middle and clap your hands loudly. If you hear a distinctive ringing immediately after clapping then the room is quite reflective to sound and will probably not be a good place for a playroom or television. Rugs are the first priority, followed by an absorptive ceiling such as acoustical tile or rough plaster.

Sound transmission through floors can be controlled by two means. ***Resilient*** ceiling suspensions can be used to prevent the passage of sound through floor frames and into ceiling materials where it will be carried to the next level. These are generally thin metal strips called resilient bars to which the ceiling is fastened, and are available at builder's suppliers or through a gypsum board products supplier. ***Massive*** floor systems can also be used to prevent passage of sound between floors. These are usually a thin (1–2 in.) layer of concrete applied to a wood frame floor before the finished floor is installed. If your building can support the weight these are very effective for reducing the passage of sound between floors (see the Construction Notes chapter). Remember that all sound control methods will work both ways. That is, any resilient or massive system will reduce the passage of sound from both sides. These systems are dependent, however, on full isolation between the floors. If a furnace duct or stair without a tight fitting door passes between floors the results will be disappointing.

Masking Sound Some people find that electronic sound generators are effective for providing a gentle masking sound which can relieve the tension generated by unavoidable household or city noise. These devices generate sounds similar to falling water or surf, which are intended to be soothing, particularly at bedtime.

Appliances and Plumbing Household appliances such as washers, dryers, and refrigerators transmit motor noise into floors which is then carried throughout the house. Placing them on concrete floors or isolating them with small rubber cushions placed under the feet will reduce noise. Furnace ducts both generate and carry noise. The furnace motors cause vibration in the ducts, which rumble, squeak, or rattle, and the duct openings allow sound to pass between rooms. Well constructed ducts that are securely fastened with screws and braced against vibration will reduce the problem. Foil backed duct insulation can be applied to the outside surface to reduce noise further. They will, however, still carry sound between rooms which are connected to them. The problem is largely unavoidable except with complicated and expensive baffling methods. Duct systems should be avoided when lessening sound transmission between rooms is critical, such as between separate suites. Never put glass fiber sound insulation inside ducts to reduce noise. The fibers will become airborne and be inhaled, and the rough surface will collect dust and odors, and possibly breed microorganisms.

Plumbing noise such as water hammer, and rumbling or rushing sounds from pipes, is caused when noisy pipes transmit sound to walls and floors. Water hammer can be eliminated by installing air cushions at critical locations such as washer taps. Transmission of pipe noise can be reduced by using suspension type pipe straps and oversize holes where pipes pass through framing. "Silent flush" type toilets are also helpful. Consult your plumber.

SECTION II

Understanding and Control of Indoor Hazards

5 UNDERSTANDING CONTAMINATION PROCESSES

There are well-known processes of pollution affecting both the global environment and our local regions. Industrial practices, which contribute to air, water, and soil pollution, as well as noise, electromagnetic, and radioactive contamination, are in the news every day. Closer to home are our personal habits, such as using a car, smoking, using pesticides and herbicides, and a long list of other practices, which are potentially detrimental to our health and to the health of those around us. Most of these involve well understood, clearly documented risks. However, the chemical, biological, and physical processes which occur in our homes are less well known, yet they can be just as detrimental to our health.

Chemical Processes Which Produce Contaminants in the Home

COMBUSTION

Burning anything in the home, whether it is a candle, a gas stove, or a fuel in a fireplace, consumes vital oxygen, and produces water vapor and various dangerous air contaminants. These range from such irritants as nitrogen dioxide, to potentially deadly asphyxiants, such as carbon monoxide, and carcinogens such as benzo pyrene. There are a number of other contaminating products, as well. (See The Indoor Hazards chapter.)

Unless these combustion products are immediately and effectively removed from the home by chimneys and vents, and a supply of air is provided to replace the gases that are removed, irritating or dangerous indoor conditions will quickly develop.

OUTGASSING

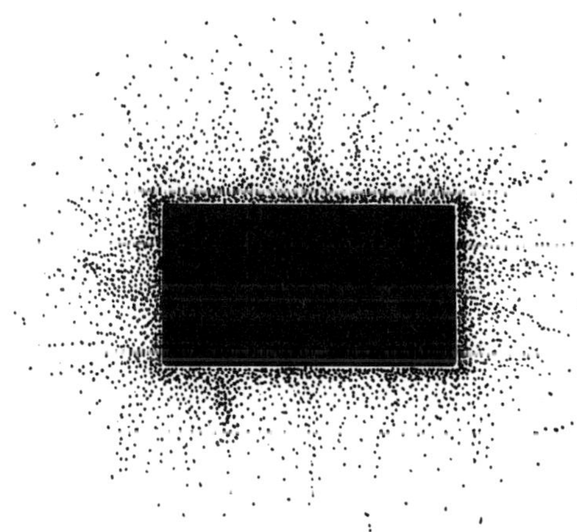

Fig. 5-1 Outgassing. *Contaminants 'outgas' from chemically unstable materials (eg. plastics, rubber, paints, adhesives, synthetic fabrics).*

This process is a form of evaporation occurring not with liquids, but with solid materials. Though we usually think of solid materials as permanent and stable because they are firm to the touch, they are all actually constantly changing at varying rates. If one could see the molecular activity on the surface of an active material, such as some plastics or paints, it would appear to be slowly boiling, releasing a cloud of gas into surrounding air. Outgassing is caused by the slow release of chemicals which are not perfectly bound (stable) within the structure of the material. These might be components of the material itself, or various additives, such as solvents, softeners, dyes, and treatments, or they may be by-products of reactions going on within, or at the surface of, the material. Examples of the latter are oxidation and evaporation caused by heat and light. (Discussed below.) *Among the most common materials which outgas harmful contaminants are some of the thousands of products made from the synthetic plastic resins. These include many kinds of plastic and rubber products, synthetic fabrics, fabric treatments, adhesives, paints, waxes, and polishes.*

IMPORTANT CONTAMINANTS IN THE HOME

Formaldehyde: This is released, for example, from formaldehyde-based insulation foams and resin glues used in wood composition board, as well as from many other sources. (See the Materials and Selection chapter.)

Other Volatile Compounds: These include toluene, benzene, naphtha, and many others, which are released from solvent based adhesives, paints, waxes, and cleaners, as well as from upholstery and plastics.

Plasticizers: These are organic compounds, including the phthalates and many others, which are added to plastics to keep them soft and flexible. (They are the source of the familiar "new" smell of an auto interior, a shower curtain, or plastic upholstery.)

Fortunately, most of the hazardous products which outgas from synthetic materials have strong odors which we can easily detect if we pay careful attention to the immediate response of our noses. The outgassing process, which is stimulated by heat and light, constantly increases the burden of indoor contamination. The resulting indoor situation requires constant and reliable fresh air ventilation.

OXIDATION

Oxidation is a chemical change affecting most materials. It is caused by heat, light, and air, as well as by electrical activity and chemical agents. *Oxidation of harmless common elements, such as carbon, will form carbon dioxide and carbon monoxide, a dangerous asphyxiant. Oxidation of such common gases as nitrogen and oxygen will form nitrogen dioxide and ozone, both serious respiratory irritants.*

The most common sources of oxidation in the home are gas ranges and other unvented flames, the breakdown of unstable chemicals in building and furnishing materials, the action of sunlight and heat on draperies and floor coverings, and the use of poorly designed or maintained electronic air cleaners or other electrical devices.

Household oxidation cannot be prevented, but it can be minimized by ***eliminating unvented combustion appliances, carefully selecting stable building and furnishing materials, preventing the exposure of unstable materials to heat and sunlight, and the careful choice and use of electric appliances.***

ABSORPTION

Contaminants in the home environment carried in air, food, and water are *absorbed* into the body by chemical interaction. Whether inhaled, swallowed, or in contact with the skin, all contaminants which are chemically soluble in human tissues will enter the blood. Once in the blood, they are carried to organs and tissues where toxic activity takes place. Some chemicals, such as many of the volatile solvents, are readily discharged again from the body. Others, such as the organochlorine compounds (common in pesticides and industrial chemicals) stay in fatty body tissues, and in organs like the liver, and are not readily discharged.

The effects of most inhaled and swallowed toxic substances are already well known, but recent research shows that bathing in contaminated water also causes absorption of toxic substances. In fact, 50%-60% of the absorption of contaminants in household water occurs through the skin. (See the Water Treatment chapter.)

ADSORPTION

Adsorption is the physical attachment of one material to the surface of another, and is not a chemical interaction like absorption. Airborne contaminants in the home, such as formaldehyde, combustion gases, and organic vapors from paints, will "cling" to available surfaces, such as fabrics and wallboard. Adsorption explains why an article of clothing or an entire home will continue to smell for a long period after exposure to smoke or paint fumes.

Adsorption is easily reversed, and an "airing out" period will usually clear up lingering odors.

Adsorption is also the process used by most air purification chemicals. Such materials as activated charcoal have a high adsorption capacity for certain gases, and will collect them until saturation, when they can be discarded.

ELECTROMAGNETIC FIELDS

All electric equipment produces electrical and magnetic fields of varying strengths and types. Because the human body operates by electrochemical activity, it has been believed for some time that electromagnetic fields influence us.

The two types of electromagnetic activity which are of particular interest in relation to human health are radio frequency fields (R.F.) and extremely low frequency (E. L.F.).

Radio Frequency: Large radio frequency fields are generated by radio, T.V., and microwave transmitters, and radar units. They can travel long distances and be readily reflected by metal surfaces.

The health effects of high R.F. levels are well known, and include neurological damage, eye cataracts, and other diseases. The effects of low levels are not well known. Until we learn more about this hazard it is wise to avoid exposure to transmitters producing R.F. Home computers, televisions, and microwave ovens also produce small amounts of R.F., and should not be used close to the body.

Extremely Low Frequency: Less is known about the effects of these magnetic fields, produced by power lines and electrical wiring (and some military communications). Some studies have definitely linked high energy E.L.F., such as that found near high power lines, with alarming physiological changes in experimental animals. Other studies make tentative links between E.L.F. from home wiring and childhood cancer. Until more is known about E.L.F. it is wise to avoid living near high power lines if at all possible. Some researchers recommend 200 feet as a safe distance from medium high voltage lines (50,000 volts), but that a 500 foot or greater distance is necessary for very high voltage lines (360,000 volts).

If your house is being wired, you can also confine a great deal of the wiring to unoccupied basements or other areas of little exposure.

Electrical Field Risks: Children and pregnant mothers are the most susceptible to electrical field hazards in the home. Bedrooms and playrooms for young children should be located as far as possible from any high voltage power lines near the home. Any woman contemplating pregnancy should also be very cautious about electric fields, because the fetus is most vulnerable to genetic damage during the first two weeks of development. Cautious researchers are now suggesting that electric blankets, computers, and microwave ovens be avoided during this period.

Biological Processes of Contamination in the Home

Various biological processes are constantly occurring around us, most of which are normal and harmless if we are in good health. For those who are sensitive or weakened by illness, exposure to some of these biological conditions can be harmful. Under some conditions, biological hazards can develop which are a danger to all of us.

INCUBATION

Bacteria and fungi are constantly with us in air, water, and food, on our skin, and clinging to surfaces in our homes. When they are in normal concentrations, a healthy person will not suffer undue effects from them. However, those of us who have been weakened by illness, or who suffer from sensitivity, can be seriously affected. Of course, if allowed to multiply, colonies of bacteria and fungi will also become a health threat to everyone.

Bacteria and fungi require certain conditions of moisture, temperature, nutrition, and light, in order to reproduce. Under ideal conditions they will reproduce very quickly.

Moisture: Reproduction and survival of most microorganisms increases significantly with humidity levels above 60% R.H. (See the Thermal Comfort chapter.)

Temperature: Common household temperatures are quite sufficient for fungus reproduction. Most bacteria will reproduce rapidly at a somewhat higher temperature, closer to human body temperature.

Nutrients: Some bacteria and fungi can grow on almost any organic material. This includes soil, food, wood, dust, natural and synthetic resins, and fibers. Even urea formaldehyde foam in the walls of homes has been shown to support fungi.

Light: The survival and reproduction of most microbes will be reduced by light. Strong light, particularly sunlight, with its ultraviolet component, has a significant sterilizing effect.

TRANSMISSION

Bacteria and viruses are both transmitted by air and by direct contact. While airborne, their survival is influenced largely by moisture, temperature, and light. Conditions similar to those for the incubation of bacteria and fungi will also increase the survival and transmission of bacteria and viruses. Very dry conditions (below 30% R.H.) also increase the transmission of disease by airborne pathogens by drying the protective mucous lining of the throat and sinuses.

Fungi proliferate by tiny seed-like spores released from colonies and carried by air currents. Many fungi and their spores are highly allergenic to some sensitive people, causing a range of reactions, from mild to severe. Estimates indicate that about twenty million people in the United States may be allergic to even small exposures to these. *The most alarming aspect of fungi is that they seem to be capable of sensitizing those of us without previous allergy problems,* if we are exposed to large doses. This makes fungi a potential risk to everyone.

DECOMPOSITION

Bacteria and fungi normally found in foods and other organic materials will, when allowed to multiply, cause changes to the host material, producing not only spoilage, but dangerous toxins as well. Food poisoning due to bacterial toxin production is a well known phenomenon, but the fact that fungi can produce carcinogenic toxins, such as the aflatoxin found in spoiled peanuts, is less well known.

CHEMICAL STEWS

Any number of these processes can occur in a house with the presence of a variety of contaminants, creating a chemical stew. The properties and effects of any single agent can be a highly complex subject, and the effects of such a stew are still virtually unknown. Synergy is one recognized factor in this chemical stew. Two or more contaminants in the environment can have a combined effect exceeding the total effect of each separate one. A familiar example of synergy is the health effects on smokers of common respiratory irritants and carcinogens unrelated to smoking. For example, anyone who smokes is much more likely to be irritated by smog, or to contract cancer from asbestos exposure or radon, than is a non-smoker.

6 THE INDOOR HAZARDS

Once outdoor air has been drawn into the home from the safest available source, there are processes which begin to change its composition in ways that can be harmful to our health. The major, and possibly hazardous, components of indoor air, where and how they are commonly produced, their toxic effects, together with physical symptoms, and their means of control, will be described in this chapter. More detailed instructions for control measures follow in the section DESIGNING THE HEALTHY HOME, and special measures for the hypersensitive in the section ENVIRONMENTAL ILLNESS AND YOU.

Gases in Our Homes

FORMALDEHYDE (HCHO)

Formaldehyde is one of the family of aldehydes, a group of simple hydrocarbons very widely used in manufacturing today. It is a highly irritating chemical with a very pungent odor not normally found in "natural" air in significant quantities. Formaldehyde is probably the most widely known indoor air contaminant, particularly because the disaster over the widespread use of urea formaldehyde foam insulation (UFFI) in the mid 1970's brought it to the attention of the general public. This insulation, approved for home use, was sprayed into the walls of a large number of older houses during this period, in order to save expensive heating fuel. Within a few years, the overwhelming number of health problems in those homes (in many cases *half* of the occupants were affected) due to formaldehyde release from the insulation forced both a ban on the product and a widespread program to remove it from homes. Formaldehyde is also present in a large number of new building materials and household products that have become widely used over the last twenty years. It is also produced by combustion.

Health hazards: Formaldehyde is a potent irritant which affects the eyes, nose, throat, and lungs, and may also cause skin reactions. Exposure has also been shown to cause headaches, depression, dizziness, and loss of sleep in cases of chronic exposure, such as in UFFI insulated homes. Formaldehyde has also been shown to aggravate minor illnesses, such as coughs and colds, and to *trigger* a number of other, more serious illnesses such as asthma. *A recent study on the toxic effects of formaldehyde concluded that one person in every five is sensitive to exposure.*

One of the most alarming effects of formaldehyde exposure is the sensitization reaction. In many cases of chemical hypersensitivity, formaldehyde exposure has been a factor in the onset of the problem. This chemical appears to stimulate an immune type reaction in people who have previously enjoyed a normal level of susceptibility to irritants in the environment. Repeated exposure to high levels, or chronic exposure to elevated levels, such as those that occur in homes treated with UFFI insulation, seems to be sufficient to trigger hypersensitivity. People who are affected this way may then go on to suffer with exposure to a wide range of common substances, such as fabrics, paints, foods, carpets, building materials, plastics, household odors, smog, and dust.

Though formaldehyde is not yet listed as a carcinogen (a cancer causing agent) by health authorities in the U.S., it *has* been shown to cause nasal cancer in rats, and very recent studies have connected it to certain human cancers. It is one of the most potent of many environmental irritants which are linked to increased cancer *risk*. These irritants cause mutations of the genetic material in tissue cells which alter their reproduction—one of the steps in the onset of cancer.

Symptoms: Eye, nose, and throat irritation, dry throat, sneezing, and coughing. Headache and dizziness may accompany these symptoms, as well as skin rash from contact with such materials as particle board and treated fabrics which contain formaldehyde. Frequent blinking, burning sensations, itching eyelids, or a dry "scratchy" feeling are signs of eye irritation due to exposure. A wide range of more serious symptoms, including heart palpitations, severe depressions, violent pains, shortness of breath, loss of sense of smell and taste, and swelling of the throat, are common among sensitive people. Heart irregularities, severe bladder problems, phlebitis (vein inflammation), and blood clotting have also been seen as reactions to formaldehyde.

Concentrations: Small background levels of formaldehyde are present in outdoor air due to combustion and other forms of pollution. These may be in the 0.01 to 0.02 ppm range. The lowest measured levels of formaldehyde *in homes* are around the 0.01 ppm range, which is below some outdoor measurements. This is a barely measurable level and a good target level when planning for low pollution buildings. Most people can smell formaldehyde at concentrations of about ten times this level (0.1 ppm), and this amount has been set as the acceptable indoor limit by governments in Canada, parts of the U.S.A., and Europe. Some homes have measured levels ten or more times higher (1.0 ppm or more), which is clearly hazardous.

There is no definite threshold level for safety which applies to everyone, but *due to the sensitizing nature of this chemical, extra caution is warranted.* This is one of the pollution situations where the whole idea of "acceptable amount" should be discarded by those concerned about prevention. *The goal for our homes should be no detectable formaldehyde in air. Serious reactions can also occur to the formaldehyde in cosmetics, dentifrice, soft drinks, beer, and other foods.*

Sources: There are so many sources of formaldehyde in the home that a complete list would fill a large volume. It appears in many adhesives, paints, fabric treatments, insulations, plastics, upholstery materials, carpets, etc. In many new homes there are more building and furnishing materials that contain formaldehyde than those which do not.

MATERIALS WHICH MAY CONTRIBUTE TO FORMALDEHYDE POLLUTION

Urea formaldehyde foam insulation
Particle board, chip board, and interior plywood
Carpets, carpet pads
Upholstery fabrics
Upholstery foam
Construction adhesive
Furniture, cabinets
Paints
Burning of gas, oil, wood
Tobacco smoke
Household waxes, oils
Cosmetics, mouthwash, toothpaste
Beverages, beer, wine
Exterior plywood
Wallpaper
Glass fiber insulation
Plaster, stucco, concrete
Fabric dyes
Fabric treatments
Wallboard

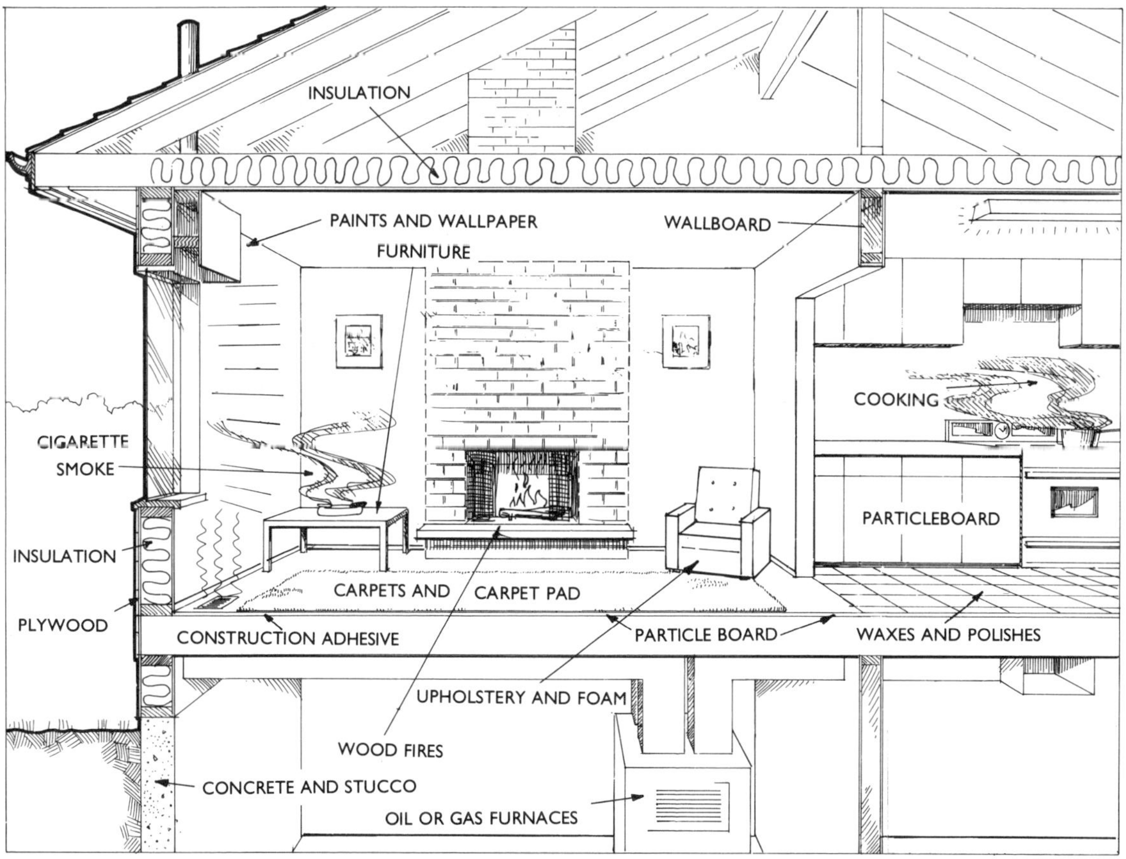

Fig. 6-1 Some Formaldehyde Sources in the Home

Formaldehyde is most often used in the resin glues, plastics, and foams that appear in many of these products. Because these ingredients are inexpensive and convenient, nearly all manufacturing industries are heavily committed to them. The second most common use of formaldehyde is as a preservative, fungicide, and stabilizer in these products and many others. This explains why it appears in products as diverse as wallboard and cosmetics. The third most common use is as a fabric treatment agent used in permanent press clothing, draperies, fireproof materials, and other fabrics.

Formaldehyde and related chemicals are also produced by combustion. Generally, the more smoke being produced by burning (from cigarettes, incinerators, and poorly tuned engines, for example), the more formaldehyde and other pollutants are being produced.

Paths of entry: Very little formaldehyde generally enters the home from outside, as there is usually little in the surrounding air. The vast majority of sources are right in the building materials, furnishings, and household products around us. The formaldehyde in these materials is constantly being released as an invisible gas which mixes with the air around us. This is called outgassing, and is a form of evaporation similar to the steam rising from hot water.

Some formaldehyde in household products evaporates very readily. This is true for cleaners, waxes, and some paints, which can more easily be controlled, as they are used in small quantities—usually with extra ventilation. However, the formaldehyde in urea formaldehyde resins, such as those used in foam insulation, particle board, and interior plywoods, evaporates more slowly. *These present the greatest health problems, both because they are used in such large quantities in homes and furnishings, and because they can remain active pollutants for months or years.* The formaldehyde in other resins, such as those used in exterior grade plywood and some fabric treatments, release their gas even more slowly.

Increased temperature and humidity increases the rate at which formaldehyde will outgas from materials. A home containing materials made using formaldehyde that is left closed up in hot weather will build up quite high levels. This contributes to the "bad air" smell that confronts you when you return. Such conditions create the worst exposures, particularly in new homes, and should be avoided. Another factor aggravating this problem is the fact that formaldehyde (and other airborne pollutants) will "cling" to surfaces such as walls, rungs, and fabrics. This is called "adsorption," and explains why it takes a long time to "air out" a building to rid it of smells after it has been closed up for some time.

Controls: The only way to control formaldehyde is by ***careful selection of the materials in our homes to avoid those which will release it.*** *There is no adequate way to protect yourself from this hazard if you live with potent sources of this chemical.* Later chapters deal with identifying materials made without formaldehyde, and those with low formaldehyde emissions. (See the chapter Materials and Selection.)

Small amounts of material, such as the particle board in cabinet frames, can be treated to "seal" in the gas. This is advisable for everyone who must live with small amounts of formaldehyde producing materials. Urethane varnish or hard plastic veneer are the preferred sealers, but samples of these must be tested first by those who are hypersensitive. A well sealed air barrier of aluminum foil can reduce the entry of formaldehyde from glued wood products in walls and ceilings.

Remaining traces of formaldehyde which cannot be avoided can be reduced by good ventilation. (See the Home Ventilation chapter.)

Notes: Our ability to smell formaldehyde and many other airborne organic compounds is most acute immediately after entering a contaminated room, and it diminishes with time. *This "adjustment" phenomenon is common with many chemical pollutants and should be regarded as a warning that first impressions are often correct.*

Mobile homes are plagued with formaldehyde problems. This is apparently due to their relatively small size, tight construction, and the quantity of particleboard, plastics, and glues used in making them. The problem is worsened by their small sized rooms and poor air circulation. This problem diminishes over time as the chemical dissipates, and is usually less acute in buildings over five years old.

ORGANOCHLORINES

Organochlorine compounds are chemical combinations of organic chemicals (containing hyrdrogen and carbon) with chlorine. Organic chemicals are known as the building blocks of life. They are also the basis for synthesis of many new compounds which do not occur in nature. When natural or synthetic organic molecules are combined with chlorine, which is a very active and hazardous chemical element, they become quite different substances and can present many health hazards.

Many pesticides are organochlorines. They are usually the most toxic compounds in this family, as well as the most persistent in the environment and in human and animal tissues.

Many liquid solvents are organochlorine compounds. They are found in cleaning fluids, and some paints, waxes, and plastics.

Some stabilized plastic resins such as P.V.C. (Polyvinyl chloride) are also members of this family. Vinyl chloride, the basis of P.V.C., is a potent carcinogen which can easily enter air or water. The potent and highly carcinogenic P.C.B.'s (Polychlorinated byphenyls) are also in this family. They are found in electrical equipment and some plastics.

Organochlorines are also formed when the chlorine in treated water combines with naturally occurring organic compounds. This results in the production of toxic gases, such as chloroform and chloramine.

Health hazards: Virtually all organochlorines are toxic, and some, such as pesticides, are highly toxic and carcinogenic; others, such as cleaning solvents, accumulate and seriously damage such organs as the liver and kidney. Most are soluble in the body's fatty tissues, where they collect and are later released into the bloodstream with toxic results.

All organochlorines are potential carcinogens, and some, such as dioxins, vinyl chloride and P.C.B.'s, are particularly potent. They combine directly with our genetic material, causing cancer.

Other organochlorines, such as the chloroform gas produced by chlorine in water, are serious respiratory irritants, and are toxic to body cells.

Symptoms Acute exposure to organochlorines will cause a wide variety of symptoms, including nausea, dizziness, skin reactions, weakness, eye irritation, nosebleed, and depression. Chronic exposure may have no immediate symptoms for many people, but may be a greater hazard, with longterm organ damage and cancer risk.

Many of these compounds have strong odors which can be recognized, but others are odorless even at dangerous concentrations.

Concentrations: A very wide range of concentrations may occur in our environment. Soils and water containing .01 ppm or less pesticide residue will present substantial risks when concentrated in foods. During their use, concentrations of cleaning solvents may reach 100–500 ppm and present serious health risks. Most are regulated by government standards and recognized as toxic in this range.

Very small amounts of vinyl chloride and P.C.B.'s are found in air and water. *These are hazardous at any level.*

Sources: Organochlorines are found with pesticide use, in dry cleaning plants, cleaning products, wood preservatives, industrial emissions, outgassing of plastics and paints, chlorine in water supplies, and many others. Industrial bleaching and the manufacturing of chemicals also produce organochlorines accidentally. As well, animal fats and meats may contain concentrated organochlorines from agricultural and industrial pollution.

Controls: Substituting safe products for those containing organochlorines in the household is an important first step. Careful choice of food supplies, reducing meats and fats in the diet, and purifying household water are also important.

Notes: In both the U.S. and Canada all household products containing organochlorines must by law be labeled HAZARDOUS and/or they must list all their ingredients. You can recognize organochlorines on labels by their chemical names containing "chloro". They will often also include a series of numbers which indicate the exact chemical structure.

Examples:

1,1,1 Tri*chloro*ethane; Tri*chloro*ethylene; Carbon tetra*chlor*ide; *chloro*benzene; hepta*chlor; chlor*dane; penta*chloro*phenol; hexa*chloro*phene.

2,4-D; 2,4,5-T (Abbreviations for organochlorine pesticides.)

Organic bromines and fluorines are often hazardous in the same ways as the organochlorines.

VOLATILE ORGANIC COMPOUNDS

This very large family of chemicals includes all the organic compounds (containing hydrogen and carbon) which readily evaporate and cause air pollution. Though at room temperature most are liquids, they will readily enter air, especially when heated. Many are also found contaminating water, and they are used as additives to solids, such as plastics.

Many volatile organics are extracted directly from petroleum oil and gas; others such as alcohols are produced synthetically by chemical methods. Most are used as solvents. They are usually intoxicants or asphyxiants (causing suffocation), and some are toxic to brain cells. They may also be explosive. All are potential hazards to sensitive persons.

This family includes alkanes, alkenes, naphthas, benzenes, toluene, xylene, ethers, mineral spirits, alcohols (methyl and ethyl compounds), ketones, aldehydes, propane, butane, polymers, and monomers.

Health hazards: Most are asphyxiants. They may cause dizziness, disorientation, or death, in large doses. Some are depressants, acting on the central nervous system and causing fatigue and muscle weakness. Most are also skin and lung irritants. Some are carcinogenic or cause kidney or liver damage. Because most are soluble in fatty tissue, they are readily absorbed, and in some cases stored, in our bodies.

Symptoms: Exposure will cause eye and skin irritation, dizziness, and muscle weakness in all people. Symptoms of exposure in sensitive people include violent headaches, nausea, loss of muscle control, heart arrythmia, and other symptoms. Most volatile organics have strong, sharp odors.

Concentrations: Many volatile organics reach very high concentrations, greater than 100 ppm, during painting or cleaning operations. Other compounds in this family, such as formaldehyde, are acutely toxic below 1 ppm. Benzene is a common solvent and is toxic above 1 ppm.

Sources: Paints, cleaning solvents, waxes, polishes, camp stove fuel, gasoline, oil, natural gas, propane and butane, dry cleaning, artificial and natural scents, and plastics.

Controls: Choose your household products carefully, and substitute with safe alternatives. (See the Home Maintenance chapter.) Air out rooms after using any necessary paints and solvents, cleaners, and polishes. Use an approved respirator mask (see the GETTING HELP section). Store fuels and solvents away from the home.

Notes: One of the most carcinogenic of organic compounds is Benzo a pyrene (BaP), an aromatic hydrocarbon produced by combustion. Incinerators, wood stoves, and auto exhaust contain BaP, as do industrial emissions, tobacco smoke, and broiled (dark) or burnt foods.

PHENOLS (C_6H_5OH)

Phenols are organic compounds derived

from coal tar or petroleum, and are used extensively in household products. The phenols include biphenyl, phenolics, and pentachlorophenol (P.C.P.). Pure phenol (also known as carbolic acid) is a potent disinfectant and antiseptic. It is widely used in hospitals and homes. It is a serious incitant to many sensitive individuals. Phenol is also used in the synthesis of plastic resins and wood preservatives, and is present in tobacco smoke.

Health hazards: Phenol and phenol compounds are highly sensitizing to skin and are suspected to be carcinogenic. Severe reactions in sensitive individuals are dangerous and can be life threatening.

Symptoms: Skin rashes, peeling, or pimples are common in all people after skin contact. Nausea, heart arrythmia, breathing difficulties, and other alarming symptoms occur in sensitive people. Phenol can be readily recognized by its strong odor.

Concentrations: Concentrations of phenols vary widely. Reactions among hypersensitive people have been observed at concentrations as low as .002 ppm in air.

Sources: Household cleaners, mildew cleaners, perfumes, air fresheners, mouthwashes, disinfectants, polishes, waxes, glues, phenolic plastics (such as hard saucepan handles), wood perservatives, and tobacco smoke.

Controls: Most of the phenols in our homes are in cleaning and disinfecting products. Choose your household products carefully to avoid them. Most products containing phenols are labeled and can easily be replaced with safe substitutes. (See the Home Maintenance chapter.)

Notes: Though phenols are everywhere in the household, they are not widely recognized as hazards. They should be avoided as carefully as formaldehyde.

RADON (Rn 222)

Radon is a colorless, odorless gas that is a serious threat to health in some regions. It is produced in certain geologic zones by the radioactive decay of naturally occurring radium. Though radon is actually relatively harmless in itself, it *is* the medium by which soil radioactivity enters the home. Once inside, radon decays into other radioactive products, the most hazardous being the polonium isotopes. These particles easily attach themselves to dust particles which are inhaled and lodged in the bronchial tubes and lungs. Once there, the isotopes release minute but very focused doses of dangerous alpha radiation into the tissues.

Health hazards: Radiation released within the body will strike genes, which may then cause the kind of genetic mutations that eventually lead to cancer. Cancer risk is usually expressed in statistical terms, and radiation exposure of this type increases the risk of developing lung or throat cancer in one's lifetime. Other factors, such as smoking, will further increase this risk.

The level of radon entering a home is dependent on three things: the amount of natural radioactivity in surrounding soils, building materials, and groundwater; the paths of entry that are open to it (such as foundation cracks and floor drains); and the direction of air flow through these paths. It is estimated that the more moderate levels found in some affected homes (1pCi/L, pico Curie per Liter, a measure of radiation intensity) could be responsible for a statistical increase in incidences of lung cancer in the order of 1 case per 10,000 pop. per year. The allowable level for homes under U.S. health guidelines is currently set at four times that level (4pCi/L).

Symptoms: There are no known symptoms of radon exposure. The known risk is a long term, statistical one.

Sources and paths of entry: Radium, the source of radon gas, occurs naturally in soils, rock formations, and groundwater, particularly in the northeastern U.S. and southeastern Canada. It is also found in other regions in connection with uranium or phosphate mining. The worst cases of radon exposure have occurred where tailings and waste from uranium or phosphate mining was used for landfill, or where it has polluted residential groundwater. In some cases mining waste has been found in the concrete used for foundations, so that a steady source of radioactive pollution was built into the home. In some regions, clay bricks, gypsum board, and concrete products, when made from soils high in natural radiation, are another source. Water supplies coming from wells drilled into rock can also be potent radon sources. The gas can reach high concentrations in poorly ventilated bathrooms and kitchens during washing.

When radon gas is released during the natural breakdown of radium, it enters the soil or groundwater around the home's foundation and finds its way into the home through cracks in the foundation, floor drains, vents, and basement windows. How easily this gas can enter a house will depend on the condition of the foundation, and on the differences in air pressure between the outside and inside. The reduced inside pressure, which comes from exhausting inside air without providing adequate incoming air to replace it, is the main cause of increased radon entry. A similar situation can also be caused by wind conditions, or by a home's natural upward airflow. (Refer to the Home Ventilation chapter.)

Concentrations: The concentration of radioactive products is a highly technical subject, but it is not difficult to compare the levels commonly found in homes with public health standards. Four pico Curies per liter of air (4 pCi/L) is the standard accepted for homes by the U.S. government's department of health. The levels commonly found vary from only 3 percent of this allowable maximum in unaffected areas, to levels 5 or 6 times this amount in problem areas. However, this "safe" standard is 4 times the level connected with a known small statistical increase in lung cancer, and only 2 percent of the levels allowed in uranium mines. Standards in Sweden for new houses and those *recommended* in the U.S. by the ASHRAE (American Society of Heating Refrigeration and Air Conditioning Engineers) are much lower than the U.S. national standard. Levels well below the accepted 4 pCi/L should be the goal for prevention in the home.

Controls: A good deal of work has been done lately in the U.S., Canada, and Sweden, to develop better controls for radon gas in homes. The most effective strategy is to ***prevent the gas entering by increasing the building's air pressure*** to levels slightly above those outside. ***Sealing foundation cracks,*** and ***providing separate ventilating air to basements*** are also helpful, as is ***outside venting of basement drains. Increased ventilation rates*** are generally useful, particularly in bathrooms, where radon released from well water can build up during showering. There is some evidence that ***air filtration and activated charcoal filtering*** will help remove radon, but this is probably less effective and more costly in the long term than proper sealing, ventilation, and air pressure control.

Notes: In regions with naturally high geological radiation, local public health authorities should be able to supply information on the radon hazard. The U.S. Environmental Protection Agency can provide information and direct inquiries to local authorities. Home measurement is recommended if there are indications that your region may be affected, and special care should be taken ***in any case*** with foundation sealing and ventilation. Where there are tailings from uranium or phosphate mining, granite bedrock near the surface, or wells drilled into bedrock supplying your water, there is cause for concern, and complete measurements should be taken in homes. Your health department should be able to direct you to a source of test devices, or recommend an independent testing service. (See the chapters Controlling Indoor Air Quality, and Testing For Contamination.)

CARBON MONOXIDE (CO)

Carbon monoxide is a very dangerous, colorless, odorless gas not normally found in significant quantities in the air around us. Carbon monoxide is produced by incomplete combustion, such as in poorly adjusted gas flames and automobile engines. It is easily absorbed by the bloodstream and rapidly interferes with normal breathing.

Health hazards: Carbon monoxide combines with blood hemoglobin, reducing the body's capacity to absorb oxygen. In very small concentrations it may cause intoxication and headache; in larger doses it will cause asphyxiation and death. Exposure to dangerous levels may cause long term neurological damage. Increased levels are particularly dangerous to people with heart and lung disorders, and with circulation problems.

Symptoms: Exposure to low CO levels may cause blurring of vision, loss of judgment, headache, nausea, and dizziness. Patients with heart and lung problems may experience aggravated symptoms. Serious exposure calls for immediate medical attention.

Sources: Unvented or improperly vented

combustion appliances such as gas or oil stoves, furnaces, water heaters, and damaged chimneys, are common sources of carbon monoxide contamination. Automobile exhaust drawn into the home from an attached garage or a busy street is another common source. Cigarette smoking, candle flames, and open fireplaces also contribute carbon monoxide fumes.

Concentrations: Very low levels, in the range of 0.5 ppm, are acceptable for indoor air. Where there are levels above 5 ppm some detrimental effects may occur after long exposure. At levels of 100 ppm (which can be exceeded in a closed kitchen with a gas stove burning) exposure should be limited to short periods, especially for those with health problems. U.S. Government standards limit allowable exposure to only one hour at levels of 35 ppm. Levels of 1000 ppm will damage health, and with lengthy exposure can cause loss of consciousness and death. A car running in a closed garage will produce this condition in a few minutes.

Controls: First, ***eliminate any unnecessary combustion appliances,*** and then make sure there is an ***adequate air supply*** and ***proper exhaust provisions*** for those that remain. ***Maintain chimneys and appliances*** regularly, and provide for an adequate ***air supply to the home free from automobile exhaust*** and other contamination.

Notes: Carbon monoxide is one of the most immediately hazardous pollutants to indoor air. Dangerous exposure may occur before one is aware of the problem, and chronic exposure may have serious effects. These effects may include reduced lung capacity leading to heart and lung problems, and loss of concentration and memory. Like carbon dioxide, this gas can be readily diluted by introducing fresh air, but unlike CO_2, carbon monoxide can cause permanent damage. Alarming levels of carbon monoxide sometimes occur due to automobile exhaust and industrial emissions. Smokers are especially susceptible to CO poisoning, due to their elevated blood levels of the gas resulting from tobacco smoke.

NITROGEN OXIDES (NO, NO_2)

Oxides of nitrogen are strong smelling, highly irritating, and toxic gases. They are responsible in part for the brown haze found in urban smog. They are byproducts of combustion and the action of sunlight on polluted air.

Health hazards: Oxides of nitrogen are highly irritating to mucous and lung tissues, and the corrosive products produced when nitrogen dioxide (NO_2) comes into contact with moist lung and bronchial membrane will cause tissue damage. With prolonged exposure lung function will be impaired. This kind of damage is seen in lung diseases such as emphysema in smokers, and in people with high exposure in the workplace. NO_2 exposure also causes depression of white blood cells, reducing immunity to disease. Nitric oxide (NO) is irritating but less hazardous than nitrogen dioxide.

Symptoms: Nitrogen oxides will cause burning sensations in the eyes, nose, and throat, and this irritation may lead to coughing fits and watering eyes. Sometimes there are also sensations of lightheadedness and intoxication. Frequent minor respiratory illness such as coughs and colds can be early signs of exposure.

Sources: Nitrogen oxides are byproducts of combustion when nitrogen, the most abundant gas in the atmosphere, is heated to high temperatures. The major indoor sources of these gases are fuel burning stoves, furnaces, water heaters, and cigarette smoke. Automobile exhaust and industrial emissions are the major outdoor sources.

Concentrations: Common indoor levels of nitrogen oxides range between .05 and .5 ppm, but higher levels are found during smog conditions. Lung tissue damage from prolonged exposure can occur above .5 ppm and extreme symptoms usually develop above 10 ppm.

Controls: ***Ventilate combustion appliances properly,*** and ***increase fresh air supply from selected sources.***

Notes: Nitrogen oxides have a strong odor that can be detected at low levels (around .1 ppm). Such levels are considerably below those considered hazardous.

SULFUR DIOXIDE (SO_2)

Sulfur dioxide is a colorless gas with a sharp odor not normally found in significant amounts in "natural" air. It is formed by the oxidation of the sulfur contained in various fuels when they are burned. Sulfur dioxide from coal burning plants and other industrial processes forms a caustic acid when combined with water. This is a major contributor to acid rain.

Health hazards: The acid irritant formed when sulfur dioxide comes into contact with bronchial and lung tissues leads to increased minor respiratory illnesses, such as colds with coughs and bronchitis. Though sulfur dioxide is not considered as destructive as nitrogen dioxide and some other irritants, it can aggravate symptoms in patients with respiratory disease. It is not lethal in the concentrations usually found in air samples.

Symptoms: Burning sensations in the throat and nose, coughing, and choking.

Sources: Major indoor sources are poorly vented stoves, furnaces, and water heaters burning fuel oils with a high sulfur content. Natural gas usually contains only small amounts of sulfur and produces little SO_2. Outdoor sources include industries burning high sulfur coals and oils, pulp mills, petroleum refineries, smelters, and Diesel engines.

Concentrations: Typical indoor concentrations range from .01 ppm to .05 ppm. These levels are not irritating to most people, but much higher outdoor levels can be found downwind from industry. Exposure to levels above .2 ppm is irritating to most people, and at much higher levels (10 ppm) it is acutely irritating.

Controls: Where practical ***replace fuel oil burning appliances with electric.*** Provide adequate exhaust for any remaining combustion appliances to control indoor build-up. Increased ventilation rates will not be helpful in many areas where outdoor levels are higher than those indoors. Some fabrics such as cotton and wool will actually adsorb SO_2 and even neutralize it to some extent. ***Wool rugs and draperies,*** where appropriate, can actually reduce indoor pollution and can be cleaned to remove chemical deposits.

Notes: Sulfur dioxide is a very great hazard to the survival of forests, lakes, and waterways. Acid rain is the result of careless regulation of industry's use of high sulfur fuels.

OZONE (O_3)

Ozone is a colorless, unstable gas with a pungent odor usually associated with electrical equipment. Ozone decays rapidly into harmless oxygen, but it can be very irritating even in minute concentrations, particularly to people with respiratory problems. Ozone is normally present in "natural" air but only in very small amounts.

Health hazards: Ozone is a respiratory irritant which causes temporary damage to mucous membranes and lung tissue. Ozone exposure also affects visual performance and judgment. It is particularly hazardous to people suffering from asthma, hay fever, emphysema, and other respiratory illnesses. High ozone levels during smog conditions are linked with an increased death rate among patients hospitalized for life threatening illnesses.

Symptoms: Ozone exposure causes irritation to the eyes, nose, sinuses, throat, and lungs, leading to running eyes and nose, coughing, and burning sensations in the nose and throat. Blurred vision and loss of concentration may also accompany these symptoms. Ozone exposure can cause serious aggravation of symptoms in persons already suffering from respiratory illness.

Sources: Ozone is produced by the action of electrical discharges on oxygen, or by the action of sunlight on chemical smog. Electrical equipment such as brush type motors (the type found in kitchen appliances, sewing machines, and power tools), electronic air cleaners, ion generators, and photocopiers, are the main indoor sources. Outdoor air may contain serious ozone levels during smog conditions, electrical storms, or near power transmission lines.

Concentrations: Indoor air concentrations of .001 ppm are quite typical for homes and not considered harmful. At about forty times that level (.04 ppm) many people begin to experience negative symptoms. Much higher levels, around 1 ppm, will cause strong reactions with alarming changes to lung and throat tissue after lengthy exposure. Levels approaching 1 ppm have been measured during smog conditions.

Controls: ***Remove unnecessary electrical equipment,*** install specific ***ventilation for ozone sources,*** such as photocopiers, and ***maintain electronic air filters*** regularly. Manufacturers' literature and test reports should be consulted if you have an older model electronic air cleaner. ***Increasing the fresh air supply*** from the best available source is also helpful.

Notes: The pungent odor of ozone makes it relatively easy to recognize. It is also fairly easy to locate indoor sources, as they are all associated with high voltage electrical discharge. Brush type electric motors which may produce ozone in the household can be recognized by the presence of small sparks inside their housings during operation. These sparks are normal and can usually be seen through ventilation holes in the unit.

CARBON DIOXIDE (CO_2)

Carbon dioxide is a colorless, odorless gas, normally present in air in only small quantities. Because it is heavier than other gases and does not mix easily, it tends to accumulate in enclosed areas and near the floor. High carbon dioxide levels are usually found with unvented combustion appliances such as gas stoves, or with poor fresh air supply. High levels are usually perceived as "stale air" or "stuffiness."

Health hazards: Carbon dioxide is a central nervous system depressant which slows responses and reduces alertness. It also stimulates the urge to breathe. At above normal concentrations it causes discomfort and drowsiness; at very high levels it will cause death by suffocation. The effects of exposure to elevated levels of this gas are believed to be temporary under most circumstances.

Symptoms: Feelings of stuffiness, drowsiness, or claustrophobia. Headache and depression may occur with higher levels; loss of consciousness and death at very high levels.

Sources: People's respiration, and combustion, are the major sources within the home. Faulty chimneys or inadequate air supply to fuel burning appliances, and poor ventilation of combustion products, are the major causes of CO_2 buildup. Uncomfortable levels will also occur in enclosed spaces with poor ventilation due to occupancy.

Concentrations: Common levels in unpolluted outdoor air are in the 350 ppm range. 2000 ppm is considered uncomfortable by most people, and 5000 ppm or above, will cause serious loss of alertness, and other toxic symptoms.

Controls: ***Replacing fuel burning appliances*** such as gas stoves with electric appliances; ***providing a fresh air supply*** and ***good ventilation for combustion appliances*** that cannot be dispensed with; ***regular care and cleaning of chimneys. Increasing the fresh air supply*** is a remedy in all cases.

Notes: Carbon dioxide is often responsible for the sensation of "stale air." It usually does not reach hazardous levels because such levels can be easily sensed before they become dangerous. Carbon dioxide is easily measured by simple devices. It is a convenient indicator of the quality of a building's fresh air supply, since many other indoor air pollutants tend to follow quite closely the levels shown by carbon dioxide.

For these reasons, CO_2 is often chosen as the gas to be monitored by the automatic sampling equipment which is sometimes used to control ventilation in commercial buildings.

The Particles

ASBESTOS

Asbestos is a mineral fiber mined from the earth. It is very fire resistant, workable, and inexpensive to produce. Until recently, large amounts of asbestos were used in building materials and fire resistant coatings, and even in some clothing. Now asbestos has been recognized as a serious threat to the health of those exposed to it in large amounts, or over long periods of time, and its use in consumer products has been severely restricted. *Asbestos is the only natural fiber that has been linked with cancer.*

Health hazards: Asbestos fibers freed from asbestos-containing products by wear or disturbance will enter the air. Particles that are small enough will be carried by air currents and will enter the throat and lungs. Once lodged there, they will stay and cause long term irritation and tissue damage. Over long periods of time, such accumulated asbestos is likely to cause asbestosis, a serious lung disease, and can lead to lung cancer or mesothelioma, a particular form of chest cancer. This problem can be aggravated by smoking, and if asbestos is eaten in food or water it can also cause intestinal irritation, sometimes leading to cancer. *The diseases caused by asbestos accumulation will not appear for twenty years or more.* Exposure to asbestos can also, in combination with other influences such as smoking, dramatically increase the risk of chest cancers.

Symptoms: *There are no immediate effects of exposure to asbestos.* Those who have suffered long term exposure may experience coughing, shortness of breath, chest tightness, and sputum as early signs of disease. Anyone with such symptoms, or those who have worked in industries handling asbestos for long periods, should, of course, be seeing their physicians for regular care.

Concentrations: Asbestos is normally present in amounts of less than 1 fiber/c.c. of air. This means that an average sewing thimble full of air would contain less than 1 microscopic particle of asbestos. Levels of 10 or more fibers/c.c. have been measured in homes near materials containing asbestos, such as old plaster or heating duct insulation, particularly when they are disturbed. *This amount is ten to twenty times the allowable levels for industry. An appropriate level for asbestos in the home is exactly none.*

Sources and paths of entry: Asbestos in building materials and household products has been closely regulated in the U.S. and Canada since 1980, or earlier for some items. The major sources in the home are such materials as plaster, ceiling tiles, insulation board, and heating duct tape, that were made with asbestos and installed previous to 1970. These materials "shed" fibers when they become worn, or are disturbed. (Many schools and public buildings in the 1940's and 50's and even later were also sprayed with structure fireproofing made from asbestos. Much of this has begun to shed fibers into the air, and must be removed at great expense.)

Another source of asbestos is the city street. Brake linings of cars, trucks, and buses contain asbestos which wears off during use. This dust collects on the street and is blown around, collecting in some areas. *The air entering the home from a busy city street can be laden with asbestos, particularly during dry, windy periods.*

Renovation and demolition of older buildings can be risky due to accumulated loose asbestos that is stirred up by the activity. Careful precautions must be taken in such cases, with dwelling areas and heating ducts sealed off from potential sources. The areas should be dampened with a water mist to reduce dust, and all present must wear good quality filter masks. The U.S. Consumer Product Safety Commission publishes a useful guide to asbestos in the home. (See the GETTING HELP section.)

Controls: ***Removing materials containing asbestos if they are crumbling*** is the only practical way to control asbestos in your home. This should be done only by qualified people with proper equipment, and using protective measures. *Never attempt to clean up asbestos with a vacuum cleaner.* It will do more harm than good by stirring up and spreading fibers.

Notes: Though some methods of "sealing" materials containing asbestos have been suggested, they are probably only suitable for small amounts.

TOXIC AND PROBLEM METALS (LEAD, MERCURY, ZINC, CADMIUM, ETC.)

These metals and others in the environment can be absorbed into the body through food, air, or skin contact. They accumulate to various degrees in organs and can become quite toxic.

Lead has been used as a gasoline additive for many years. Recent efforts to replace it with other compounds are finally progressing in the U.S. Once a common base for paints, lead was also used in water pipe and plumbing fittings. It has been replaced by other materials in most of these uses and is now closely regulated, except for its continuing use in soldered water pipe.

Mercury is very toxic and used in such industries as metals smelting, papermaking, and chemical processing. Chemical compounds of mercury find their way into water ways and are absorbed by plants and animals.

Zinc is commonly used to coat steel to reduce rusting. Many household items, such as furnace ducting, stovepipe, and tools, are zinc coated, and will release dangerous zinc fumes if heated to high temperatures. Some zinc coated items also may find their way into the kitchen, where they can release zinc if used in contact with food.

Cadmium is used in plating household hardware and in paint pigments. Old refrigerator shelves plated with cadmium have been known to poison people when they were used as broiler racks or barbecue grilles.

The aluminum in cookware is very chemically active, and will readily combine with many foods. The metal is also very soft and easily scraped off into food. Though it is not considered a toxic metal, it easily combines with foods during cooking, forming chemicals whose effects are not well understood.

Health hazards and symptoms: In cities, our most prevalent toxic metal problem is with lead. Lead from leaded gasoline engine exhaust accumulates in the body, causing degeneration of nerves and brain tissue. This is particularly serious in children due to their small size in relation to the dose, and can cause poor mental and physical development and other illnesses. Lead from old paints is also a serious problem in old buildings.

Mercury poisoning causes nervous symptoms such as trembling, loss of muscle control, and headaches, as well as nausea and hair loss. Like lead, mercury accumulates in our bodies and is not readily expelled.

Zinc is a necessary trace mineral that our bodies require in small quantities, but is very toxic in larger doses. The main hazard is inhaling the fumes from the heated metal. (A well-known problem for welders in their work.) Sharp chest pains and shortness of breath follow inhalation of zinc fumes.

Cadmium poisoning is serious and causes nausea, headaches, and blurred vision.

Elevated levels of aluminum in brain tissue has been linked with Alzheimer's disease, though it has not been found to be a cause. The debate over this continues.

Sources and controls: The most serious quantities of lead come from vehicle exhaust in inner city areas. Though unleaded gasoline will eventually relieve this problem, leaded gasoline is still burned in most areas. The lead is carried short distances from highways and deposited on streets, buildings, and plants. It can enter our homes directly or be deposited on the food we eat. ***Ventilation air should not be entering your home from the street side, particularly if you live near a busy urban street or highway.***

Plants or fruits grown near a busy roadway should not be consumed, nor water that comes from highway runoff. Such water should also not be used for gardening.

In old buildings with lead paint, children playing on the floor can pick up dangerous amounts of lead shed from peeling walls and ceilings. Old paint which may contain lead should be removed by scraping, and carefully collected for disposal. *A good dust mask is necessary while doing this.* (See the GETTING HELP section.) *Keep children away until cleanup is complete.*

Lead from solder in water pipes is also a source of exposure. This can be eliminated by ***changing to copper pipe with mechanical joints.***

Mercury can leak from broken thermometers and fluorescent lamp tubes. ***Dispose of these with care.***

Do not use zinc coated implements in the kitchen, or where they are exposed to high heat. If you have a wood stove or furnace, stainless steel or heavy uncoated steel are the best materials for the pipe which leads to the chimney.

Old refrigerator or freezer racks are

often cadmium plated, and should never be used for cooking. Store food only in approved containers of glass, stainless steel, or hard plastics. Metal containers not approved for food storage may contain toxic metals which can enter the food stored in them.

Use glass, stainless steel, or enamelled steel cookware instead of aluminum.

AIRBORNE MICROORGANISMS

Bacteria and viruses released by people carrying illness can spread disease when they are carried through the air and inhaled by others. Fortunately, few really dangerous diseases are transmitted this way, and these organisms have a very short life when they are drifting in the air. Air temperature and humidity have an effect on the time that bacteria and viruses can survive outside the body. Generally, moderate conditions of about 40% to 50% relative humidity at comfortable room temperatures are best for reducing the spread of airborne microorganisms. (This is covered further in the Thermal Comfort chapter.)

Health hazards and symptoms: The most important factors in the transmission of illness by these pathogens are the health of the person exposed and the amount of exposure to a sick person. The symptoms of respiratory illness and flu caused by viruses are well known.

Concentrations: Bacteria and viruses are all around us wherever we are, and most do not cause disease under ordinary circumstances. However, where conditions allow them to reproduce freely there are serious health risks with exposure to particularly virulent strains or elevated numbers.

Sources and paths of entry: Close contact with someone carrying illness is the prime means of transmission by these organisms. Under some circumstances in the home, however, certain bacteria can also multiply outside the body and increase the incidence of illness. *One example is humidifier fever, where warm, damp conditions inside a poorly maintained humidifier can cause the spread of organisms to cause flu-like symptoms or even pneumonia.*

Controls: Some viruses and most bacteria are dependent on high humidity in room air for their survival, but low humidity causes dryness of the linings of the nose, throat, bronchia, and lungs, and increases the risk of becoming ill. For this reason ***40% to 50% relative humidity is usually considered ideal to control the spread of pathogens.*** Humidifiers, air conditioners, heating ducts, and all surfaces in the home where constant dampness persists, can be a breeding ground for pathogens. ***Proper maintenance and moisture control is essential to a healthful home.***

AIRBORNE BIOLOGICAL ALLERGENS

For those who react to them, airborne substances from plants and animals which cause allergic reactions are by far the most common biological hazards in our homes. Pollens, fungi and their spores, animal dander, and house dust, *can all be very harmful or even lethal to people with hypersensitivity. Some things, such as fungus spores and animal dander, can also sensitize people who have not been reactive before.* People who have previously enjoyed freedom from hypersensitive reactions may begin to develop symptoms after prolonged exposure and should be cautious. This may happen with a moldy carpet, for example, or dog and cat hair.

The onset of hypersensitivity is a very complex medical problem that involves general health, individual makeup, diet, and exposure to both biological and chemical sensitizers in the environment. While personal care and diet are the starting points in treatment and prevention, *control of those incitants in the home which aggravate the problem is fundamental.*

Types of biological allergens:

Pollens These tiny grains released by trees, plants, and shrubs, are carried great distances by winds. Some, such as ragweed, are very prolific and affect a large number of people.

Fungi Molds, yeasts, mushrooms, and mildew spores are generally invisible, but sometimes appear as a tiny cloud of dust when they are disturbed. Any part of the fungi, alive or dead, including the invisible spores, can be allergenic.

Animal dander All animals shed hair, feathers, and tiny flakes of skin throughout the year. They collect on surfaces or become airborne, and are allergenic to some people.

Dust Common house dust is made up of fibers shed from numerous sources, including fabrics, furnishings, soil, and plant materials. These dirty fibers are normally home to microscopic spider-like mites which are irritating to some people.

Health hazards: All these things are made up of complex proteins, as are all living things. Our bodies are equipped with a sophisticated protective immune system that recognizes "foreign" proteins as not belonging in or near us. In hypersensitivity, our immune system reacts also to common proteins, like those found in plant pollens, as if they were foreign, leading to various degrees of illness, and even to life threatening reactions.

Symptoms: The most common symptoms of exposure to these allergens are sneezing, coughing, shortness of breath, congestion, running nose and eyes, and other respiratory difficulties. Skin problems include itching, burning sensations, and rash. A wide range of other symptoms including palpitations, fainting, internal pains, confusion, and loss of muscle control can also be caused among reactive people. (See the section, ENVIRONMENTAL ILLNESS AND YOU.)

Concentrations: Small background levels of biological allergens are normal and not harmful to any but the most sensitive. While not usually measured, higher concentrations are recognized as the usual trigger for reactions.

Sources and paths of entry: Most pollens are produced outside, though some houseplants can create problems. Airborne pollens enter the home through any opening, including furnace and air conditioning intakes. Fungi grow in any damp area, indoors or outside, and spores are spread by any disturbance, including housecleaning, normal foot traffic, or air movement. Animal dander is spread by contact with animals and air movement. All of these substances can be carried indoors on clothing, particularly animal dander.

The heavier particles of house dust settle out and appear as dust films or balls, and the lighter particles, carried by air movement, are more likely to remain suspended in the air.

All of these particles will be disturbed by housecleaning. Sweeping and portable vacuum cleaners (as compared to centrally installed ones) are particularly bad for stirring up allergens and increasing the amounts in the air to be inhaled.

Controls: ***Restricting the entry of biological allergens into the home is the first line of control for these substances.*** For many allergy sufferers, it is necessary to keep doors and windows closed during the pollen season, to filter incoming air, and to maintain dry conditions. Relatively safe chemicals, such as borax or vinegar, can be used to destroy colonies of molds. Offending surfaces, such as damp carpets, should be removed.

Thorough ***housecleaning with a built in vacuum*** is the preferred method for controlling the dust and other particles that are inevitable indoors. ***A slightly dampened mop or cloth is very effective*** for cleaning smooth surfaces. (See the Home Maintenance chapter.)

Notes: As exposure to large doses of fungi or their spores may cause sensitization in otherwise healthy people, *fungus control in the home is a concern to all.*

OTHER PARTICLES

A vast range of non-biological particles are also present in indoor air. Some are small enough to be suspended in the air and then inhaled. These present a health hazard to everyone. The most common are from smoking, engine exhaust, industrial emissions, agricultural chemicals, and construction. Particles of harmful liquids (aerosols) are also contaminants that can be inhaled. They are produced by various household products, such as spray cleaners.

Health hazards: Inhaled particles become lodged in the sinuses, bronchia, and lungs. Some can be absorbed and eventually discharged by the body, but others, such as pesticides and asbestos (see above), cannot. The most hazardous are the carcinogenic components of smoke, and such substances as asbestos and some industrial chemical discharges.

Other substances, such as glass fibers, silica dusts, carbon from smoke, and construction dust, though not considered carcinogenic, can cause lung diseases such as emphysema. Inhaling any sort of particles will at the very least reduce lung function and eventually increase heart strain.

Symptoms: Coughing, shortness of breath, congestion.

Concentrations: Particles less than 10 microns in diameter (.01 mm or .0004 in.) are considered respirable (small enough to pass through into the bronchia and lungs). The largest of these are visible in bright light, or in heavy concentrations such as smoke or dust clouds, but the smaller, most easily inhaled particles, are usually invisible. The total suspended particles in indoor air usually ranges from 25 to 150 mcg/M3 (micrograms per cubic meter). Heavy smoking, construction, and other disturbances can raise this to 750 or more. The recommended range is less than 100.

Sources and paths of entry: Smoking, construction (sanding, plaster). Particles are stirred up by air movement, circulated by furnaces.

Controls: Avoidance of these articles is the only safe control. Wearing a proper dust mask during construction and cleanup is essential. (See the Home Maintenance Chapter, and the GETTING HELP section.)

7 CONTROLLING INDOOR AIR QUALITY

Any effort to control environmental quality must start with an understanding of the potential problems in your home. To understand air quality, to know what contaminants may be affecting your home, and to learn what health hazards they might present is a necessary beginning. The specific methods of reducing your health risk can then be applied. What follows is an introduction to the methods of controlling these factors. The special needs of the environmentally sensitive are covered in the section ENVIRONMENTAL ILLNESS AND YOU.

In many cases increased ventilation will improve air quality, but a more comprehensive approach will usually require three steps to control pollution problems.

- *Locate the source of contamination and remove it, if possible.*
- *Isolate, "seal," or otherwise neutralize those sources that cannot be removed.*
- *Dilute any remaining traces of contamination with increased ventilation.*

There are five major kinds of contamination to be considered:

- Products of combustion and respiration (CO_2, CO, water vapor, etc.).
- Chemical contaminants from building materials and other sources in the immediate environment (formaldehyde, radon, etc.).
- Chemical contaminants from fabrics and furnishings (organic chemicals, synthetic resins, adhesives, formaldehyde, etc.).
- Chemical contaminants from household and garden products used or stored indoors (paints, solvents, cleaners, polishes, pesticides, etc.).
- Biological contaminants: pollens, microbes, spores, house dust, etc.

Combustion Products

UNVENTED GAS AND KEROSENE HEATERS

These are the worst sources of combustion gases indoors. *Do not use them under any circumstances.* The only possible exception to this might be temporary uses with large amounts of fresh air supplied. These appliances, which are generally portable and without outside vent pipes, discharge all of their noxious combustion products into the

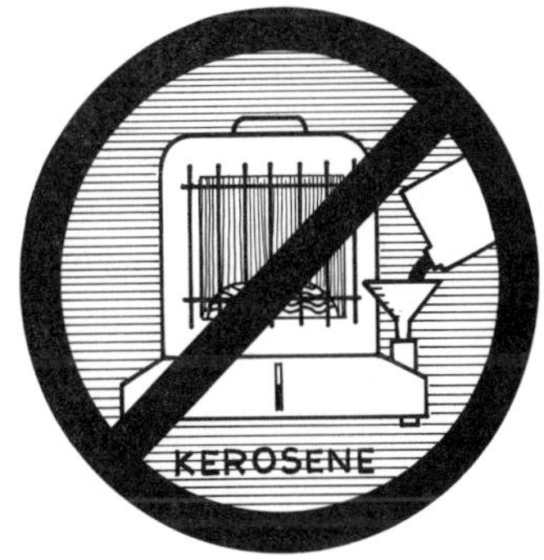

Fig. 7-1 Kerosene Heaters Are Unsafe

room air. Numerous cases have been reported of carbon monoxide poisoning (as well as house fires) caused by unvented portable heaters. They are still in use in large parts of rural America, though this practice is slowly diminishing. All fuels used in homes should only be burned in safe, approved, outside vented heaters, with safe, well maintained chimneys.

GAS RANGES

These are the second group of offenders, as they are generally not directly ventilated and must rely on kitchen fans or open windows for exhaust. A gas range operating in winter in a closed, or semi-closed kitchen delivers carbon dioxide, carbon monoxide, nitrogen dioxide, water vapor, and traces of other harmful gases to the room air. Studies have shown that a conventional gas range operating for 20 minutes in a semi-closed kitchen can produce health threatening levels of these dangerous contaminants.

Recent innovations in gas burning appliances, such as ceramic burner inserts, have helped to reduce the amount of nitrogen dioxide produced by the flame, but ***electric cooking appliances are definitely preferable*** from a health and safety standpoint, and should be the preferred choice when possible. If you must use a gas range, ask your utility company or appliance dealer about pollution control devices, such as electronic ignition and the forthcoming ceramic inserts. *Any* kitchen range (gas or electric), should be ventilated by a fan-operated range hood ***vented to the outside.*** This will remove the products of combustion and cooking, which can be a health risk if allowed to remain indoors, as well as causing offensive odors. Range hoods without outside vents are ineffective and should not be used. (See the Kitchen chapter.)

UNSAFE CHIMNEYS

These are the third cause of toxic combustion gases entering the home. A fuel burning furnace, heater, or water heater must be connected to a sound chimney which is free of fire hazard, leaks, and potential for reverse draft. The chimney must exit from the roof at a location where it cannot vent gases toward nearby opening windows, and it must be large enough for the appliance which is connected to it. Do not use old brick, stone, or concrete chimneys without a thorough inspection, as they may be unsound, or may not have appropriate fireproof liners rated for their intended use. Chimneys may also "backdraft" (flow in reverse), allowing dangerous gases to reenter the home. This condition is common for brief periods during the normal on-off cycling of a furnace or water heater, and may continue for a few seconds or more until the chimney warms up, when normal draft can be re-established. Though this may be acceptable in leaky homes, ***preventing backdraft is essential if the house is to be tightly sealed,*** or if building airflow is to be altered. (See the Testing chapter.) This would be the case, for example, if ventilating fans are to be added. (See the Home Ventilation chapter.) Any fuel burning appliance must also be provided with a fresh combustion air supply. (See the Home Heating chapter for details.)

REDUCING CONTAMINATION FROM COMBUSTION

Where fuel burning appliances are the only available choice, isolation may be especially useful if there is anyone with hypersensitivity problems in the home. The health of some sensitized people is jeopardized by even the slightest amounts of natural gas, propane gas, or fuel oil vapor in the air. Where these fuels are the only choices available, take steps to isolate the appliance from the home. One approach is to ***build a fireproof, airtight room in the house around the offending furnace and water heater, and ventilate this room to the outside.*** This room must be designed to provide fresh air to the appliance for combustion, and, of course, must be carefully built to all building and fire code regulations. This is an expensive and complex option, and should not be undertaken without expert advice.

Another method is to ***remove the appliance to a separate furnace room in a detached building.*** This approach is more successful than a furnace room within the home. It can be readily applied to liquid based heating systems where no room air need be exchanged between the house and furnace room. Such a system will pipe hot water or anti-freeze mixtures to radiators in the house, or to radiant panels in floors or ceilings. It can also provide household hot water.

Caution: Dilution is not an appropriate solution to the problem of dangerous combustion gases. *They must not be allowed to enter the home.*

Chemical Contaminants from Building Materials

Many building products produce chemical contaminants which are harmful to health if allowed to build up inside our homes. To control contamination from these sources it is necessary to carefully select building materials for new construction or renovation, and to remove existing materials which are potential sources of contamination.

Of the many contaminants identified in Section I, formaldehyde is the most prominent, both because it is very common, and because it has a potentially debilitating, sensitizing effect on some people. (See Formaldehyde in the chapter The Indoor Hazards.)

FORMALDEHYDE

The most potent source of formaldehyde in building materials (other than urea formaldehyde insulation) is usually in *pressed-wood products*. The glue used to bond *particle board, chip board,* and some plywoods will emit this gas for lengthy periods after installation. *Because many construction adhesives, carpets, carpet pads, wallboards, paints, and upholstery materials also contain formaldehyde, you must carefully select materials to reduce the potential formaldehyde load of your home.* Exterior grade plywoods, for example, are usually safer than particle board for interior use, but they do cost more and do not have the same wear resistance for certain uses, such as floors. However, where there is someone hypersensitive in the home, all glued wood products should be avoided. Fortunately, some carpet fibers and pads are not treated with formaldehyde, and oil base paints are often safer than acrylic latex once the initial drying period has passed. (See the Materials and Selection chapter for details.)

Reducing Formaldehyde Contamination: If you have small amounts of pressed wood in cabinets and furniture which cannot be avoided, contamination can be reduced by sealing them. These materials can be *sealed* with a layer of formica, or with two or more coats of a varnish, such as urethane, to reduce the levels of free formaldehyde released into the air. A chemical solution of 8% sodium bisulphite has also been tested in experimental homes for neutralizing small amounts of formaldehyde residue in building materials, but it cannot be used without expert advice. Some companies specializing in UFFI removal can do this. (See the GETTING HELP section.) Unfortunately, many other materials containing formaldehyde, such as some carpets, and rubber carpet pads, fabrics, upholstery, and adhesives, cannot be effectively isolated and should be avoided in a health conscious home.

Fresh air ventilation will help to control unavoidable traces of formaldehyde. Air contamination research for NASA has shown that spider plants (*Chlorophytum elatum* var. *vittatum*) will remove small amounts of formaldehyde from air. From 20 to 60 plants are needed to really clean the air of a 1500 sq. foot home that does not have a serious formaldehyde problem. However, even a small number of plants can make a difference in smaller homes with problems, such as mobile homes.

Other indoor chemical contaminants that may come from building materials include asbestos, radon, solvents and aromatic chemicals, and synthetic resins.

RADON

Radon is a colorless, odorless gas produced by naturally occurring radiation in rock and soils. Radon can enter homes through joints and cracks in foundations or through drain openings. It can also be carried by water from deep wells or released from bricks and cement products as well as natural gas.

The radioactive by-products of radon become attached to dust particles and are inhaled. Once lodged in the lungs these radioactive particles can cause cell damage. *Approximately 5–10% of all lung cancers are related to radon exposure.*

Some concrete, brick, and gypsum board may have significant radon levels. Natural stone, particularly granite, may have high levels. If you live in a radon area, such as Pennsylvania or parts of New York state and Colorado, or in southern Ontario or Quebec in Canada, do not use local building materials such as stone and concrete in large quantities inside the home. If large portions of your house are stone, concrete, or brick from these areas, they should be carefully sealed on the inside with cement mortar, and an impermeable air barrier. A fireplace, chimney, or masonry wall inside your home is unlikely to be a radon hazard. Most radon comes from soil and water outside the home, finding its way in through openings and cracks in foundations. Radon from deep well water will also build up in bathrooms during bathing.

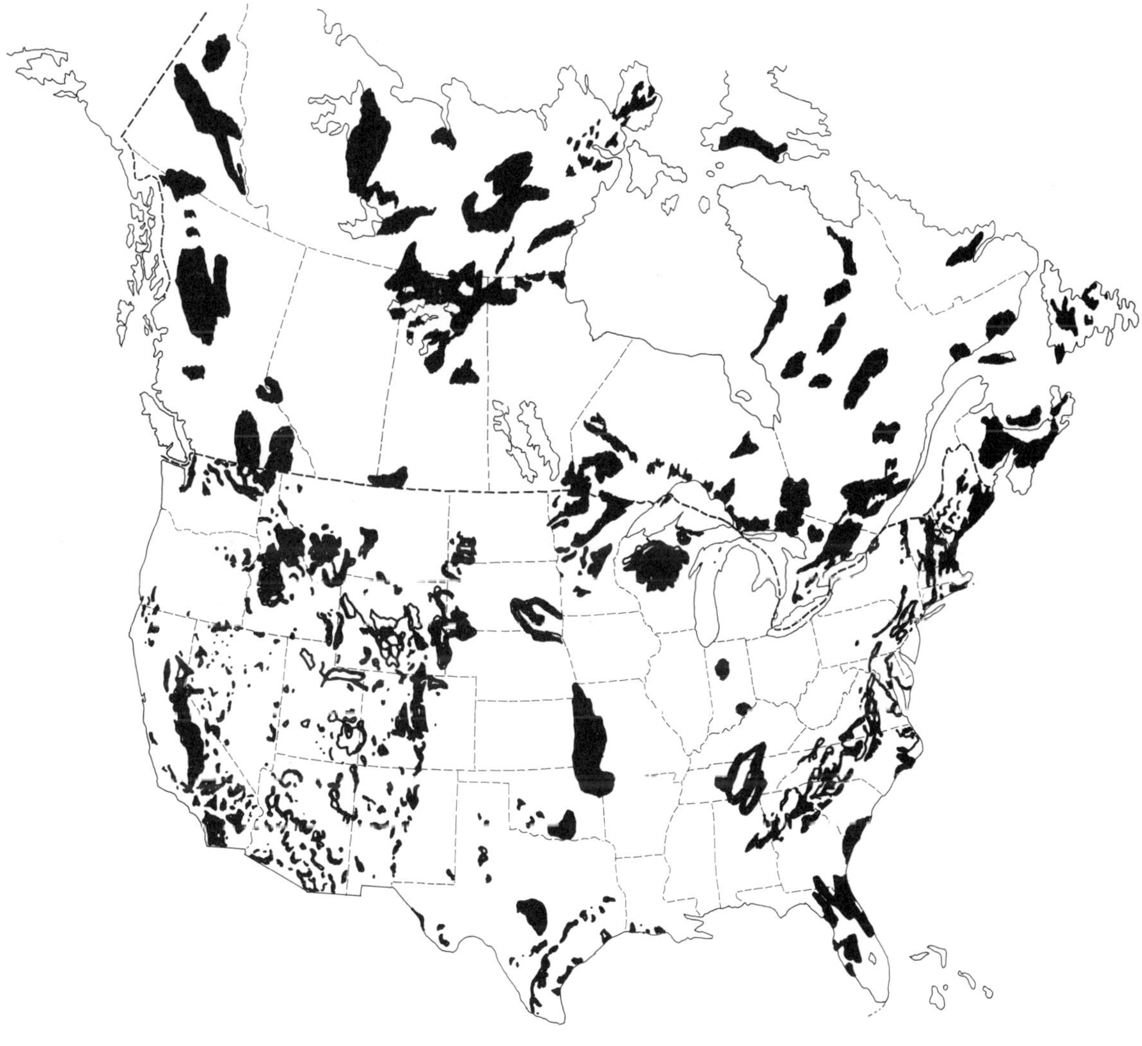

Fig. 7.2 Areas with Potentially High Radon Levels *The shaded zones indicate known areas where uranium occurs. Soil or rock in these areas, including granite, phosphate, and shale, may produce radon. If you live in one of these areas there is a greater chance of radon exposure in your home (though radon problems can also occur outside these zones). Test for radon particularly if you have a basement, unventilated crawl space, or a drilled well. (See the chapter Testing for Contamination.) Sources: U.S.E.P.A; Energy, Mines & Resources, Canada.*

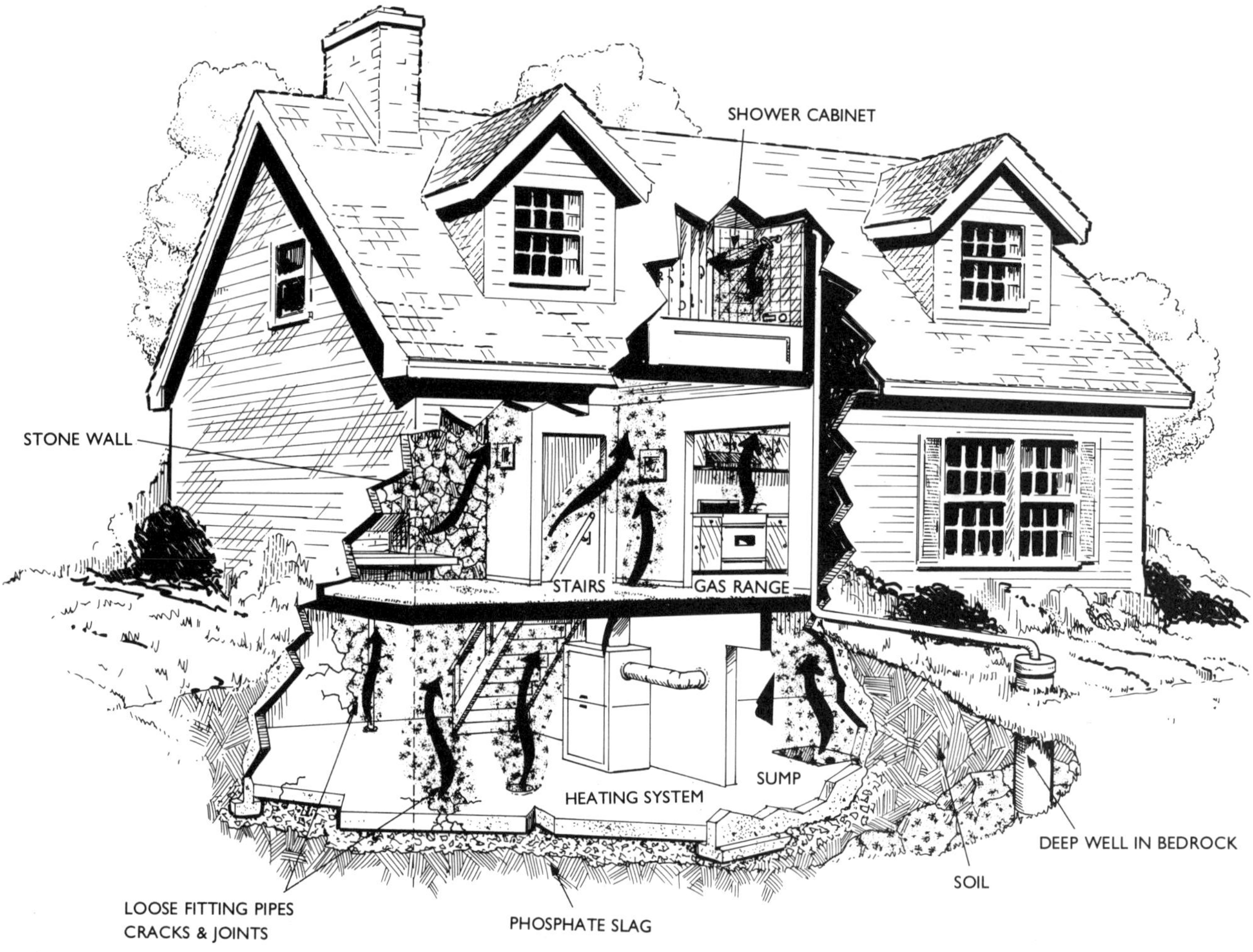

Fig. 7-3 Radon Sources and Paths. *Radon from* Soil *and* Groundwater *enters the basement through* Cracks and Joints *or* Sumps, *and is drawn upward into living spaces by airflow or through* Heating Systems. *Radon is also released from wellwater during bathing or washing, and from stone, brick, and cement.*

Preventing Radon Entry

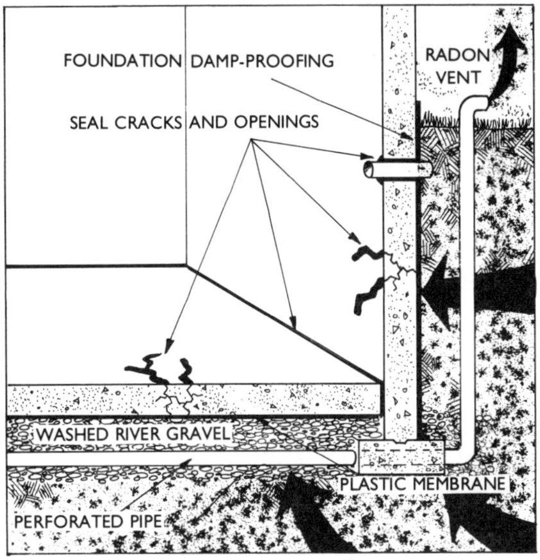

Fig. 7-4 *Seal all basement cracks and openings with caulking and cement, and treat walls with* Damp-proofing. *(For prevention measures for new construction, see the Construction Notes and Basement chapters.)*

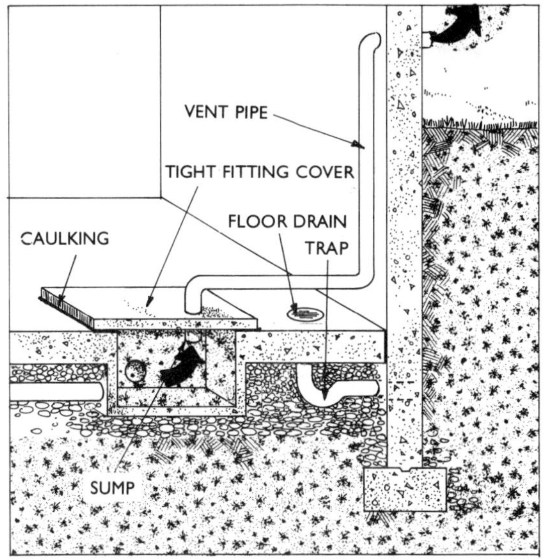

Fig. 7-5 *Groundwater in sumps should be vented to the outside, by placing a* Tight Fitting Cover *over the sump with* Caulking, *and connecting it to a* Vent Pipe. *Protect* Floor Drains *with a* Trap.

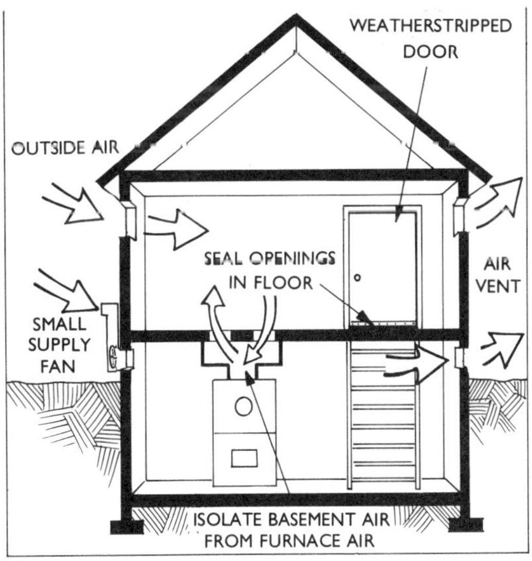

Fig.7-6 *Radon in basements can be reduced and prevented from entering living spaces by: pressurizing the basement with a* Small Supply Fan; *sealing basement stairs with a* Weatherstripped Door; *isolating the furnace by sealing any basement air returns; ventilating the living areas separately.*

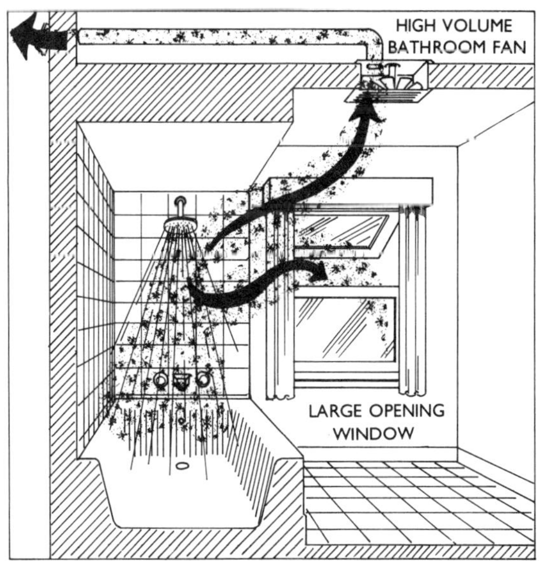

Fig. 7-7 *Radon released from deep well water can be removed from bathing and washing areas by good ventilation. In extreme cases, a special water filter may be required. (See the chapter Water Treatment.)*

FABRICS, FURNISHINGS, AND FINISHES

Many household items and articles of clothing, cosmetics, and soaps, may cause problems in hypersensitive people. This is true of most synthetic products and even some "natural" ones. The human immune system, once it has become overreactive and begun to respond to the slightest irritants instead of just protecting us from disease, can react with the most frightening and bizarre symptoms to the most common sorts of exposure. (See the section ENVIRONMENTAL ILLNESS AND YOU for a medical explanation and a personal account.) Whatever our present health condition, these materials around us in our homes are our close companions with which we spend half our lives or more. They should be chosen with caution. Contaminants released from materials in close contact with our skin may be responsible in the long term for subtle irritation, actual health problems, or even sensitization reactions leading to hypersensitivity. (Many of these will be discussed in later chapters.)

Some of the more frequent offenders which affect indoor air are clothing, bedding, carpets, draperies, and upholstery materials. Many of these are made from synthetic fabrics or contain chemical treatments which release tiny fibers or gaseous chemicals into the air. Even natural materials, such as cotton and wool, are often treated to prevent wrinkling or staining, to fireproof or mildew proof them, or to change their texture and washability. These treatments may contain formaldehyde, irritating synthetic resins, perfumes, dyes, and many other chemicals which can be breathed, or absorbed through the skin, in quantities sufficient to irritate even those who do not generally have hypersensitivity problems.

The best rules for choosing these materials are to avoid *anything*, whether synthetic or natural, which has a peculiar odor, and to read carefully the labels on all products, selecting those with the simplest and most readily recognized contents. This strategy is more critical for the more intimate items such as cosmetics and underclothing and bedding, and decreases in importance with the more distant items such as outside building materials. Remember that not all synthetic items are "bad" and not all natural materials are "good." Some people with sensitive skin find certain synthetics such as acetates very tolerable while wool may be highly irritating. Even some 100% cotton, wool, or silk products are loaded with dyes and chemical residues that make them unacceptable to many. The source of cotton may also be critical, because very toxic chemical defoliants and pesticides may have been used on it. The hypersensitive person must learn to judge the effect of all these materials by self-testing (described in the Materials and Selection chapter).

Problem materials are not readily isolated. They may be allowable in some rooms such as living rooms, but should be removed from rooms where we spend a great deal of time, such as the bedroom. (See the Sanctuary chapter.)

The effects of many problem materials can be diluted by improved ventilation and conventional filtration. Chemical components, such as formaldehyde, can be reduced by special filtration. (See the Home Ventilation chapter.)

SOLVENTS AND AROMATIC CHEMICALS

Paints, soft plastics, sealants, and adhesives are the major sources of these chemicals. Paints and varnishes are made up of various resins and fillers, which are dissolved in toxic chemical solvents, most of which evaporate from the surface into the air during curing. Some sealants, such as caulking used around windows, and soft plastics, such as upholstery covers, are kept soft and flexible by the action of these toxic chemicals, which were mixed with them during manufacture. These petroleum distillates are readily absorbed by the body. Many are retained in fatty tissues and can reach levels which will cause chronic illness.

Products that release quantities of these chemicals into your home are nearly all recognizable by their pungent odor; some can be identified by their labels. *When selecting materials always include sniff testing of samples of these items, both before and after curing.* Good ventilation will dilute the effect of those which cannot be avoided. "Flushing" with copious amounts of fresh air during their drying and curing periods will reduce the buildup of contaminants in the air. "Baking" these materials by raising room temperatures or using heat lamps during drying will speed up curing. (See the Materials and Selection chapter for further details.)

SYNTHETIC RESINS

Over forty types of synthetic resins are used in the manufacture of plastics and synthetic fabrics. Many, such as those used in the hard plastic veneers covering kitchen counters and tables, are extremely stable and do not break down readily or release any chemicals into your home. Others, such as those in vinyl coated wallboards, many synthetic carpets, soft upholstery, plastic floor coverings, and numerous others are less stable, and will release contaminants into your home. (See the chapter Materials and Selection.) *As there are no appropriate means for isolating these materials, choose carefully.*

All of these contaminants can be diluted by increased ventilation. None can be removed with conventional filtration, but their effects can be reduced with special air purification devices. (See the Home Ventilation chapter.)

Household and Garden Products

So many toxic chemicals are found in common household and garden products that to try to describe them accurately would fill volumes. It is wise for all of us to minimize our use of chemical products around the home, and to take care with storing and using those we consider necessary. The following products may contain health threatening agents if not used with care.

PESTICIDES

Most pesticides are hazardous chemicals and should be avoided in the home. There are safe, effective ways of controlling house and garden pests which do not contain these chemicals, and which are often easier and cheaper to use. A good book on the subject is *The Encyclopedia of Natural Insect and Disease Control,* by Roger B. Yepsen, Rodale Press, 1984.

POLISHES, WAXES, ETC.

Many of these contain solvents and dyes that can be dangerous if absorbed through the skin or inhaled.

SPOT REMOVERS, DRY CLEANING AGENTS

Many contain solvents and propellants which can be very hazardous to health if used indoors.

CLEANERS

Laundry products, scrubbing powders, glass cleaners, toilet cleaners, etc. Many of these can be hazardous if spilled, used improperly, or inhaled. Even the seemingly benign items such as dish soap can be irritants to the hypersensitive, and care should be taken with their selection, use, and storage.

PAINTS, OILS, AUTOMOTIVE PRODUCTS

Many of these are corrosive to the skin or hazardous if inhaled.

STORING HAZARDOUS PRODUCTS

An outdoor shed or separate garage is a great asset in storing those necessary items that are potential hazards. Paints, solvents, automotive products, and many others can be more safely stored this way than in cupboards or on basement shelves. Check labels to see which items might have to be protected from freezing if that is a problem in your area. *Never store fuels such as gasoline or flammable solvents such as paint thinner in your home.* Not only are they a fire hazard, but even small amounts of the fumes can make sensitive people ill.

Store products which must be kept inside for convenience or to preserve them at room temperature in a carefully controlled fashion. Secure shelves or cupboards may be adequate, but safer measures may be needed under special circumstances. If there is someone hypersensitive in your home, be extremely cautious with the use of any chemical product. Each one should first be self tested by the affected person. (See the Materials and Selection chapter). Indoor storage can be made safer by providing airtight cupboards that are vented to outside air. Where there are young children in the household, lock all storage areas securely. (See the Storage chapter.)

Biological Contaminants and Dusts

These household contaminants are either natural organisms and their by-products, or small fibers shed from common household materials. All are in the form of small particles which can be circulated by air movement. They include pollens, molds, mites, animal dander, bacteria and viruses, and house dust from a wide variety of sources. The smallest particles are generally carried the furthest by moving air and are most readily inhaled; the largest settle out most quickly and are less likely to be inhaled.

There are two types of hazard from these materials, pathogenic and allergenic.

Pathogenic materials are organisms, such as bacteria, viruses, and some fungi, which are generally recognized as causing disease. They will affect everyone to some extent, and increased exposure is generally assumed to increase the risk of disease. Allergenic materials cause immune reactions in people who are sensitive to that particular item. *Immune reactions can range from uncomfortable in minor cases to life threatening in extreme cases.* Increased exposure does not necessarily mean increased reaction, but prolonged exposure can increase sensitivity to some items and lead to new sensitivities, as well.

VIRUSES AND BACTERIA

The hazardous varieties come from people who are carrying illness, and can be carried between people by air currents. For example, the bacteria which cause some types of pneumonia can be transmitted in this way. Viruses are fundamentally different from bacteria, but some can also spread illness when carried between people by air currents. The kinds of viruses associated with flu and the common cold, for example, can be transmitted in this way.

Contrary to some popular beliefs, better housekeeping and personal hygiene probably do not have much effect on the transmission of illness by bacteria and viruses under normal circumstances. The general health and resistance of the individual, and the amount of contact with carriers, are the most important factors. Fortunately, these organisms have a very short life outside of the body and are more likely to die when drifting in the air than to land on someone and infect them. The one factor which we can control that makes some difference is the humidity of household air.

At common room temperatures, most airborne organisms will die more quickly when the relative humidity (R.H.) of the air is between 40% and 60%. This range is also preferred for best comfort and for other health reasons. It is also best for the storage of furniture and books (see the Thermal Comfort chapter).

FUNGI AND MOLDS

Fungi are a large group of small, plantlike organisms which include molds, mildews, some plant diseases such as rusts, and mushrooms. Some microscopic fungi are associated with human skin diseases, and the spore "seeds" released from common molds are known to be highly allergenic and can cause serious distress in sensitive people. All homes contain some fungi and this is not cause for concern. But some may support large colonies of these organisms, and may have quantities of airborne spores which can cause health problems.

Fungi can only grow in damp conditions, and do not require light or much heat. They can feed on many building materials including wood, paints, and adhesives, and can grow very rapidly in damp, dark, warm places. The most common place for mold problems is in basements, where porous or cracked foundations allow moisture to enter. This problem is aggravated by carpets or wall coverings which trap moisture. Another common cause of mold growth is poor insulation of walls, ceilings, and floors over unheated crawl spaces. In this case the inside surface may become so cold that it will cause condensation of the moisture in warm room air. This sort of problem usually shows up as damp spots which become discolored by mildew. Mold problems caused by dampness also occur around bathtubs, sinks and toilets, leaky pipes, and in unheated storage spaces. In very hot, humid climates mold problems may be very severe, and may call for special measures such as dehumidification.

Mold problems can be easily identified by the appearance of stains or musty odors, peeling paint, and the growth of crusts of sometimes colorful fungi colonies. These colonies can be temporarily stopped from growing by the application of a solution of borax (see the Home Maintenance chapter) but will return if damp conditions persist. Moisture control is the key to controlling fungi. (See the Thermal Comfort chapter.) Problem growths in your home can be cleaned up by removing any carpets or wallcoverings that have become damp and musty, scrubbing walls, ceilings, and floors with a borax solution, and taking steps to stop dampness. Fungus colonies can release large amounts of allergenic spores when disturbed, so take precautions when cleaning up. The room to be cleaned should be cleared of all furnishings and closed off from the rest of the house. This includes temporarily blocking heating vents and keeping doors tightly closed. Damp sponges are best for cleanup of affected areas. *Do not use a portable vacuum, particularly if there are hypersensitive people in the home, as this may spread spores everywhere.*

Cleanup and dampness control will reduce the airborne spore count if your home has a fungus problem, but will never eliminate it entirely. This sort of problem cannot be solved by isolating it, but must be treated directly and minimized. Good air filters will reduce the severity of any remaining amounts once cleanup is complete. (See the Home Ventilation Chapter.)

POLLENS, HOUSE DUST, MITES, AND ANIMAL DANDER

Pollens are, of course, the most prevalent airborne allergens. Hay fever, and more severe forms of allergy to plant materials, affect nearly 15% of the population, in some cases so severely that life can be miserable for months out of every year. Airborne pollens from grasses, shrubs, trees, and flowers find their way inside through open doors and windows, or are carried in on clothing or hair. Pets sometimes bring large amounts of pollen indoors.

House dust is made up of small particles and fibers that have been shed from fabrics, soils, people, furniture, and everything else that comes into your house. These particles generally quickly settle onto the furniture and floor. Mites are tiny animals related to spiders, invisible to the unaided eye, but everywhere around us in house dust. Their presence is the major reason why house dust causes reactions among allergy sufferers, even when pollens and house pets are not present. Animal dander is the hair and skin shed by domestic animals that mixes with the dust in our homes. All of these are potentially allergenic, particularly the pollens and animal dander; they can be controlled by good housekeeping.

Controlling what comes into your home, and regular dusting and vacuuming, are the best ways to manage these problems. If you have allergy problems at home, use a damp cloth to pick up dust so that it is not spread. If possible, install a built-in vacuum system, to reduce the dust disturbance of vacuuming. (See the Home Maintenance chapter.) Permanently fastened carpets, and street shoes worn indoors, are the two most common factors which make thorough house cleaning and allergen control difficult. Dust mites cannot be easily controlled by cleaning, but control of humidity in your home will reduce their numbers.

Another factor related to house dust is that such household pollutants as the radioactive by-products of radon (stastically linked with cancer) become attached to dust particles and are carried into the lungs. Reducing dust levels will reduce the paths by which contaminants can affect your health.

ASBESTOS

Asbestos may be found in insulation materials, particularly in the metal ductwork of old heating systems, in some wallboard and plasters, and in the heat shields of stoves and fireplaces. It is also used in shingles, and in some floor tiles, and ceiling panels. Asbestos removal can be tricky and hazardous. If you have asbestos in your home seek expert advice on its removal. *Do not handle any substantial amount of material containing asbestos without evacuating your home, and wearing a high quality filter mask.* (See the GETTING HELP section.) *Do not attempt to clean up asbestos waste with a vacuum cleaner. This will spread the fibers everywhere.*

Asbestos products, particularly soft ones, slowly disintegrate, shedding small asbestos fibers which, when inhaled, lodge in the lungs and bronchia and cause irritation and disease. There are ways to reduce this shedding if small amounts of asbestos products must remain in the home. For example, asbestos tape on metal chimneys or heating ducts which cannot be removed can be sealed with a layer of heat resistant foil tape. Small amounts of asbestos board, like the insulating heat shields behind furnaces, can be sealed with a heat resistant paint, such as aluminum engine paint. *There are no safe and effective methods for sealing any large quantities of asbestos board, ceiling tiles, duct insulation, etc.* These must be removed if they are deteriorating.

Small remainders of most of these indoor contaminants can be diluted with improved ventilation. Those that are particles, such as asbestos, can be partially trapped with effective air filters. Radon is more difficult to control once it has entered the home, and is not as readily "diluted."

SECTION III

Designing the Healthy Home

8 THE HOUSE AND ITS SITE

The region and climate are also raw materials for the house.

Those of us fortunate enough to live in a region we have chosen, have various reasons for preferring a particular climate or terrain, some of which may be health related. These reasons may include pollen conditions, outdoor air quality, temperature, and humidity.

Unfortunately, many cherished myths about regional health benefits do not withstand the test of personal experience. Many hay fever victims, for example, have moved to the desert in order to escape seasonal afflictions only to find that desert air can also be loaded with allergenic plant materials. Many others have moved to rural locations, dreaming of clean environments, only to find agricultural chemicals and industrial emissions in the air, or a severe problem with unsafe housing or contaminated water.

Whether we have chosen our location or not, we all find ourselves in some relationship, negative or positive, with the environment outside our homes, and must rely to a greater or lesser extent on the house itself to moderate those conditions.

THE HOSTILE ENVIRONMENT

Where outdoor conditions throughout large parts of the year cause discomfort or health risks due to pollen, air contamination, extreme temperatures, and noise pollution, the home can be designed as a more "closed" environment to "control" outside conditions. This sort of home might have:

- Fully mechanical ventilation, with filtration and, possibly, air purification.
- Complete air conditioning and humidity control.
- Double or triple glazed windows, tight fitting doors, and garden buffers to reduce noise.
- A fully enclosed sunspace or greenhouse.
- Shade trees or windbreaks to protect the house, improve comfort, and reduce energy demand.

THE COMPATIBLE ENVIRONMENT

Where outdoor conditions are compatible with our health and comfort throughout much of the year, the home can be a much more "open" place which embraces outside conditions. This sort of house might have:

- Natural ventilation.
- A garden or courtyard as an outdoor living space.
- Trees, shrubs, and pools to temper conditions for outdoor living.

AIR QUALITY

Both regional and local factors affect the quality of available outdoor air. The regional factors are pollen from agriculture and nature, plant odors (e.g. terpenes from coniferous trees) urban contamination (smog, auto emissions, etc.), industrial emissions, dust from agriculture or from the regional geography, humidity, and prevailing winds. The local factors are pollen from garden plants, automobile exhaust, agricultural chemicals, house and garden chemicals, local industrial or other contamination, and local air movement.

PLANNING THE HOME SITE

Those of us living in detached houses have the opportunity to influence environmental conditions by the way we use the building site and yard. In addition to views, neighbours, sunlight, yard, and garden requirements, and all of the other factors which usually influence site planning, there are other considerations important to planning the home for health and well being. (Apartment dwellers must rely on strategies inside the building. See the chapters Home Ventilation, Controlling Indoor Air Quality, Sound, Materials and Selection, and Home Maintenance.)

NATURAL AIR MOVEMENT

A well placed home gains a great advantage from natural ventilation. In many regions, prevailing winds during the warm season are from one or two distinct directions. Orienting the home with these directions in mind will be most advantageous for healthful cross ventilation. Opening windows placed on opposite sides, in line with wind directions, are very effective. Be aware that air movement may be moderated or re-directed by trees or building features. Use small flags or banners to help indicate wind behavior around the home.

The hazardous effects of local automobile emissions decrease sharply with distance from the roadway. House air drawn from a rear yard, side yard, or from high above ground level is likely to be far less contaminated.

GARDEN BUFFERS

Shrubs, trees, and ponds can provide a natural buffer between the home and street, reducing contamination, visibility, and noise. Dense trees or hedges, such as low evergreens, or solid board fences,, are helpful in reducing the entry of noise into the yard from the street. Carefully placed screen walls outside of the home can also reduce the admission of noise through doors and windows.

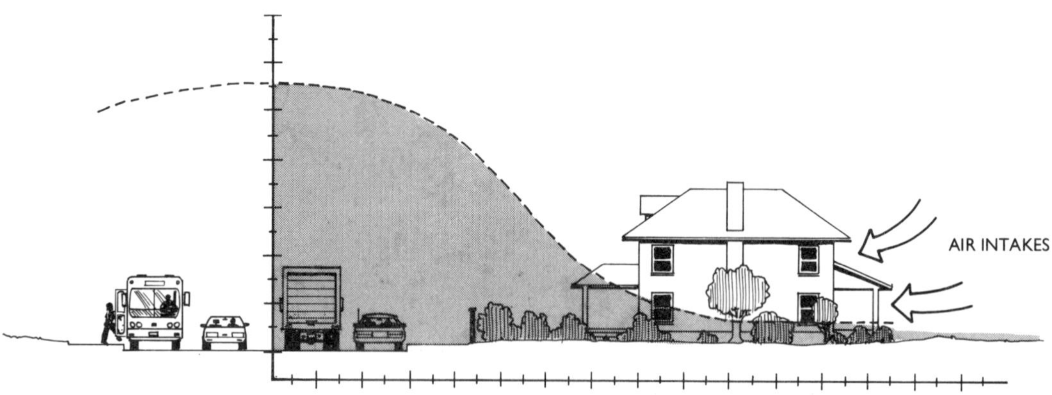

Fig. 8-1 Local Air Contamination from Automobiles. *Local automobile air pollution decreases rapidly with distance from the road. Where possible, plan home ventilation so that air intakes are in the back yard, away from streets.*

CONTROLLING DAMPNESS

Chronic dampness near buildings will encourage unhealthy fungus growth, and will also be damaging to the structure. Dampness and fungus spores can be risky particularly for the sensitive individual.

• Restrict and prune back vines and shrubs growing against any walls which receive little sunlight. This is particularly critical in damp climates.

• Restrict tree growth overhanging the building.

• Ensure that all surface drainage is sloped away from the building.

• Around foundations, provide a broad, porous border, such as washed gravel, for drainage. (See the chapter Construction Notes.)

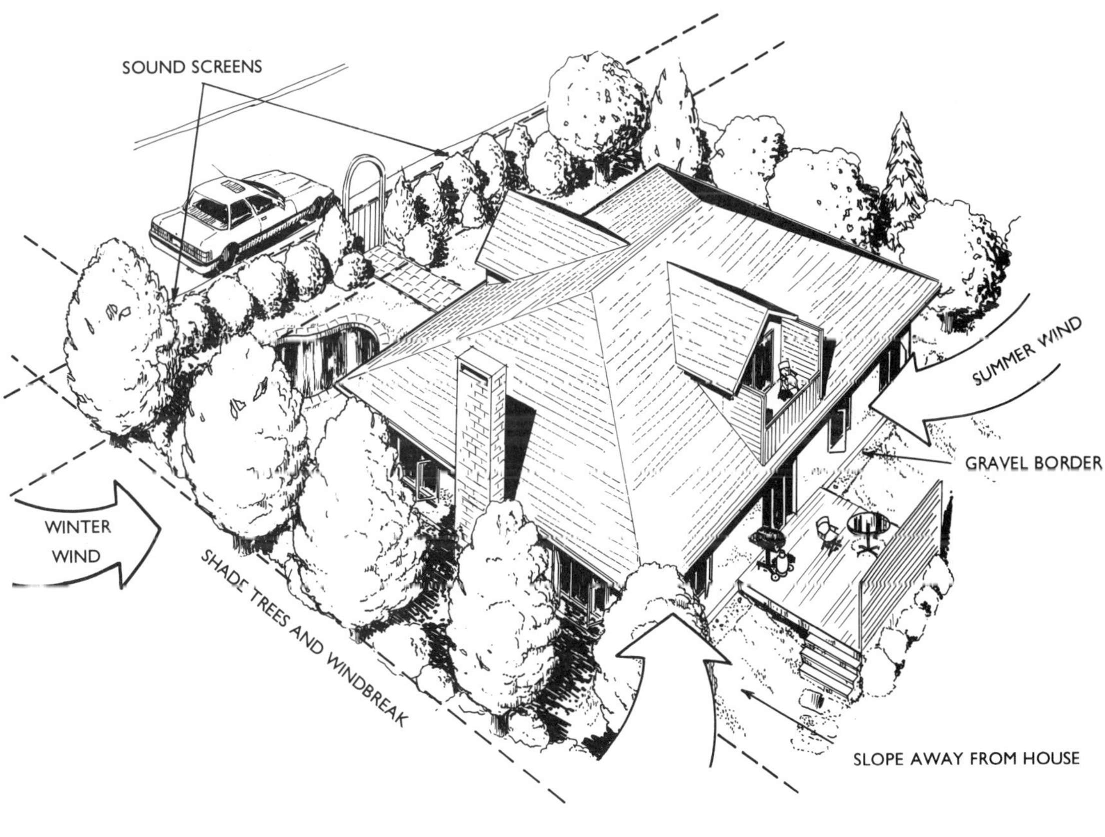

Fig. 8-2 The Site. *Careful site planning can provide the best shade, natural airflow, drainage, and sound buffers for your home.*

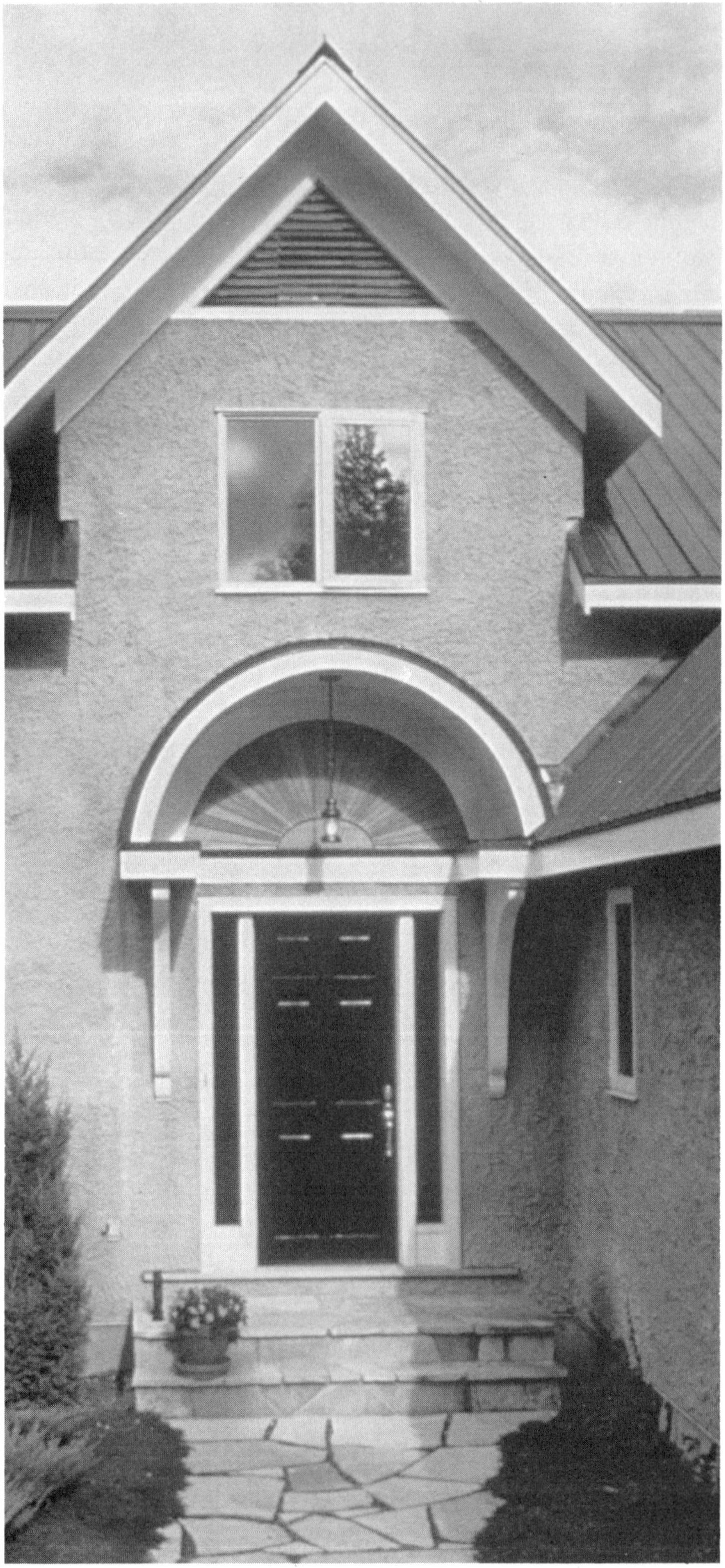

Entrance to a specially designed, clean air house. Photo © 1986 Jim Merrithew

9 THE ENTRY

The entry is the place of welcome that was once a prominent feature of our homes. The vestibules of another era and the "mud rooms" of our country homes have largely disappeared in urban settings, and with them have gone a comfortable and convenient transition place between outdoors and indoors. In the health conscious home, the entry can help to keep out soil, pollens, and other substances, as well as to save heating and cooling energy. In some homes, the Asian tradition of removing street shoes at the door prevails, and the entry serves as a place for exchanging shoes and house slippers.

An entry can be:

- A bright and pleasant area for changing and storing coats and shoes.
- A secure air lock, with inner and outer doors to save energy and reduce the entry of contaminants. An air filter can even be placed here.
- A place for drying wet outdoor clothing.

Helpful Features in an Entry

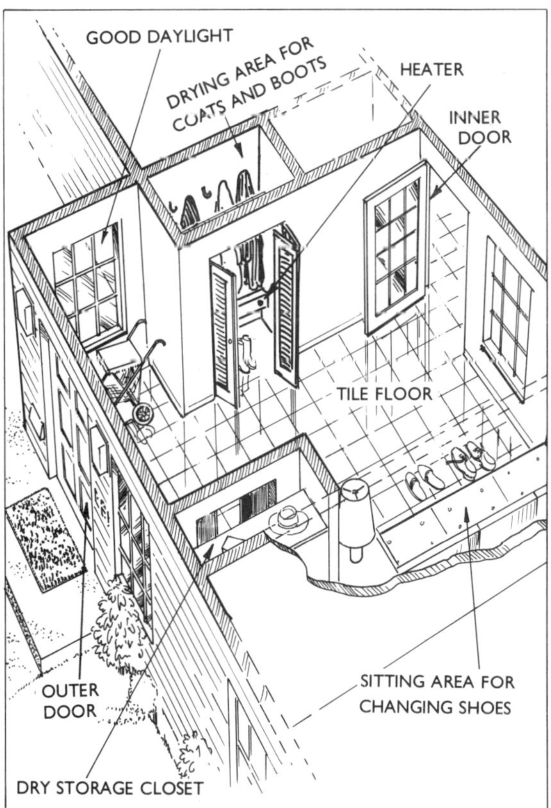

- A convenient hanging and storage area for coats, and a seating area for changing shoes.
- Both inside and outside door mats.
- A small heater where shoes and coats can be dried.
- A durable floor covering, such as ceramic tile, or hard vinyl tile, if acceptable to anyone in the home with chemical sensitivities.
- Tightly fitted doors with good weatherstrips.
- Obvious shoe racks and available house slippers if you wish to have people leave street shoes there.
- A good source of daylight and ventilation.

Fig. 9-1 The Entry. *The entry can be a bright place of welcome, as well as an airlock and a place to store and dry outdoor clothing and footwear.*

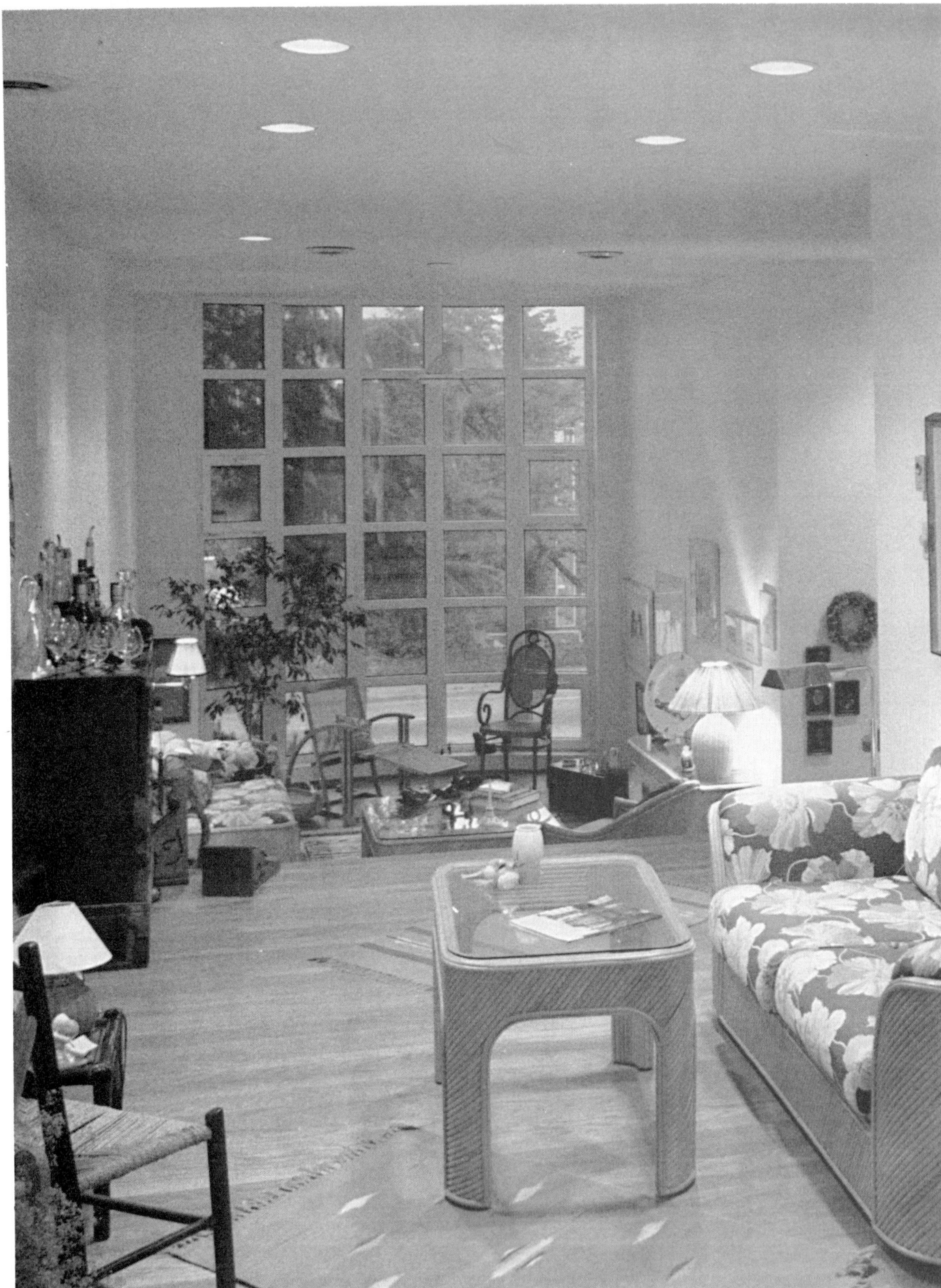

Living room designed with health conscious principles. Design by D. McIntyre and E. M. Sterling. Photo: Brian Dust

10 THE LIVING ROOM

Well planned and well furnished living spaces can have both bright, pleasant places for gatherings, and more secluded areas for quiet retreat. A living room may have a variety of furniture types and groupings, a variety of windows and views, and good adjustable lighting. It may also have varied levels, different floor coverings, and many other features which contribute to adaptability and interest.

The important considerations for health and well being in the living room are its ventilation, lighting, finishes and furnishings, and its traffic flow.

VENTILATION

When the outside air quality is acceptable to everyone in the home, good cross ventilation from windows and doors is an effective and simple means of ventilating living spaces for health and comfort. A large opening window or outside door located on the side of the room oriented toward the desired wind during the warm season, and a similar opening on the opposite side, is a good, workable arrangement. When planning or renovating, gather wind information by observation, or from neighbors.

When pollens, air contamination, or extreme temperature or humidity make outside air inappropriate for ventilation, a mechanical filtration and heating/cooling system is required. These may be central installations or window mounted units. (See the Home Ventilation and Home Heating/Cooling chapters.)

LIGHTING

For most people, good daylight (light from the sky not including sunlight) is an important feature of living spaces. The most even daylight comes from northern exposures, and the most variable on a daily basis, from the east and west. Both sunlight and daylight are available in the southern sky, dependent on season, time, weather conditions, and latitude. Available daylight will penetrate most deeply into a room through tall windows that reach the ceiling as nearly as possible. Light colored ceilings and walls will also assist by reflecting light.

Sunlight is a valued commodity in living spaces, particularly during the cold season. South and east exposures are usually the most appropriate for sunlight, while west exposures are prone to overheating on summer afternoons. Planning for exterior shading, such as awnings, roof overhangs, or trees, will help to admit sun when it is desired and to exclude it when it is not. Adjustable metal blinds are an effective, attractive means of controlling inside daylight and sunlight. Horizontal blinds have the advantage of being adjustable to redirect strong light upward or downward to reduce glare. Chemically stable metal or enamelled metal blind materials will not outgas and cause air contamination, as plastic, treated paper, or fabrics are prone to do, particularly when they are subjected to sunlight and heat.

FINISHES AND FURNISHINGS

In traffic areas, such durable floor finishes as ceramic tile, slate, marble, or hard vinyl tile (where tested and found acceptable), will reduce wear and aid cleaning. Keeping traffic areas clean is an important strategy for reducing contamination from pollen, soil, and dust.

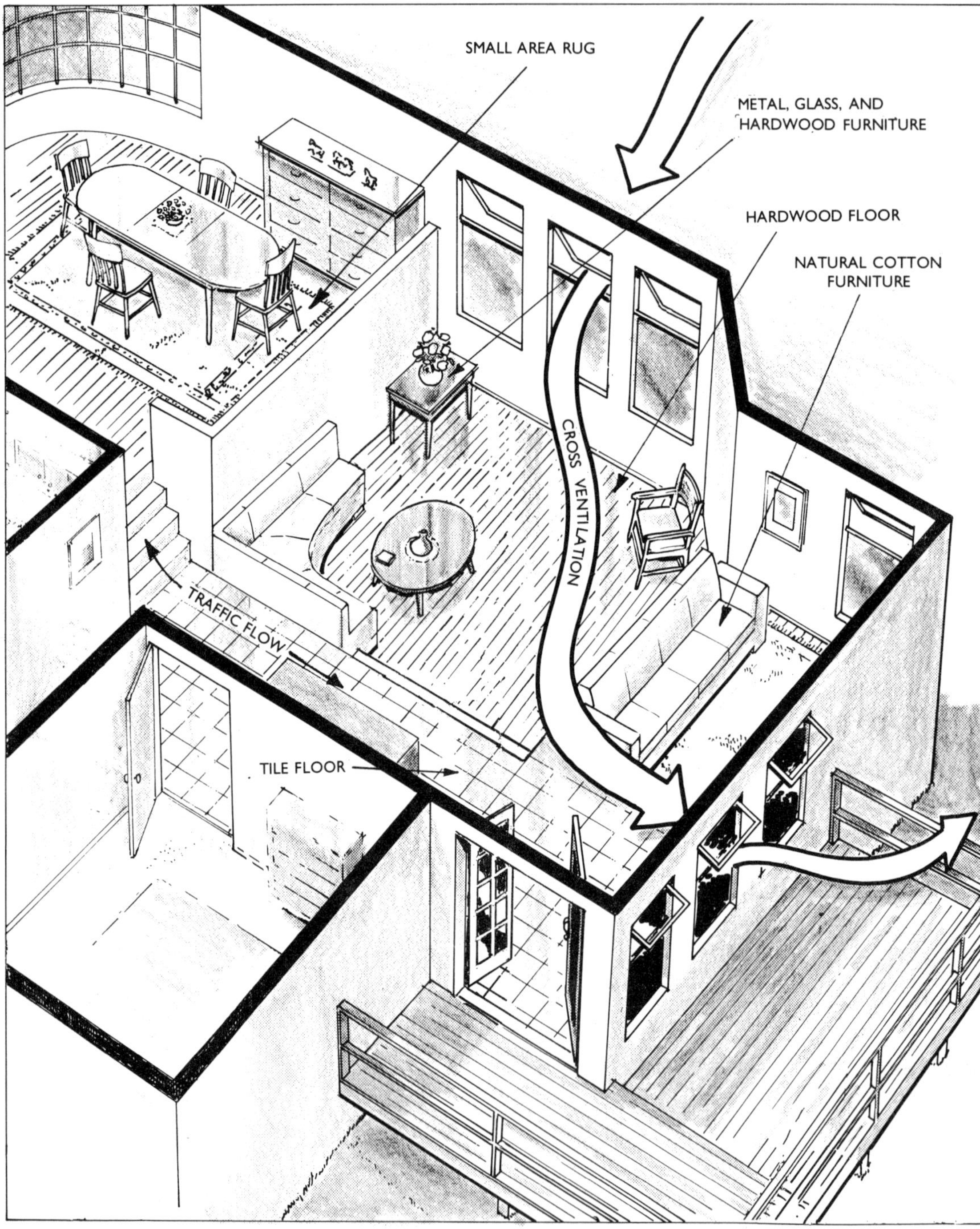

Fig. 10-1 The Living Room. *The living room should be separate from traffic flow and provide good daylight and ventilation.*

Cautious use of area rugs made from fibers (such as untreated cotton) that are acceptable to any sensitive persons in the household can soften and add warmth to the decor. Wall to wall carpets, and fabrics made with questionable components, can introduce contamination and cleaning problems.

Careful selection of furnishings will reduce the risk of contamination from such sources as particle board furniture frames, foamed plastic fillings, and irritating synthetic upholsteries. Furniture made with cotton fabrics on metal or hardwood frames is often acceptable to sensitive persons.

TRAFFIC FLOW

In family households, good traffic flow is particularly important for reducing irritation from intrusion and interruption. This is achieved by designing living areas to be separate from entries, kitchens, and main corridors. In small houses or apartments, careful furniture placement can create a separation between sitting areas and traffic areas to achieve much the same thing.

MAINTENANCE

A built in vacuum is very effective for cleaning with minimum dust disturbance. (See the Home Maintenance chapter.) Damp cloth dusting and damp mopping are also effective.

The use of cleaners and waxes should rarely be necessary in living areas, but when it is, they should be carefully tested for individual sensitivity. Small area rugs and removable washable upholstery covers can be laundered or cleaned elsewhere, and then well aired before their return. Many carpet and upholstery cleaners are harmful to the environmentally sensitive. They should only be used if individually tested and approved. (See the Home Maintenance chapter.)

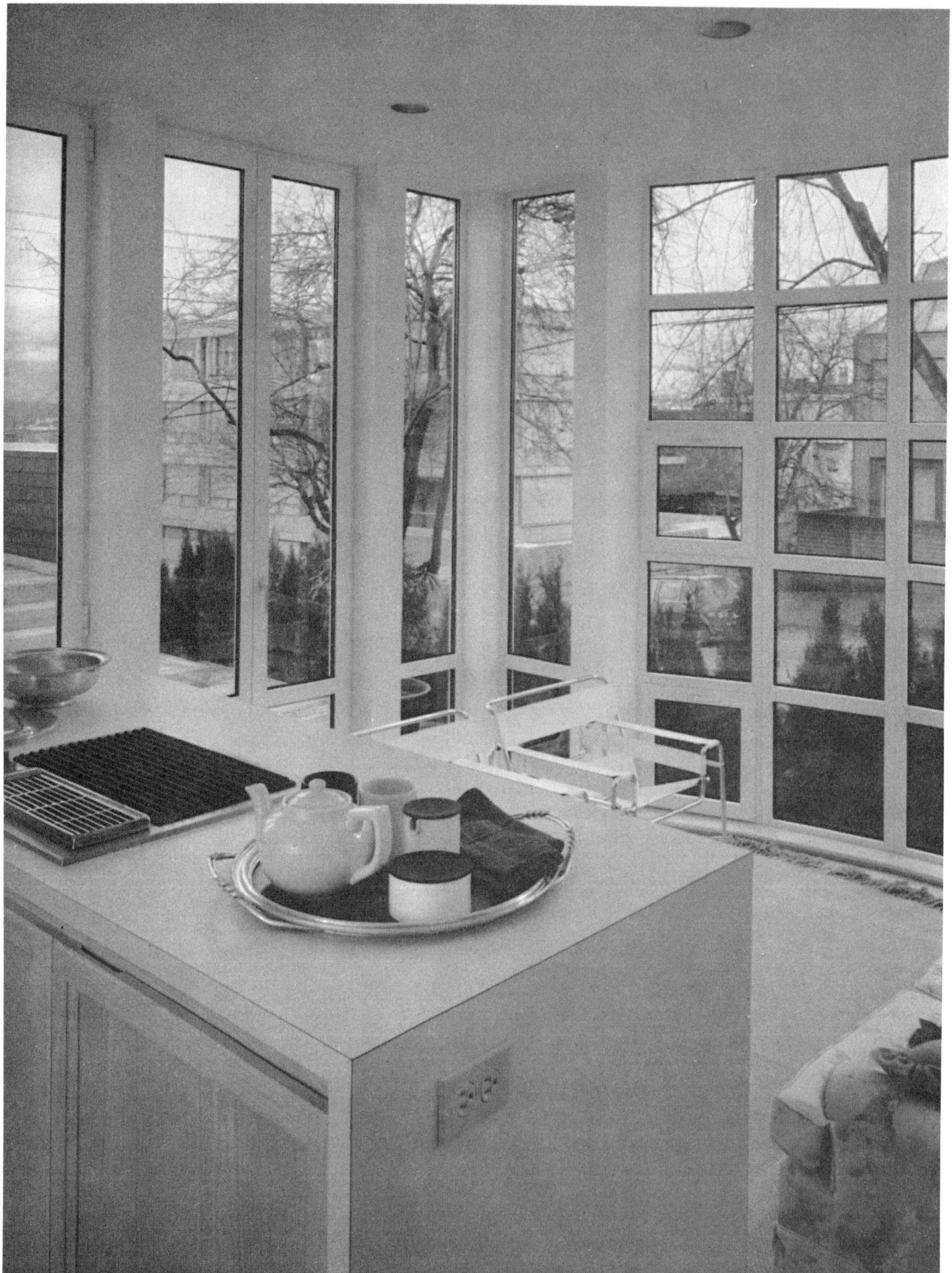

A bright, airy kitchen, with electric range ventilated below to the outside. Design by D. McIntyre and E. M. Sterling. Photo: Anthony Fulker Photography

11 THE KITCHEN

The kitchen is in many ways the most important room in the health conscious home. Good working conditions, reduced exposure to contaminants from cooking and appliances, and safe food storage and preparation conditions, are just a few of the concerns for the kitchen. Air quality in the kitchen is particularly important to the environmentally sensitive.

VENTILATION

The kitchen is a potent source of odors and air contamination that can affect both those working there and others anywhere in the home. The major sources of air contamination in kitchens are ranges, particle board in cabinets, cooking food, appliances, and trapped moisture and food wastes. It is important to reduce these sources of contamination, and to maximize ventilation.

Ranges: Gas ranges are major contributors of many dangerous air contaminants, such as carbon monoxide and nitrogen dioxide. *It is practically impossible to provide enough combustion air supply and direct exhaust for open flame cookers to eliminate air contamination.* It is also difficult to eliminate the small amounts of gas which escape into room air when a burner is lighted, or when it leaks. Electric ranges are much safer and simpler to control, as actual cooking and spills on burners are the only major sources of odors and contaminants. In addition, it is possible to use large amounts of ventilation air, since there are no flames to disturb.

A range ventilator or hood with outside exhaust for any kind of stove is essential to air quality control. The most effective and quietest have remote mounted blowers, where the blower and motor are mounted on

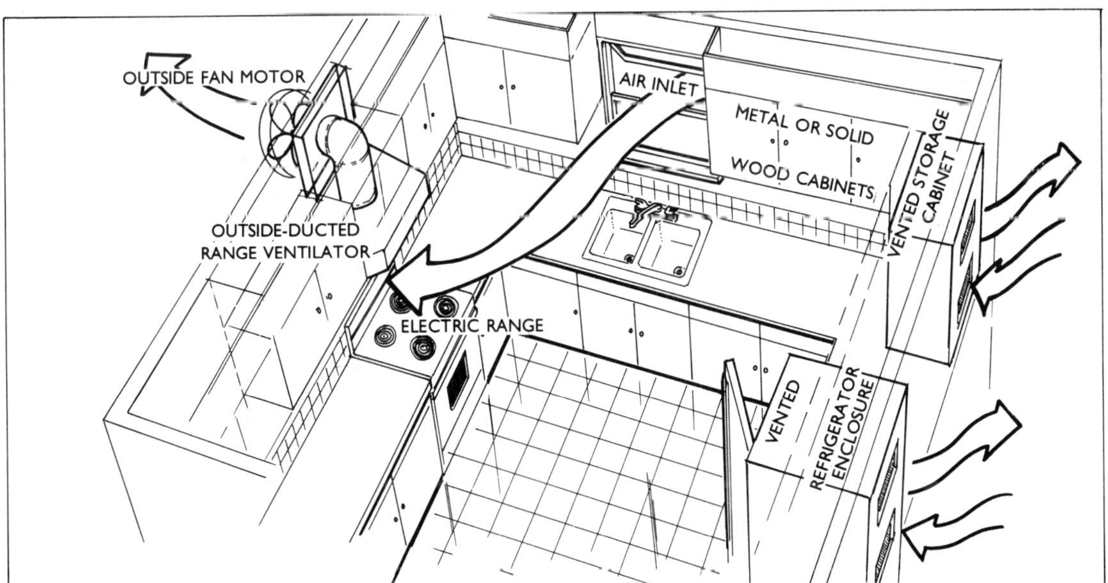

Fig. 11-1 Kitchen Ventilation. *An* Outside-ducted Range Ventilator *is essential to kitchen ventilation. Those with an* Outside Fan Motor *are quietest and most efficient.*

an outside wall and connected to the range or hood by a metal duct. Wall mounted fans designed for the kitchen are also effective.

Cooking: *Cooking food with high heat produces a large number of noxious and potentially hazardous air contaminants.* Burning fats, proteins, and sugars release respiratory irritants, and some suspected carcinogens as well. Slow cooking methods, steaming, and other ways of lowering cooking temperatures will reduce air contamination, and also lessen the necessary reliance on ventilation.

Air Supply: A source of intake air for the kitchen is needed to replace air exhausted during fan operation. An open window or door is often enough. *Failure to provide an air supply during exhaust fan operation will upset the air pressure balance in the home, and cause infiltration of potential contaminants.* In a tightly sealed or energy efficient home, this can create hazards, such as reverse drafting in chimneys, and infiltration of auto exhaust. (See the Home Ventilation chapter.)

Cabinets: Most commercial kitchen cabinets made in the last 15 years were made with frames of particle board—a source of formaldehyde gas in varying degrees. The health hazards from this gas are numerous, and it is particularly offensive to many sensitive people. Some older cabinets will probably have given off most of their formaldehyde load, and will emit comparatively little. (This may take from six months to several years from the time of manufacture, depending on the composition of the board and the temperature and humidity of the kitchen. High temperature and humidity generally accelerate this process.) Some very new cabinets are now being made with low emission board which produces less formal-

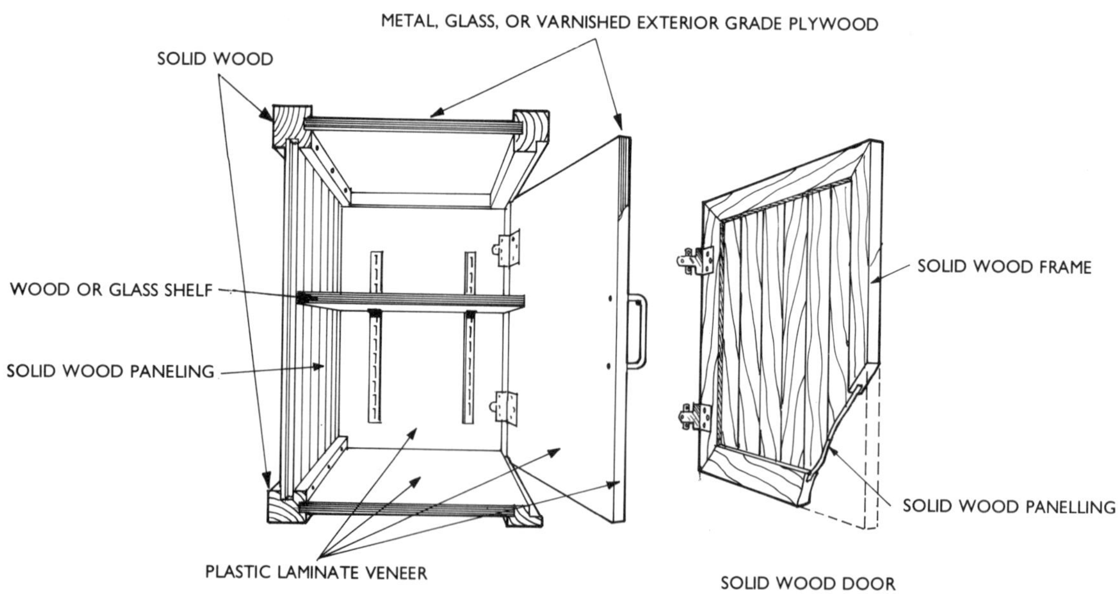

Fig.11-2 Solid Wood Kitchen Cabinet. *Metal or solid wood cabinets will reduce the air contamination load in the kitchen.*

dehyde. (Check manufacturer's information or the classification stamped on the board. The labels "Exposure 1" and "Exterior" classifications indicate low emission levels). The most problematic cabinets are likely to be those made without low emission material in the past 5 years.

To reduce formaldehyde emissions from cabinets:

• Use solid wood, metal, or exterior grade plywood for cabinet frames.

• Seal the surface of any remaining particle board with plastic veneers, or with a waterproof gloss paint (such as alkyd or enamel), varnish, or a wood sealer.

• Ensure proper ventilation, especially during outgassing of new products. (See the Home Ventilation chapter.)

Appliances: Even such small appliances as toasters and countertop electric ovens often produce large amounts of odor and gases that may be irritating to the environmentally sensitive. Because of this, the same sort of ventilation through open windows or kitchen fans needed for ranges should also be maintained for small appliances.

For some with extreme sensitivity, the ozone produced by small motors, such as those in kitchen blenders and mixers, can be highly irritating. Where necessary, these should be used only with caution and proper ventilation. Reactions have been reported to the plastic parts found on most refrigerators, and to the small amounts of heated dust, oil, or refrigerant that may be found on the outside of the unit. Where this is a problem, the refrigerator can be mounted in an outside ventilated enclosure, and sealed from the kitchen air. *Remember that refrigerators need cooling air circulation around the coils and the motor for safe, effective operation.*

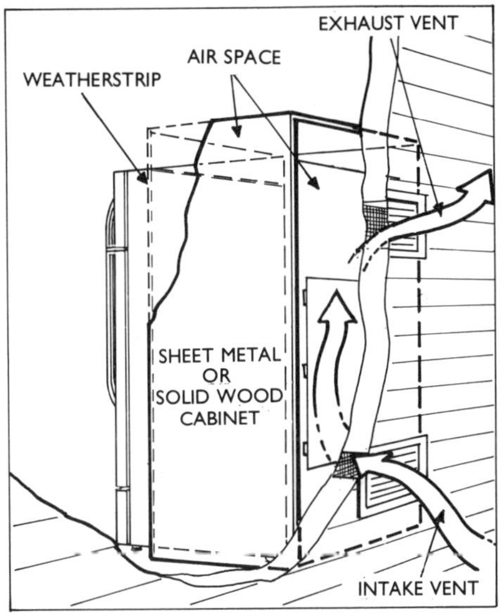

Fig. 11-3 Refrigerator in Outside Ventilated Cabinet. *For those who are sensitive to the plastic parts and oil in refrigerators, the unit can be built into a ventilated* Sheet Metal or Solid Wood Cabinet. *Commercial refrigerators are also available with remote mounted compressors.*

KITCHEN SURFACES

Floors, wall coverings, work surfaces, and the joints between them, are critical areas in the kitchen for maintaining clean, non-toxic conditions. Hard, smooth surfaces with well sealed joints are less likely to collect the moisture and food wastes which lead to cleaning problems and contamination.

Floors: Ceramic tile set in cement mortar with cement based grouts is a durable, safe, and beautiful answer to the problems posed by kitchen floors. Special cement based grouts (usually called "acid resistant grouts") are available that are formulated to resist kitchen food spills. Their contents should be carefully checked, however, and should not be used if they contain fungus retardants. If carefully applied, they will give a good seal between tiles. The alternative is to use a conventional cement based grout, and then to seal it with 5% silicone sealer. However, the silicone has a petroleum base similar to the base in oil paints and should not be used where there is chemical sensitivity.

A less costly and very satisfactory floor is a finished cement slab. This type of floor is made with a layer of conventional concrete with a finished topping layer applied, usually with color added. However, as this type of finish usually requires a seal or wax, these products must be carefully sampled for sensitivity reactions.

Hard vinyl composition floor tiles made with very stable plastics are a satisfactory solution for many people. The adhesive used to fasten them, however, is a potential irritant and must be self tested. Sheet type or cushioned plastic floor coverings, and carpets rated for kitchen use, are generally strong sources of chemical contamination, and not acceptable to the environmentally sensitive.

Wall coverings: Hard plastic laminates and ceramic tiles are both durable and beautiful finishes for splash areas at the back of kitchen counters, and for behind ranges and at the back of storage cupboards. Consider also installing these wall coverings in such areas as the lower cupboards where garbage is held, in order to ease maintenance.

Though very irritating during their application, durable, water resistant oil paints are acceptable to many people once they have dried and cured. This process can be accelerated by extra heat and ventilation. They make excellent and beautiful finishes for walls and ceilings. Many paints, however, contain fungicides, tints, and other chemicals which are unacceptable to sensitive people. Before a final choice is made, a well cured sample of a paint, such as an alkyd enamel, should be carefully tested to determine any sensitivity. (See the chapter Materials and Selection.) Careful application with brush and roller, and a few days of alternating heat and ventilation, seem to be most effective for minimizing odors. Spray applications tend to spread fine particles where they are not wanted, often require extra solvent which increases noxious fumes, and may not produce a surface as smooth and durable as one produced with brush and roller application.

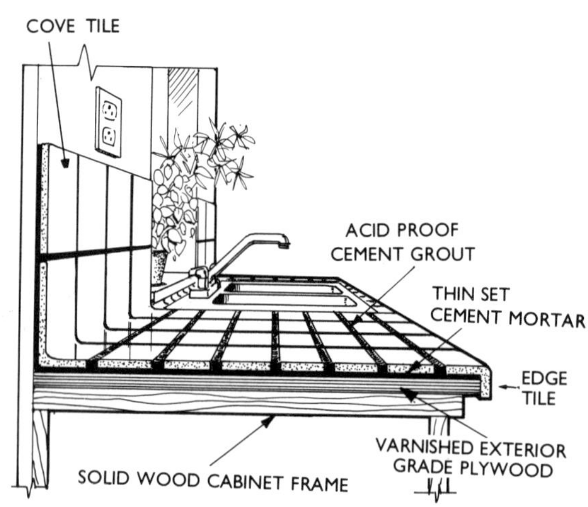

Fig. 11-4 Ceramic Tile Counter Top. *All joints and edges must be sealed and protected from damage.*

Joints: Many ceramic tiles are available with special cove (inside corner) and outside corner pieces which are used to form a clean and neat joint between surfaces. These require only the usual grout treatment to make a permanent seal. Other finishes, such as the plastic laminates, will require some form of caulking where they join, to prevent moisture and food waste collecting. Trapped food and moisture will harbor fungal and bacterial growth and produce odors. Silicone caulking (which is often acceptable to even very sensitive persons after the initial curing period of a few days has passed), is a very durable material for this purpose. Some silicone bathroom caulking (sold as tub sealer) is treated with fungicide, however, and should be avoided if sensitivity is suspected, or if you wish to be especially cautious.

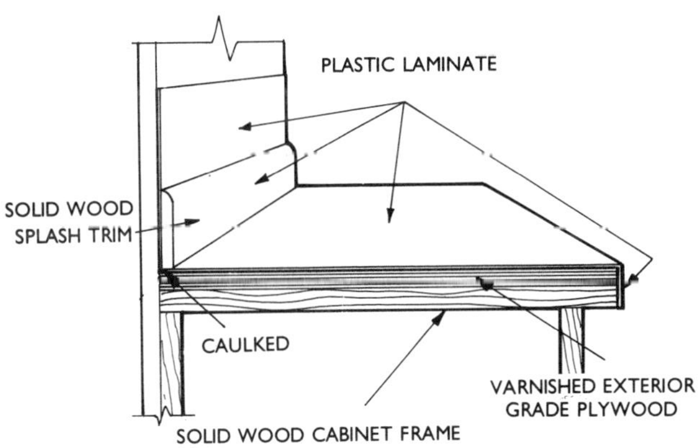

Fig. 11-5 Plastic Laminate Counter Top. *All joints must be caulked to prevent moisture entry.*

Contact Exposures: Food preparation surfaces, storage containers, cooking vessels, and cabinet interiors are all potential sources of direct food contamination. Porous surfaces, such as wood cutting boards, (particularly those built into cabinets), readily absorb moisture and food waste, easily becoming sour and mildewed, as well as attracting insects. Portable cutting surfaces made from hardwood or plastic are recommended, as they are more easily cleaned and kept dry, as well as being more adaptable than those which are fixed in place. However, anyone with chemical sensitivity should test for acceptability, as they may contain toxic glues where they are joined together.

Some food storage and cooking implements made from soft plastics and corrodible metals may introduce contamination into food if they are not handled carefully. The most stable and therefore recommended materials for these purposes are glass, ceramic, and stainless steel. Soft plastics, galvanized or other plated metals, and iron or copper pots, may react with foods, causing odors, discoloration, or dangerous contamination.

Cabinet interiors may also contaminate food that is not stored in tightly sealed containers. For many years some plastic and paper shelf coverings were impregnated with a pesticide to control kitchen insects, until residues of the chemical were found in food stored there. Bare particle board cabinet interiors may also impart odor and contaminaton to food. Reduce this by thoroughly sealing the surfaces and edges with a heavy urethane varnish, or oil base paint. Store cleaners and other household products in a separate cabinet, away from food storage areas. An outside air vent in this cabinet, if it is well sealed, will ensure that hazardous fumes will not leak into the house.

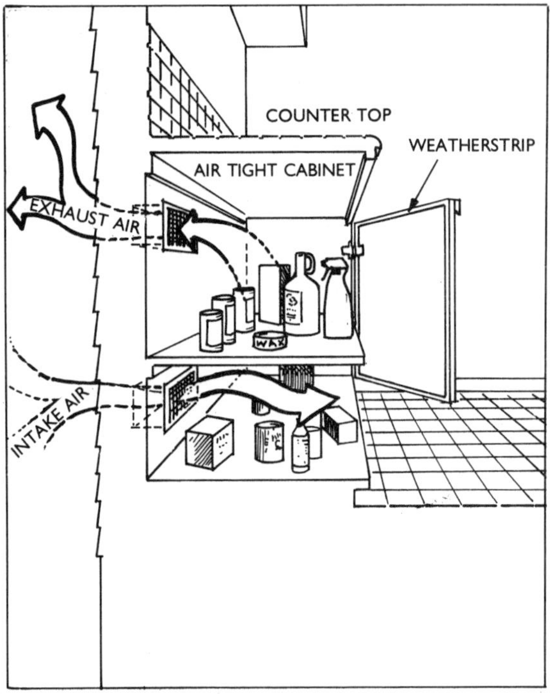

Fig. 11-6 Kitchen Cabinet Ventilated to Outside. *Soaps, cleaners, and waxes can be stored in a separate cabinet isolated from room air.*

KITCHEN LIGHTING

The traditional kitchen ceiling fixture, mounted at the center of the room, is inadequate for many tasks, and often unappealing as well. This type of lighting tends to emphasize the floor and cabinet fronts, while not providing enough light directly on the work surface. A simple and inexpensive remedy is to use a small lamp, of the type designed to mount directly under the upper cabinets. This sort of lamp, either a miniature incandescent or a compact fluorescent tube type, will illuminate the work area directly, improving kitchen safety and visual appeal. An overhead lamp, if mounted on the ceiling above the usual working position, is also effective for directly lighting the work area. Valance lights or wall wash type indirect lighting, which contain lamps mounted behind reflective shields, can be used for an effective background light in kitchens.

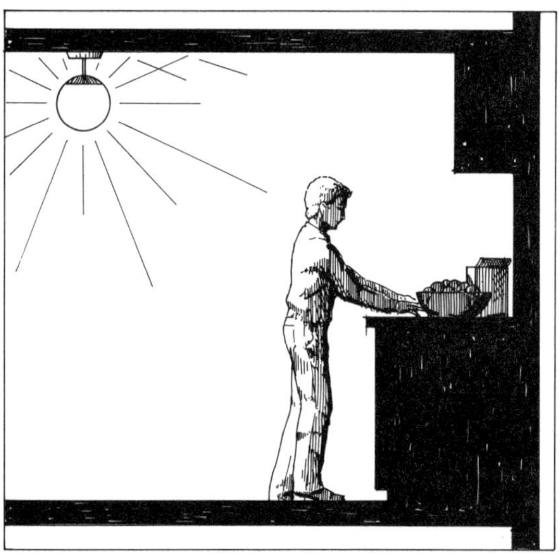

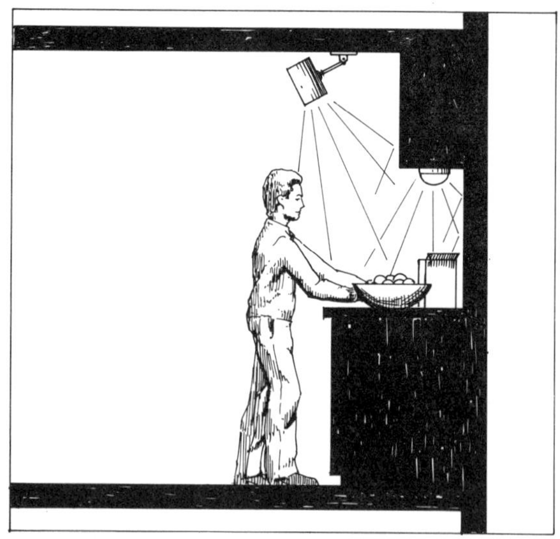

Fig. 11-7 Kitchen Task Lighting

Poor task lighting. A central overhead lamp causes shadow on the work area.

Good task lighting. A direct overhead lamp, or under-the-cabinet lamp, lights the work area effectively.

12 THE SUNSPACE/GREENHOUSE

The therapeutic value of sunlight and daylight are well known. A room of light in the home can be an inviting and healing place, particularly in northern climates where weak winter light does not reach far into the home through conventional windows. Its benefits are both physiological and psychological, but it brings more subtle aesthetic pleasures as well.

The Sunspace

The sunspace is distinctly different from a greenhouse, in that it is fully incorporated into the living space, and is not necessarily divided from the house with a separately controlled climate. The sunspace will, of course, provide good conditions for many plants, and a greenhouse can also be a pleasant place for people, but a sunspace will not be controlled specifically for plants as is a greenhouse.

A room, or a part of one, if it has an easterly, southern, or westerly exposure not heavily shaded by outside obstructions, can be converted into a special place to go for light and sun when one does not wish to be outdoors. It can also be a source of light and cheer, influencing the entire home. However, for both comfort and safety, the sunlight must be very carefully controlled.

Relatively simple and inexpensive renovations to an existing home or apartment, such as the addition of a glass door or large window, skylights, or a "greenhouse window," can all transform an area into a sunspace. In cases with the appropriate exposure, an apartment balcony can be readily made into a sunspace (or greenhouse) by adding a glass enclosure to the exit door. A factory made greenhouse unit can be used.

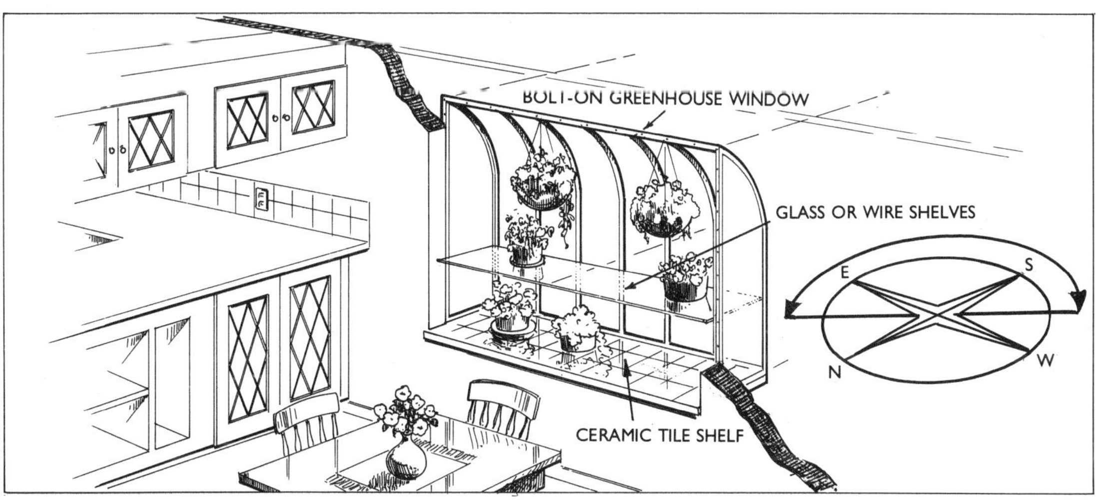

Fig. 12-1 A Greenhouse Window. *An apartment or room can be transformed by light. A greenhouse window is a simple and effective device.*

THE GLASS AREA

The glass area in a sunspace must serve a number of purposes. It must admit daylight and sunlight, yet allow control of glare, excess heat, and damage from excess ultraviolet light. It must also permit control of winter heat loss and any condensation problems, as well as the entrance of noise where this is a problem. For safety and security the glass must also be protected from breakage.

LIGHT AND HEAT

Tall windows which reach the ceiling or connect directly to skylights will admit the most penetrating light. South facing windows have the advantage over skylights of admitting more sunlight in winter, when the sun is low, and less in summer, when the sun is high. Compared to windows, skylights admit more sunlight when the sun is high, and will more readily cause overheating. For this reason large skylights are inadvisable in regions with strong summer sun. This is particularly so for southern exposures, unless they are equipped with sun control devices. External control devices such as louvers are the best.

Interior horizontal metal blinds can be used to control glare and excess sunlight, but they will not control overheating from sunlight as effectively as external shutters or louvers. There are many blinds systems with special frames to fit skylights.

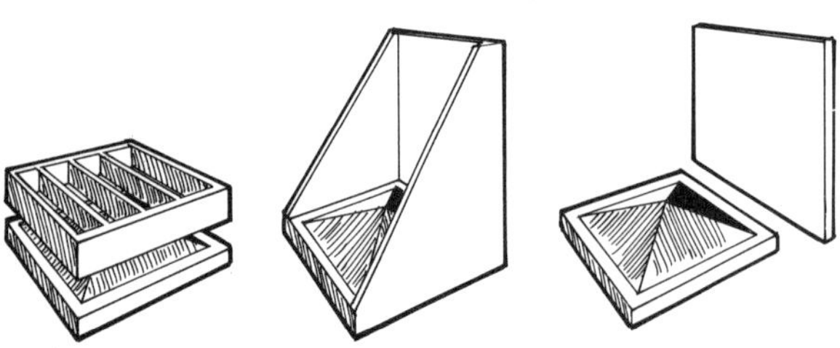

Fig. 12-2 Shading Devices for Skylights

GLASS TYPES

Solar control glass is available which will admit much of the sun's light while rejecting much of its heat. Such a glass may be necessary to reduce excess heating, particularly where poor house design has resulted in too much unsheltered glass facing south or west. However, as they often create a dark and gloomy mood on winter days, when daylight is weak, they should be used only when absolutely necessary.

Ultraviolet (u.v.) light from the sun can be a serious health hazard even indoors. Excess exposure to this high energy, invisible light causes sunburn and increases the risk of skin cancer. Ultraviolet light also causes the rapid deterioration of building and finishing materials, increasing outgassing and air contamination. (See the chapters Understanding Contamination Processes and Materials and Selection.) Fortunately, most common types of glass reject 95% of the sun's ultraviolet light, preventing its admission to the home. Many plastics, however, do not. Some of the plastics used in skylights and safety windows will admit substantial amounts of this light. In addition, when heated, these plastics may outgas air contaminants. They can be used to advantage in greenhouses where extra ultraviolet light is needed for certain plants, but they are not advisable in rooms which receive a great deal of sun and are connected directly to living spaces.

Breakable glass is a life-threatening hazard if used in skylights or in floor to ceiling windows. Always use tempered safety glass, or wire reinforced glass, for skylights, doors, or windows which begin less than 12" from the floor. This building code requirement is sometimes disregarded by inexperienced builders, or when glass is being replaced.

Heat loss, which causes discomfort, and inside condensation, are cold weather symptoms of glass's poor insulating quality. The use of single panes is rapidly disappearing in northern regions due to high heating costs, and is also being replaced by double or triple glass in warm climates to reduce cooling loads. Double or triple glass, either in factory made sealed units or when created by adding storm sash over windows, will not only save energy, but will improve comfort, and reduce such condensation problems as fungus growth and structure damage. Temporary plastic sheet window coverings can be effective for saving heat and stopping drafts, but should be used on the *outside*. They are potential sources of contamination and should not be in your home, particularly when exposed to strong light. Insulating shutters, which tightly cover windows and skylights at night, are also a highly effective means of saving energy. Multiple glazing will also transmit considerably less noise than single, and can be used to reduce objectionable street noise or other noise. (See the Sound chapter.)

Sunspace Materials

The sunspace is a particularly crucial area for careful materials selection. Due to strong light levels, potential heat buildup, and outgassing potential, such stable materials as ceramics, masonry, concrete, metals, and glass are recommended. Wood generally will not stand up well in sunspaces.

FLOOR

A concrete floor with a sealed finish (see the chapter Materials and Selection), or ceramic tile covering, are ideal materials for a sunspace. The heat storage capacity of concrete and tile will keep the room cooler during early sunlight hours, and then retain heat to be released overnight, saving energy and increasing comfort.

If you wish to convert a room in a house with a wood floor to a sunspace, consider placing a thin layer of concrete and/or ceramic tile on the wood floor, if the building's structure will support the weight. (Verify this with an architect, engineer, or your building inspection department.) If you do not wish to use concrete or tile for the entire floor, consider using it only for the floor and windowshelf areas directly inside the windows receiving most of the sun. (See the Construction Notes chapter.)

WALLS

Untreated plaster is one of the most stable and beautiful of wall coverings, and one that is generally acceptable even to the very sensitive. Though painted gypsum board is

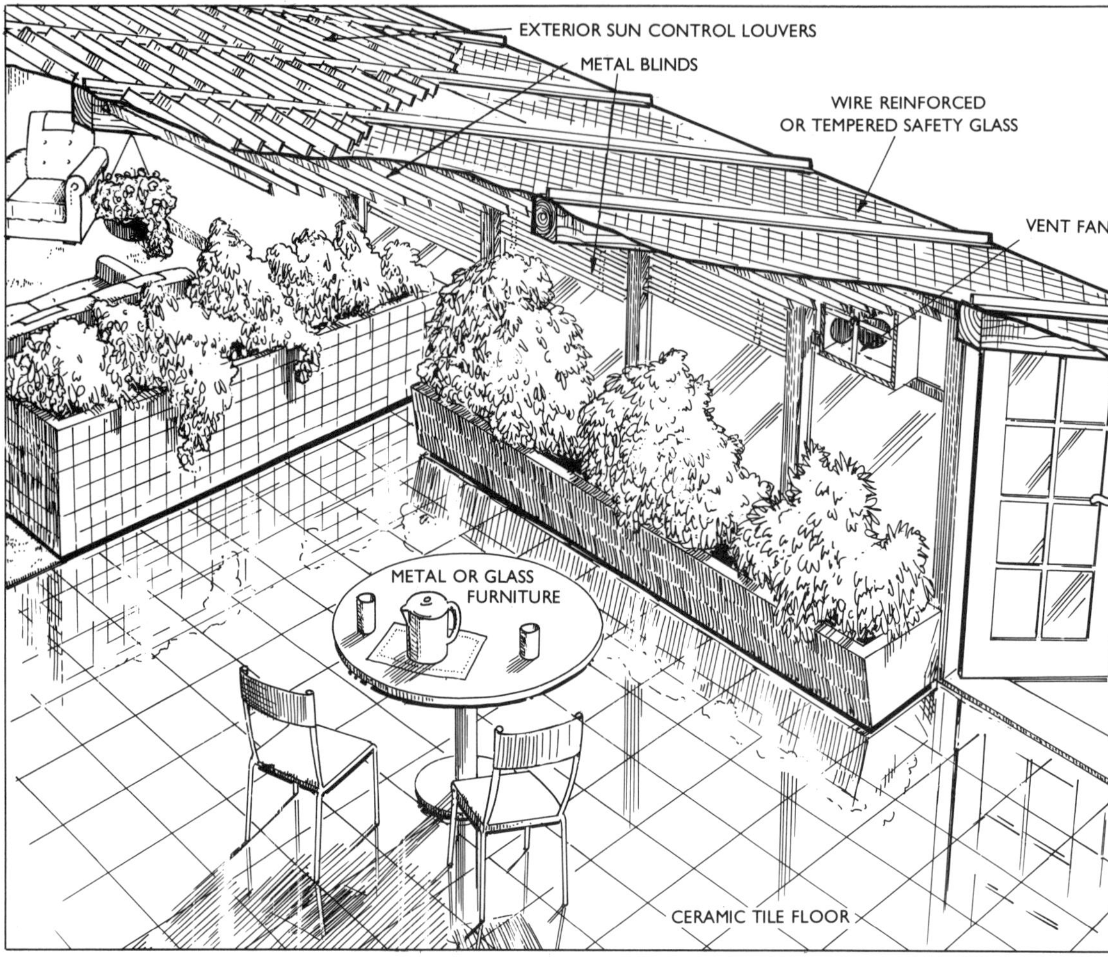

Fig. 12-3 The Sunspace. *The indoor sunspace can provide healing year-round natural light, as well as solar heat and a good environment for house plants.*

less costly, it may not be tolerated by some people. (See the Materials and Selection chapter.) Consider also a ceramic tile or brick "wainscot" wall covering reaching 3 or 4 feet up the wall for beauty, durability, and heat storage.

WINDOW SASH

Metal or enamelled metal window frames are the least likely to deteriorate, outgas, or support dampness and fungus contamination. Solid vinyl sash is also quite stable, and may be tolerated by most people, but it must be tested by the environmentally sensitive—particulary while exposed to sun and heat. Wood sash, in spite of its beauty, is often not acceptable to the environmentally sensitive because it may outgas wood resins, especially when heated. Such wood windows will also require ongoing maintenance. In addition, unless custom made, *it is difficult to obtain any that have not been treated with an unacceptable chemical wood preservative.*

FURNISHINGS

Metal furniture, glass and ceramic table tops, and hard plastic laminates are the most durable and acceptable for the sunspace. Hardwood or wicker may also be acceptable once the finish has cured, but they may suffer bleaching and cracking due to sunlight exposure. Soft plastics, synthetic upholstery materials, treated drapery fabrics, carpets, and paints should be avoided throughout the home, but particularly in the sunspace.

VENTILATION

At least two opening windows, preferably on opposite sides of the room for cross-ventilation, are a minimum requirement for the sunspace. Due to the potential for overheating, a large vent window, or a wall mounted exhaust fan located high up to remove excess heat, is recommended.

EXIT

If at all possible, the sunspace (or greenhouse) should include an outside door, providing easy access onto a balcony, patio, or garden, which can be kept open and screened for summer use. The exit and screen door can then be used to assist sunspace or whole house ventilation.

The Greenhouse

Plants in the home are widely accepted as a living decor which contributes a soft, pleasant, and healing atmosphere. Just as we give flowers and plants to people who are ill, healthy houseplants remind us all of well-being and regeneration. House plants can also literally freshen indoor air (see the chapter Controlling Indoor Air Quality), as well as providing subtle fragrance and even a source of food.

Though some plants are perfectly comfortable with the same indoor climate that suits us, in order to thrive many require elevated temperatures and humidity. In fact 65% R.H. (relative humidity) and 75°F., the upper limits for human comfort and health, are actually the lower limits for tropical plant survival. For this reason, a greenhouse with a separately controlled climate, preferably easily accessible to living spaces, is the ideal way to live with plants year-round while providing them with optimum conditions. The greenhouse, like the sunspace, can also be a special retreat in the house, providing solar heat, good light, and other benefits.

In addition to the sunspace requirements, there are some special features and hazards to consider for the greenhouse.

HUMIDITY AND HEAT

The greenhouse will require an airtight enclosure, separated from the living space by tight fitting doors, so that heat and humidity can be independently controlled. Automatic heaters, ventilators, and water mist humidifiers are valuable for maintaining ideal conditions in a greenhouse.

VENTILATION

Good cross ventilation is essential in the

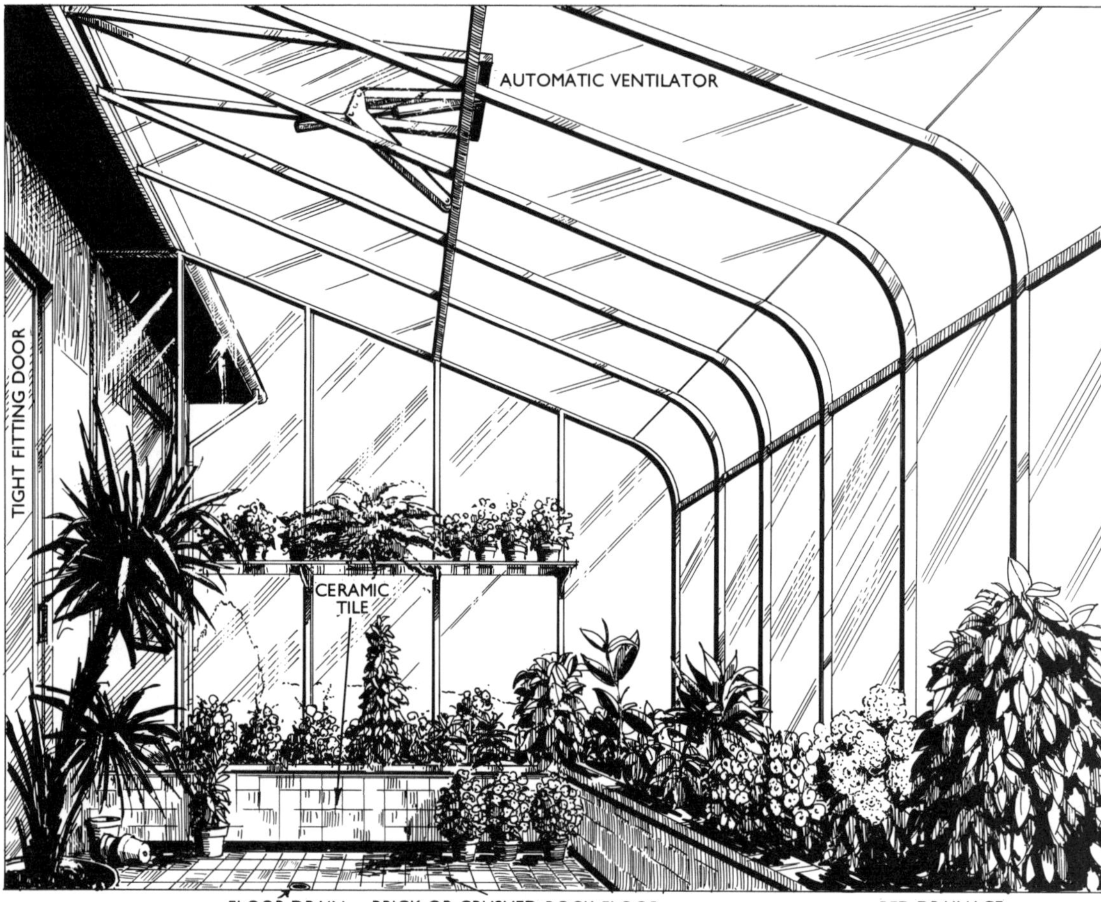

Fig. 12-4 The Greenhouse. *The greenhouse will require climate control separate from the house. It must be well ventilated, preferably with an* Automatic Ventilator, *and isolated from the house by a* Tight Fitting Door. *Good* Bed Drainage *and* Floor Drains *are also essential.*

greenhouse to prevent overheating. Many good automatic devices, such as reasonably priced temperature operated vents and electric fans, are available from garden supply stores and greenhouse manufacturers for this purpose.

DRAINAGE

Floor drains, and drainage built into beds and planters, are essential in the greenhouse for preventing standing water. Poor drainage will damage plants and may cause fungus growth.

PASSAGE

A passage door into the living space, such as a French door, will provide pleasant views of the greenhouse from inside, as well as an opening for heat and air exchange between house and greenhouse, as desired. This should be a tight fitting door, to prevent migration of undesirable moisture and heat.

ALLERGENIC PLANTS

Very careful selection of indoor plants is essential when there is asthma, hay fever, or any suspected plant sensitivity in the home. (It is virtually impossible to control the movement of pollens, odors, and dust into the living areas from a connected greenhouse.)

FUNGUS

The growth of unwanted fungus in the greenhouse, which can spread to the house, is a serious problem. Because humidity is high, moisture will readily collect in cracks and on porous surfaces which support fungus growth. To minimize this problem, make use of sloped surfaces to prevent trapped moisture, install good drainage, seal all cracks, and ensure that good light and free air circulation are available throughout the greenhouse.

GREENHOUSE PLASTICS

Many greenhouse systems use plastic panels, which can become sources of air contamination, as well as admitting excessive ultraviolet light. Though some flowering and fruit bearing plants require more ultraviolet light than will pass through glass, plastic will become a health risk with regular exposure. Check with your supplier to find out if your greenhouse material admits 20% or more ultraviolet light, and if it does, be aware that your skin must be protected as if you were outdoors. Before purchasing it, any plastic material must first be self tested by the environmentally sensitive. This should be done with a sample while it is warm and exposed to sunlight.

13 THE BEDROOM/RETREAT

We spend one third or more of our lives in our bedrooms. Those of us who do not require a "sanctuary bedroom" (see the Sanctuary chapter) may nevertheless be concerned with preventive health. If careful thought is given to the furnishing and finishing of the bedroom, it can be made a place of relief, relatively free from unwanted exposures, where we may rest better.

The key areas of potential exposure to irritants in the bedroom are the bedding, ventilation, heating and cooling devices, furniture, and floor and wall coverings.

BEDDING

After clothing, bedding is the most intimate material with which we spend many hours in contact. Bedding can contain many allergenic items which can be severely irritating to allergic or environmentally sensitive people. These often include:

- -Feathers
- -Rubber or plastic foams
- -Some synthetic and natural fibers
- -Fabric stain repellents, and wrinkle resistant treatments.
- -Fabric mildew retardants
- -Detergent residue
- -Fabric fireproofing treatments
- -Fabric softeners
- -Scents
- -Dyes

A careful choice of bedding materials is important to all of us. Irritating conditions can readily develop in seemingly benign materials due to heat and moisture, which will affect even those of us who have had no previous sensitivity problems. Many people who are sensitive to some or all of these items find that an untreated cotton futon bed, with untreated cotton covers, is the least irritating bedding available. Be sure that the cotton bedding contains no synthetic foam layer (for fire proofing). It may do so, even if sold as "all cotton." Some synthetic fibers, such as certain acetates and polyesters, also seem to be widely accepted by people with environmental sensitivities.

VENTILATION

A small, but constant source of clean outdoor air is necessary in the bedroom to replace the oxygen consumed by breathing, and to reduce carbon dioxide contamination. In older buildings the leakage around windows and doors is sometimes adequate for this purpose, but in tighter structures an opening window will be necessary. Very large volumes of fresh air from wide open windows are also often desirable in warm weather to assist natural nighttime cooling.

Cross ventilation in a bedroom is very desirable, particularly in warm climates, but is usually only available in rooms located on building corners. The use of fans to assist ventilation is a comfortable and healthful cooling method in those regions and seasons when outdoor air is acceptable and air conditioning is not necessary. Thorough and regular dusting will be necessary, however, particularly with the use of a fan, to prevent the aggravation of dust allergies by airborne particles.

HEATING AND COOLING

Many people find that a minimum amount of bedroom heating and cooling is best for the throat and sinuses, leaving them more "clear headed" in the morning. Excessive bedroom heating or cooling can cause dryness, stale air, and increased dust exposure. Radiant heat systems which do not move air by fans are less likely to disturb or "fry" dust, and will produce less skin dryness due to air motion. Ceiling or floor mounted radiant panels produce little air movement, and present no "fried dust" or cleaning problems. Liquid filled radiators are less expensive and more adaptable for those living in rented homes or apartments. (See the Home Heating chapter.)

FURNISHINGS

Solid wood or metal furniture is less likely to produce room contamination than pressed wood or plastic products.

FLOOR AND WALL COVERINGS

Wall to wall carpet, the pads used beneath it, and the adhesive sometimes used to fasten it, are all ready sources of chemical and biological contamination, and are difficult to clean. Factory made wood parquet floors and sheet vinyl or rubber floor coverings are likely to contain toxic chemicals, waxes, or adhesives which produce odors and contamination. Bare floors of hardwood planks, ceramic tile, finished cement, or hard vinyl composite floor tile (if tested and found acceptable) are the least objectionable floor coverings. Area rugs are the most versatile and easily cleaned soft floor coverings, and are available in a range of synthetic and natural fabrics, some of which may be acceptable even to the environmentally sensitive. However, be cautions of dyes used in rugs, as they may be hazardous for chemically sensitive people. Chromate and analine dyes are worst. Lighter colors and natural dyes tend to be safest.

Alkyd oil paints or some latex paints for walls and ceilings are acceptable to many, once they have cured, though this may take up to nine months in extreme cases. They must be carefully self-tested for lingering odors and individual sensitivity as they may contain unacceptable fungicides. The addition of 1 cup of sodium bicarbonate per gallon of paint will reduce lingering odors. Special hypo-allergenic paints, such as casein paints made from milk, are usually acceptable in bedrooms. (See the Materials and Selection chapter.)

14 THE BATHROOM

The three main concerns for health conscious design and maintenance of the bathroom are dampness control, ventilation, and water contamination. Bathroom maintenance, and contamination control from other sources, are also important considerations.

Chronic dampness in bathrooms encourages the growth of fungus, which can cause health problems, particularly for the environmentally sensitive. (See the section ENVIRONMENTAL ILLNESS AND YOU.) Dampness also causes persistent odors, and the deterioration of building materials, interior fixtures, and furnishings.

High ventilation rates in bathrooms are essential for odor and dampness control. Ventilation is also important for radon control in those bathrooms using water from deep wells in rock formations containing radon. This water is a potent source of dangerous radon gas, which will collect in a closed bathroom during bathing. (See Radon, in the chapter The Indoor Hazards.)

Over half of the pollutants that we absorb from contaminated water come from the water we bathe in. These pollutants enter our bodies through the skin and lungs. Chlorine and industrial pollutants are the most serious concerns.

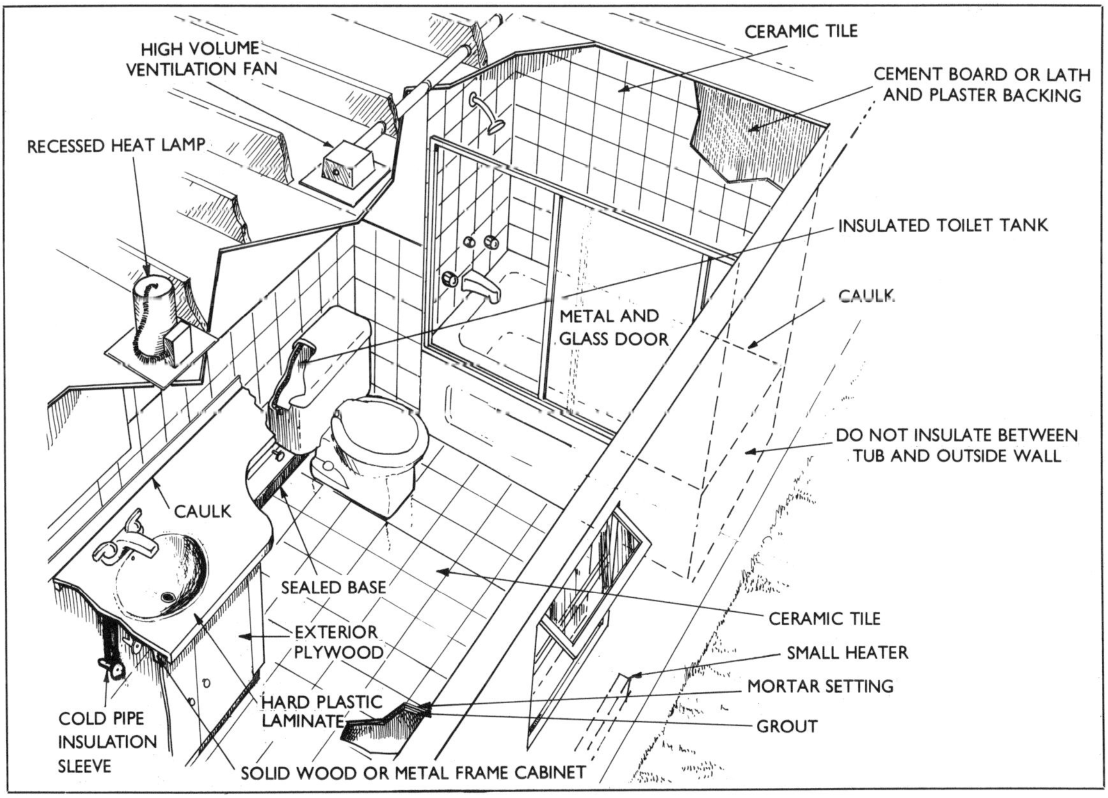

Fig. 14-1 The Bathroom. *Ventilation for moisture control, a source of rapid heat, insulation of cold surfaces to reduce condensation, and careful sealing of cracks to prevent trapped moisture, are the major concerns in the bathroom.*

DAMPNESS CONTROL

• Carefully caulk and seal all seams around tubs, shower doors, baseboards, and sinks. Plain silicone sealant is acceptable to many sensitive persons after it has fully cured. (See the Materials and Selection chapter.)

• Where possible, use tight fitting metal and glass shower doors to reduce spills. Plastic shower curtains may introduce odors and chemical contamination.

• Use such waterproof materials as ceramic tile or hard plastic laminates not only around tub enclosures, but behind toilets and sinks as well.

• Use an insulated toilet tank liner, cold water pipe insulation, and insulation under the tub, to reduce "sweating". Plastic foam toilet tank liners are usually safe because they are underwater. Commercial type fiberglass pipe insulation may be more acceptable for some people than the plastic foam types.

• Heat lamps are safe and effective for warming bathers, but may not be adequate for drying the bathroom. In cold or damp climates it will also usually be necessary to have a properly installed small heater, which can be safely left on to dry the room.

• The presence of daylight, where possible, helps to prevent the growth of fungus.

VENTILATION CONTROL

• A large opening window, or a high capacity vent fan specially designed for bathrooms, is essential for removing moisture laden air, odors, and potentially, radon.

AIR CONTAMINATION CONTROL

• For cabinets, use metal or solid wood frames or *exterior* plywood tops and doors to reduce formaldehyde exposure.

• Ceramic tile set in a cement grout is the most stable and durable (therefore most acceptable for sensitive persons) floor and wall covering. The preferred grout is the cement based waterproof type. Other types must be waterproofed with a 5% silicone sealer, but this is a petroleum based product which may not be well tolerated by sensitive individuals.

• Wall and ceiling paints should be the most durable and waterproof types. Though alkyd oil paints are petroleum based, they are often well tolerated by sensitive persons once the solvent has evaporated and the paint has fully cured. Curing may be accelerated by extra heat and ventilation after painting. Latex base paints are not as durable, and though they may be less offensive during the drying period, many latex paints are not well tolerated by sensitive persons in the long term due to prolonged outgassing and the presence of fungicides. (See the Materials and Selection chapter.)

• Bathroom windows with metal or hard plastic frames are often easiest to dry and keep clean. Wood frame windows in bathrooms will require careful painting and extra maintenance. They are not recommended.

WATER CONTAMINATION CONTROL

• Water treatment to improve water quality and reduce the absorption of water contaminants through skin while bathing may be necessary in regions with water contamination problems. (See the chapter Water Treatment for how-to instructions.)

BATHROOM MAINTENANCE

• Regular cleaning of tile joints, window frames, and other points which might trap moisture and support fungus growth, is essential. Vinegar or borax solutions may be used to safely remove and retard fungus growth. (See the Home Maintenance chapter.)

• Bathing enclosures which receive strong light, and are left open to dry after use, are less likely to grow dangerous fungus.

• To prevent mildew, clean and dry bathmats regularly.

15 THE BASEMENT

Basements are a very common source of contamination in homes. Some of the health problems that can originate in the basement are: oil and gas leaks, excessive dampness and fungus contamination, radon gas, flue gases from ineffective chimneys, sewer gases, residual pesticides, dusts, insects and rodents, and leakage from stored household and garden chemicals, including paints, solvents, and cleaners.

The potential health problems from basements are so pervasive that some health conscious home designers are recommending their total avoidance wherever possible. Instead, they recommend ventilated crawl spaces, or slabs built directly on the earth. Such considerations are particularly significant when designing homes for the environmentally sensitive.

Controlling Basement Contamination

OIL AND GAS LEAKS

Nearly all oil burning appliances will leak small amounts of fuel. This fuel can saturate concrete floors, creating a source of oil fumes that persists long after the leak is repaired or the appliance removed. Detergent cleaning, followed by sealing the affected area with a heavy floor paint or a thin layer of new concrete, can reduce the problem.

Remember that replacing a gas range with an electric one is only a first step in eliminating aggravating gas fumes from the home if there are sensitivity problems. Tiny gas leaks are also very common in furnaces and water heaters, and are not easily detected. *Though these leaks are small, they can seriously affect the environmentally sensitive.* Gas valves and burner controls are the most common points for leaks. You can test for them by applying soapy water and watching for bubbles, or with a careful sniff. Your local utility company has sophisticated electronic "sniffing" equipment and should respond quickly if called to investigate gas odors. Large gas leaks are, of course, an emergency, and must be professionally investigated immediately.

FUNGUS CONTAMINATION

Basements are a common area for fungus contamination, due to dampness and lack of light. *Fungi and the spores released from their colonies are serious allergens affecting many people, particularly the environmentally sensitive.*

Sealing basement leaks, and dampproofing walls and floors from the outside with cement based sealants and plastic sheets, preventing the accumulation of dirt or other potential nutrients for fungi to grow on, and maintaining a source of light (preferably daylight), will reduce the proliferation of fungus. *Basement carpets are a particularly serious potential breeding ground for fungi.* If used, these must be carefully maintained and kept dry. Absorbent wall coverings, such as wood fiber board or gypsum board, which

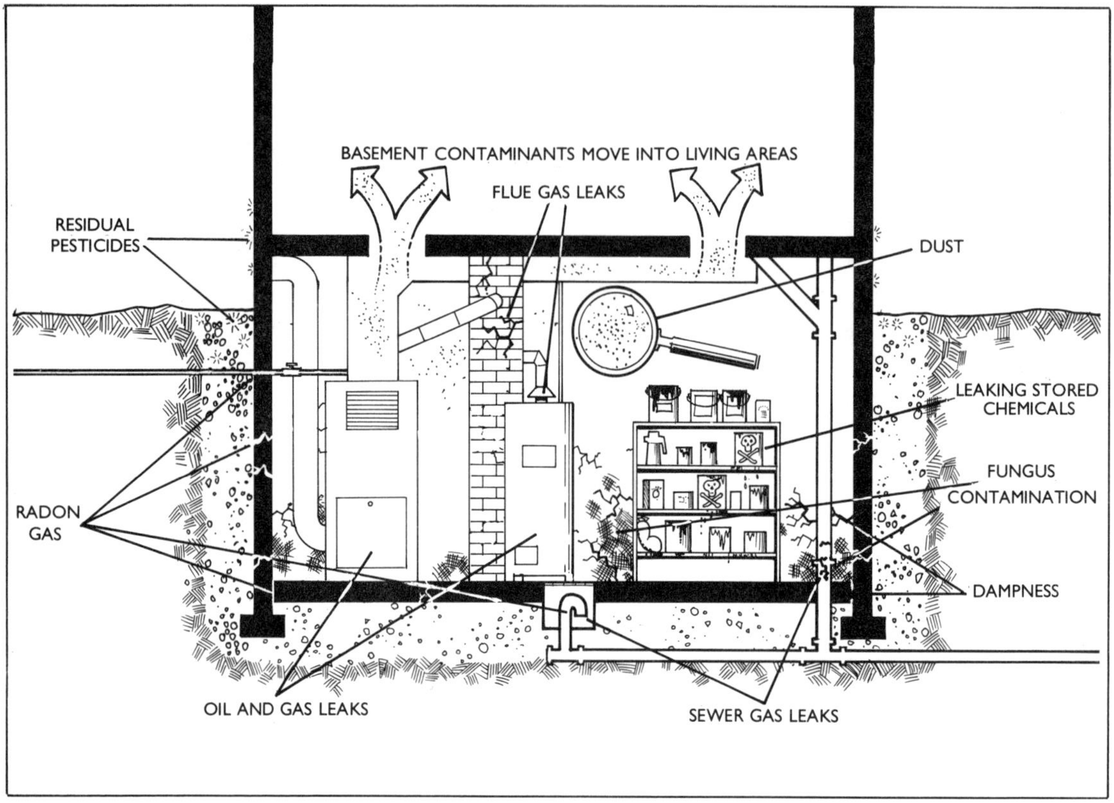

Fig. 15-1 Common Sources of Contamination in Basements

have not been sealed with an impermeable finish such as alkyd paint, are also potential sites for dampness and fungus growth. In some cases it is necessary to maintain a heater or dehumidifier in the basement to control moisture damage and fungus growth.

RADON GAS

Radon gas is a natural radioactive element found in soil and water that can enter basements through cracks and drains. Radon exposure increases the risk of lung cancer. *Radon control is focused on the basement.* (See Radon in the Controlling Indoor Air Quality chapter for more information.)

FLUE GASES

Chimneys serving furnaces and water heaters in basements are a common point of dangerous flue gas entry into the home. Make sure that the chimney's condition is sound, and that combustion appliances and fireplaces receive outside air at all times to supply their flames, and to reduce the flue gas hazard. Superinsulated homes will need special attention to supply air for any fuel burning appliances or fireplaces. (See the chapters Home Heating/Cooling and Testing for Contamination.)

SEWER GAS

Gases from sewers, which can sometimes enter basements, are a nuisance and a potential hazard. This situation usually only introduces unpleasant odors, but there have been cases of explosive gases entering homes via sewers. Basement sumps and floor drains are sometimes connected to the sanitary sewer (the same pipe serving toilets and other plumbing) by a special check valve or by a water filled trap. *If this valve (located in the basement sump) malfunctions, or the wet trap becomes dry, a bacteria laden odorous gas will enter the home.* This can also occur if unused or little used sinks, toilets, or tubs are not occasionally run to renew the water seal in the trap. A visual check and "sniff test" of sump and drains will often determine if there is any problem. Have sumps or drains which gurgle or bubble when a toilet is flushed elsewhere checked by a plumber.

Sewer pipes in basements can also cause contamination in the home if they become cracked or leaky due to house settling or corrosion damage.

RESIDUAL PESTICIDES

In some areas residual (long life) pesticides are applied to soils around the house, wood frame walls, concrete walls, and basement floors, for control of termites and other pests. Many products, such as chlordane, which is now banned, may persist in soils and buildings, though they were applied years before. This can easily be so in the home or apartment in which you live, if you were not directly involved during construction. Such residual toxins can find their way into food, air, and water, and are among the most serious poisons to accumulate in the body.

There are alternative ways of pest control, such as sheet metal shields to prevent termites from entering, which are highly effective and will not contaminate your home. (See the Home Maintenance and Construction Notes chapters, and the GETTING HELP section for references.)

DUST CONTROL

Bare concrete walls and floors are a constant source of irritating dust. Sweeping or vacuuming a dry concrete basement floor will raise very large amounts of dust, which can find its way into the rest of the house. Finishing concrete floors with durable materials such as concrete paint or hard vinyl composition tile (if self-tested and found acceptable) will reduce the dust problem. Painting concrete walls, or finishing them with insulation and wallboard, will also help.

INSECTS AND RODENTS

Inside pests in the basement, such as cockroaches, ants, silverfish, mice, and rats can all be controlled effectively with safe methods not requiring poison. (See the Home Maintenance chapter.)

LEAKAGE OF STORED CHEMICALS, PAINTS, ETC.

These are potential health and fire hazards and should be stored outside, or in safe, ventilated cupboards. (See the Storage chapter.)

BASEMENT VENTILATION

Due to all of the potential contamination hazards in basements it is a good precaution to isolate the basement from the rest of the home with a tight fitting door, and to provide it with separate ventilation and exhaust. If you have a central forced air furnace which serves both the basement and the upper floors, check with a heating contractor to find out if you can heat and ventilate the basement separately.

Radon entry, for example, can be reduced by slightly pressurizing the basement if you have a forced air furnace. This is usually done by providing a warm air outlet from the furnace to the basement and at the same time not allowing any basement air to return to the furnace. (To prevent basement air entering the furnace do not use any air return opening in the basement duct.)

16 STORAGE

A number of stored household products such as paints, solvents, fuels, oils, waxes, polishes, and cleaners, can release significant amounts of vapors or odors which can affect the environmentally sensitive. Of course, many of these are also fire hazards. Two special storage arrangements designed to reduce household contamination and fire hazards are described below.

STORAGE CUPBOARDS VENTILATED TO OUTSIDE

This type of storage is located inside the home but receives ventilation air directly from outside via a small sheet metal duct (2" to 4" dia.) passing through the wall with a screened vent cap on the outside. The vent cap will prevent rodents, insects, or rain from entering.

The cupboard is built to be relatively airtight, with exterior plywood parts, glued joints, and weatherstripped doors. A secure lock or latch is important if there are small children in the home.

This sort of cupboard is better protected from freezing than a storage arrangement which is detached from the home. It is most appropriate for non-inflammable items, such as the waxes, polishes, and cleaners which are regularly used in the home. (Note that some items, such as latex or casein paints, must be protected from freezing. Check the label.)

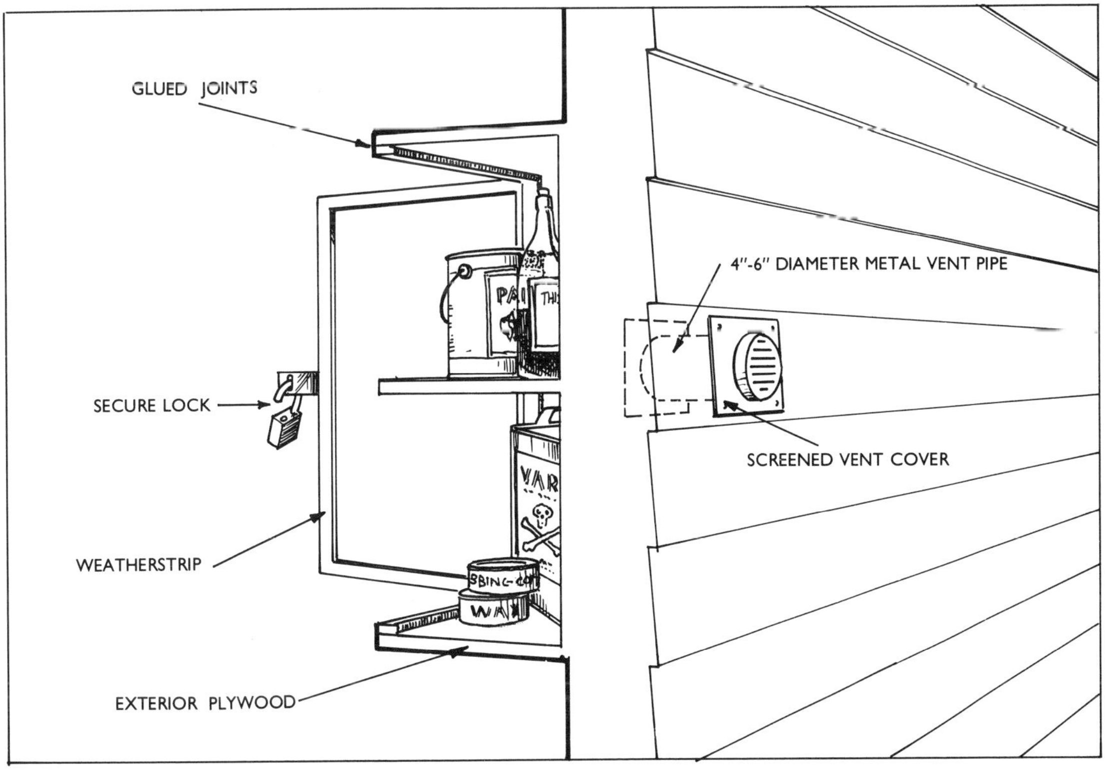

Fig. 16-1 Outside Ventilated Storage Cabinet

STORAGE DETACHED FROM THE HOME

This type of storage should be located outside the home away from windows and doors, where it is completely isolated. It is most appropriate for volatile fuels, and solvents which are inflammable and do not require protection from freezing. A metal garden shed is particularly suitable for this kind of storage.

Apartment dwellers who wish to store irritating or hazardous products outside should consider a simple weatherproof box which can be placed on a balcony or roof terrace.

17 THE GARAGE

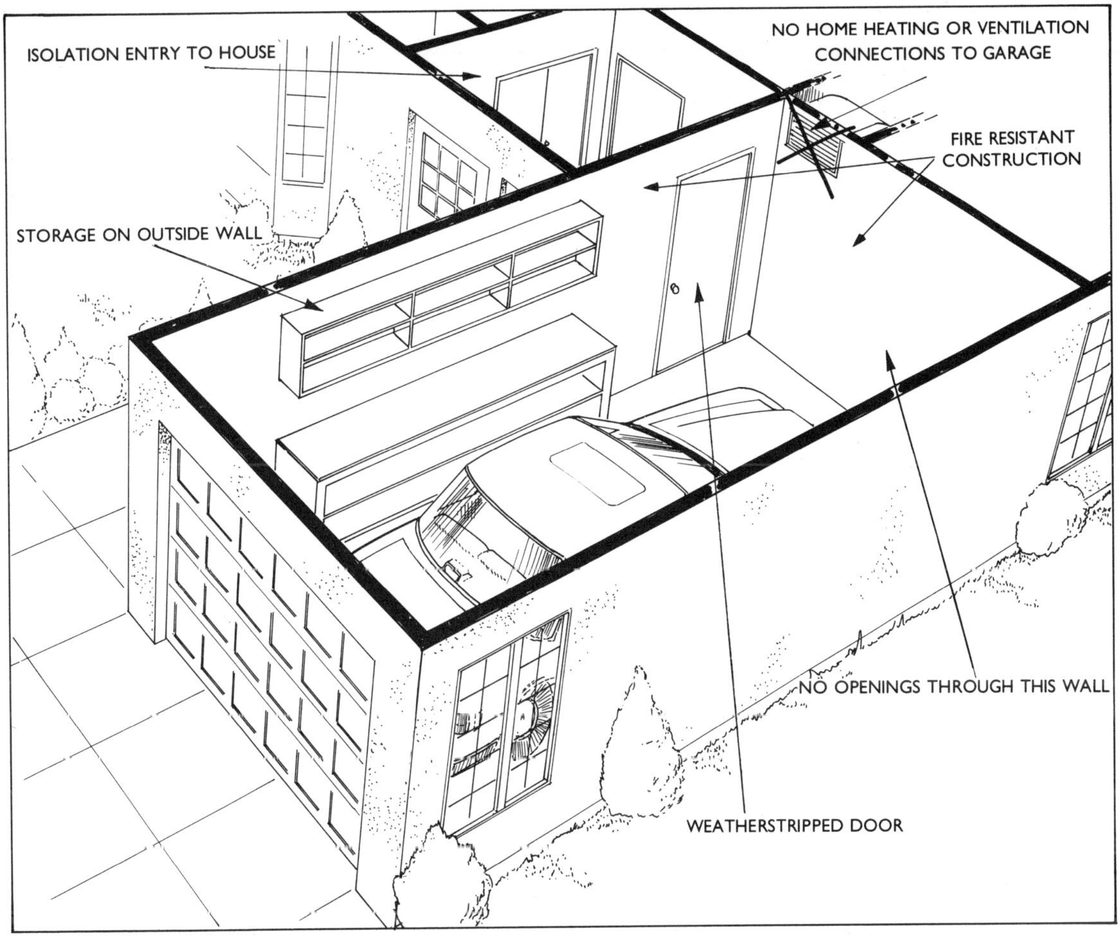

Fig. 17-1 The Garage. *Isolating the garage from house air is essential for maintaining safe conditions.*

Completely separate ventilation of garages, workshops, and outside storage rooms is essential to prevent living area contamination from these sources. Complete fire separation is also a critical safety measure that is usually covered by local fire codes, but often violated in practice.

Auto exhaust, and vapors from such storage items as paints and fuels, are just a few of the many types of contamination that may enter the home from garages or storage rooms. In order to reduce their passage into the home the following things can be done:

- Minimize the amount of common wall between the home and the garage or storage room. If possible, they should be entirely separate structures.
- Treat any common wall or ceiling and floor as if it were an outside surface, sealing it thoroughly, and covering it on the garage

side with such fireproof materials as two layers of fire rated gypsum board.

• Use a double door entry vestibule to the living area where possible.

• Do not operate auto or lawnmower engines for extended periods in these areas; do not handle volatile solvents, fuels, oils, or paints in these areas. Whenever possible, do these things outside.

• Ensure that there is no furnace duct, ventilation opening, or any other air passage leading from these areas into the home.

SECTION IV

Systems for a Healthy Home

18 HOME VENTILATION

Good home ventilation is essential for healthful, comfortable indoor air. For the environmentally sensitive, carefully controlled ventilation, with air purification where necessary, is essential.

Ventilation here refers to the movement and change of air for the purposes of maintaining good air quality. Air movement is also related to comfort, and is important for effective cooling and heating. (See the Home Heating/Cooling chapter.)

The amount of ventilation in the home is sometimes measured for purposes of research and testing. This figure, expressed in air changes per hour (ACH, discussed below) or cubic feet per minute (CFM), indicates the rate at which the air in the home is replaced by outside air. The actual proportion of this ventilation air required to expel the carbon dioxide produced by breathing and to replace the oxygen is really quite small. In a typical 1,000 square foot house or apartment occupied by three people, with a typical ventilation rate for conventional construction (.5 ACH), only about 15% of the air change is required for respiration. *The remaining 85% of the ventilation will control odors and contamination from all other inside sources.* Reducing these sources of contamination will dramatically improve the air quality. Once this is done, almost any reasonable ventilation rate will provide good conditions for health and comfort, and actual measurements will not be necessary.

THE CONTAMINATION LOAD

The total contamination from all sources in a home produces a "contamination load." These can include unvented combustion, the home's building and finishing materials, cooking, and people's activities. Removing the sources where possible, and directly venting those which cannot be avoided, such as kitchen stoves, will reduce this total load. (These and other strategies are discussed in the chapter Controlling Indoor Air Quality.)

DILUTING CONTAMINANTS

Outside air is generally used to dilute unavoidable contaminants. Where the outside air is acceptable to everyone in the home it can be introduced directly and allowed to mix with room air. Where pollens, or other outside contamination, make it unacceptable, it will have to be treated with filters and sometimes "air purifiers" before it can be used. (See Air Treatment Devices, below.) The amount of outside air required to maintain the best conditions for comfort and health throughout the home will depend on the size of the "contamination load," (including the number of people, combustion, cooking, bathing, building and furnishing materials), the size of the home, and the rate at which the air mixes.

All buildings allow some degree of uncontrolled airflow through cracks, and poorly fitted doors and windows. This two-way airflow, known as "infiltration" and "exfiltration," is a common means of "unintentional" ventilation. Often, in northerly regions, this sort of air leakage is the only source of fresh air in a conventional home in winter. However, *ventilation by air leakage is not a safe and effective means of providing fresh air,* because it cannot be controlled. For example, the home's natural upward air movement tends to draw air in through cracks both in the basement and at ground level—*the zones where the risk is greatest that such contaminants as radon, pesticides from soil, and auto exhaust will enter.* Airtight homes have a potential health advantage because they require controlled "intentional ventilation," provided by opening windows, fans, or sophisticated air purification equipment. The air comes from known sources and can be delivered in known quantities to known locations in the home. (See Mechanical Ventilation and Air Treatment Devices, below.)

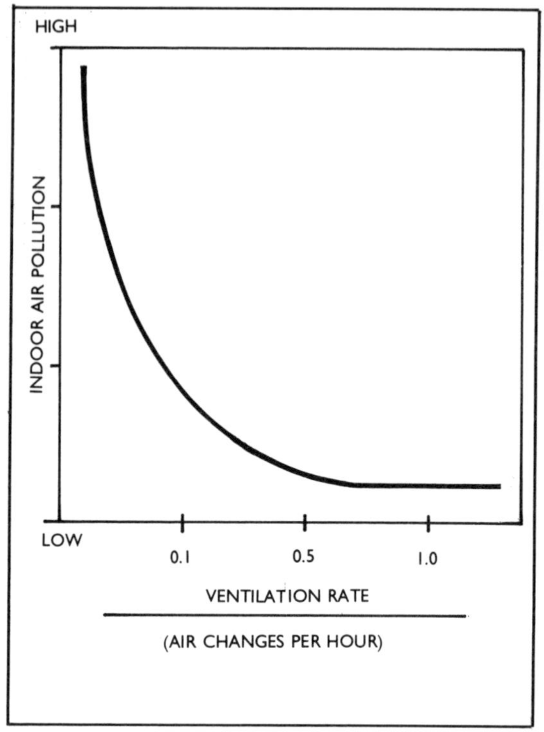

Fig. 18-1 Ventilation Rate and Air Quality. *For any given home contamination load, increased ventilation will improve air quality. Reducing contamination sources will improve air quality without increased ventilation.*

HOUSE SIZE

There is a direct relation between the interior volume of your home and the level of air contamination from inside sources. A large home, with a certain number of indoor contamination sources, will have proportionately cleaner air than a smaller home with the same contamination load. For example, mobile homes are known to have more air quality problems than permanent houses, and their small size is one factor. (Mobile homes are usually built with large amounts of particle board, plastic, and glue, which increases their contamination load as well.)

The rate of air changes in your home is usually expressed in air changes per hour (ACH). This figure indicates the number of times the entire air volume of your home is replaced by outside air each hour. If the contamination load remains the same, then increased ventilation will improve air quality.

CLEANING AIR

Good air quality is generally maintained by constantly removing contaminated indoor air and replacing it with clean outdoor air. *This is, of course, dependent on having clean outdoor air available.* Where there are pollens or dusts, they can be removed by filtration. If, however, there are irritating gases in the air, such as ozone and nitrogen dioxide, they must be removed by chemical air purification or "scrubbing."

In some circumstances dramatically increased ventilation is very useful for "flushing" the building. After painting, waxing, or polishing, increased air change will dilute and eventually dispel fumes.

Both filtration and air purification are used to preclean air before it enters the home. They can also be done *inside* the home to clean contained and recirculated air. One example of filtration is the filter in a common warm air furnace, which removes some of the dust from air before heating. The portable room air purifier which circulates room air through chemical scrubbers is another. (See Air Treatment Devices, below.)

UNDERSTANDING NATURAL VENTILATION

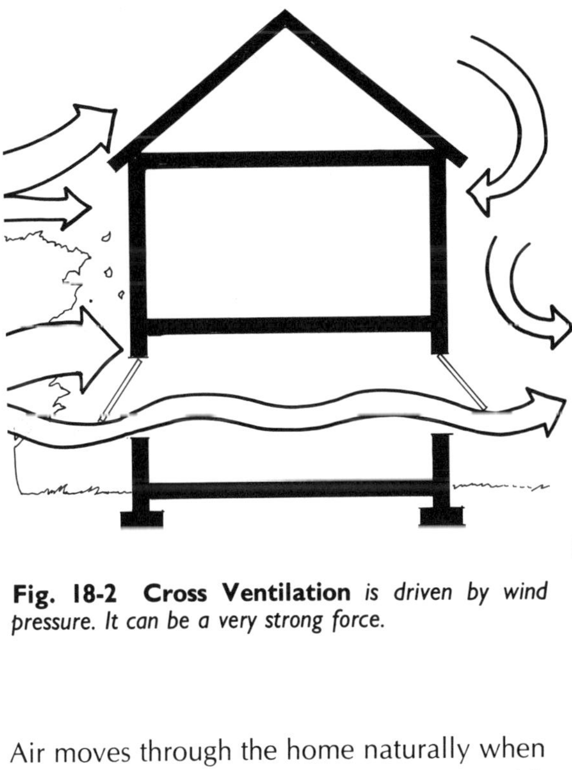

Fig. 18-2 Cross Ventilation *is driven by wind pressure. It can be a very strong force.*

Air moves through the home naturally when it is driven by temperature and pressure differences. For natural air to move horizontally across one floor of a house requires some wind to be effective. This is cross-ventilation. A breeze blowing against one side of the building causes a slight air pressure increase there. Airflow around the building causes a slight pressure drop on the other side, in the same way that an airplane wing works. As a result, any opening on the upwind side of the house will bring air in, and this air will pass through the house and attempt to escape on the opposite, downwind side. This can be quite a strong force, causing doors to slam and papers to blow around, particularly when the wind varies in speed or direction, creating rapidly changing pressure differences.

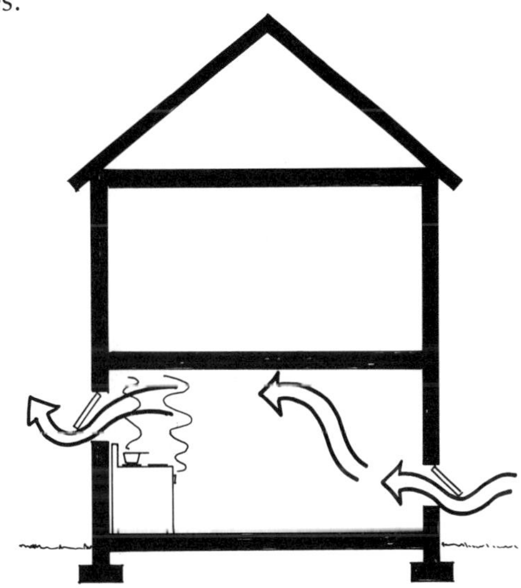

Fig. 18-3 Simple Ventilation *is driven by internal heating. It is a weak force.*

Heating the air in the home will move it a small amount by convection. Here, buoyant heated air (less dense than cooler air) rises to the top of a room. Though this is a relatively weak force, it can be used to ventilate a single floor by allowing warmer air to exit through a high opening. As air leaves the room, it tends to draw new air in to replace it. If a lower opening is available to admit air, a small airflow will be established.

The "stack effect" describes air's natural tendency to migrate upwards when enclosed in a vertical column. If this column rises a substantial distance, such as up the stairwell of a multi-storey home, and there is heating going on within that column, this can provide quite a strong force. This can be used to advantage in a multi-storey home, or in a single storey home with an attic, to provide effective natural ventilation.

Such simple devices as solar air shafts can utilize this effect to ventilate buildings with free energy. Here, a stack is heated by sunlight, or waste heat from the home, causing a strong upward airflow just like the airflow in a chimney. This causes reduced air pressure at lower levels and draws toward it new air to replace the air drawn upward. However, to be safe, this new air must come from uncontaminated sources.

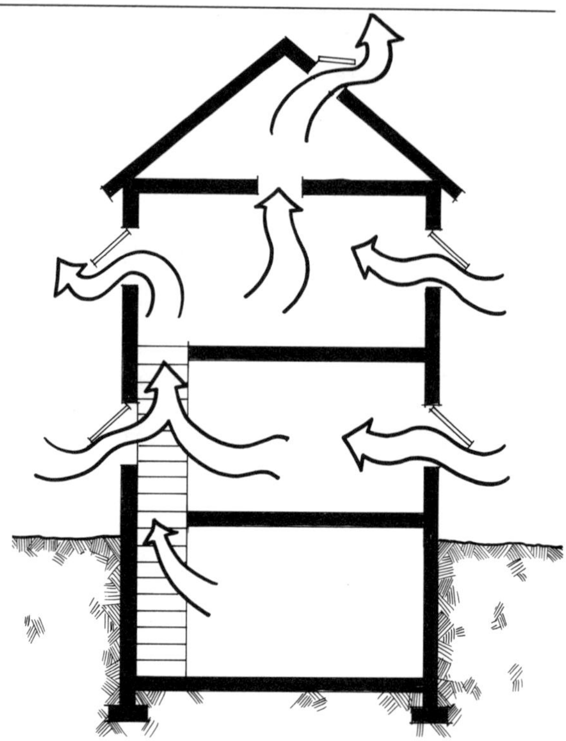

Fig. 18-5 Cooling with the Stack Effect. *The stack effect can be used for comfort cooling by providing exhaust openings in the upper floor, and intakes in the lower.*

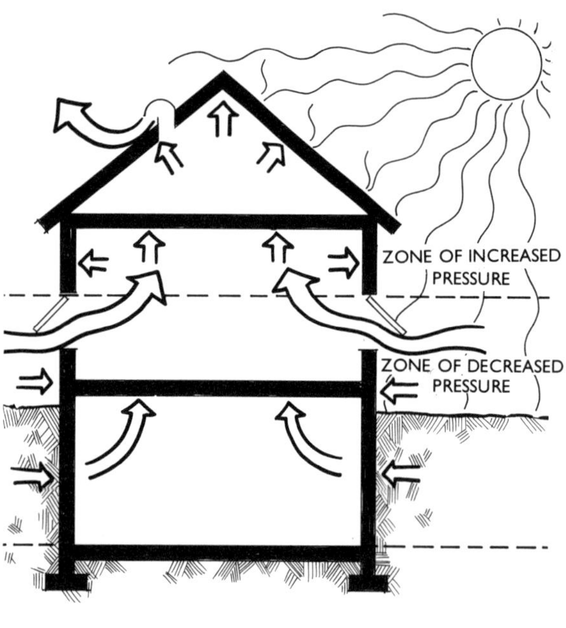

Fig. 18-4 The Stack Effect *is driven by heating in a multi-storey building. It can be a strong force.*

Both natural forces, such as the stack effect, and mechanical forces, such as a vent fan, create air pressure differences between the inside and outside of a house. These tend to move air in uncontrolled ways through the small cracks mostly around doors and windows. *It is estimated that the total amount of small openings and cracks in an average, unweathersealed home would add up to a hole one foot square.* Air moving in through such cracks (infiltration) is caused when the air pressure inside is reduced by upward airflow, or by an exhaust fan. Exfiltration is air leaking out when inside air pressure is increased by heating, wind, or supply fans.

Uncontrolled infiltration is a serious potential health hazard. It can bring with it insulating materials, formaldehyde, radon gas, asphalt fumes, microorganisms, and many other dangerous contaminants.

TIGHT HOUSES

Increasing a building's tightness by weather-sealing doors and windows, improved air/vapor barriers, and other advanced building methods, will make it necessary to arrange a ventilation system, either natural or mechanical. *There is not enough accidental leakage in a tightly constructed building to assure an adequate outside air supply for safe indoor air.* The advantages of this situation are that the ventilation air can be controlled, that it will be drawn from a known source, and can be delivered in known quantities. On the other hand, a major health concern with sealing a building is that many of the products used for gaskets, weatherstrips, caulking, and vapor barriers, themselves produce contaminants. Formaldehyde and other volatile compounds are two common offenders in these products. (See the chapter Materials and Selection for safer products.)

ADVANTAGES AND DISADVANTAGES OF NATURAL VENTILATION

Advantages

- It is free.
- It is quiet.
- It needs no maintenance.

Disadvantages

- It cannot be treated or filtered.
- It is difficult to control.
- It is not adequate in some climates (particularly in houses without enough openings).
- It may cause discomfort due to drafts and interfere with heating control.

MECHANICAL VENTILATION

Fans of various types can be used either to force air into the home, remove air from it, or to recirculate inside air. They are necessary for any common type of filtering, cooling, or air purification.

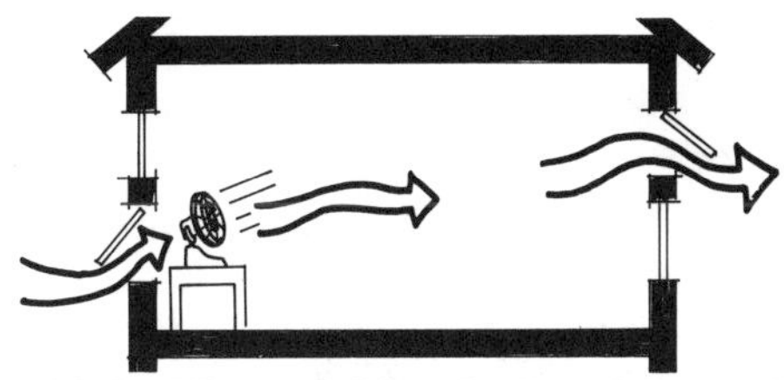

Fig. 18-6 Through Ventilation. *A fan is often required to boost through ventilation.*

Supply fan: Air may be brought into the home by a supply fan. The resulting slight elevation in indoor air pressure will tend to force air out through any available crack or opening. *For successful ventilation when using a supply fan, take care to ensure an adequate exit path for the air.* Most often a simple portable supply fan is used to increase the movement of outside air into the home. However, effective home ventilation is not usually achieved with supply fans alone.

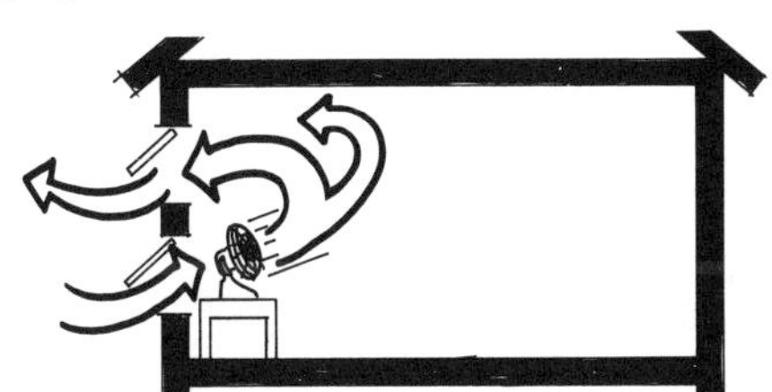

Fig. 18-7 Short Circuited Ventilation. *Without an outlet, through ventilation is ineffective.*

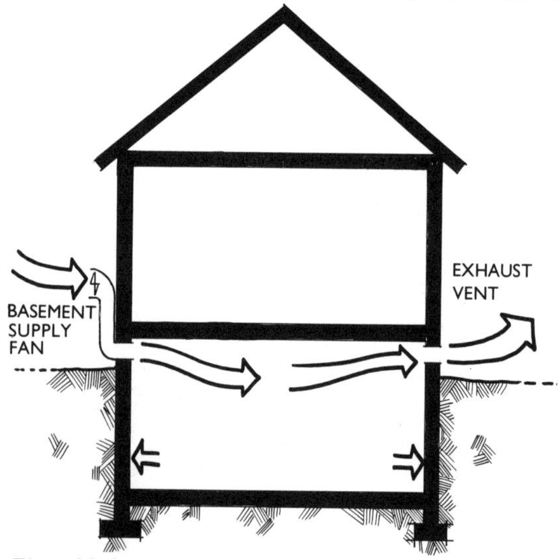

Fig. 18-8 Basement Ventilation by Supply Fan. *A* Basement Supply Fan *and an* Exhaust Vent *can be used to ventilate the basement separately, for moisture control and radon reduction.*

ADVANTAGES AND DISADVANTAGES OF SUPPLY FANS

Advantages

• They draw air from a known outside source.

• Positive inside pressure tends to force contaminants out.

• Positive inside pressure tends to reduce cold drafts from cracks.

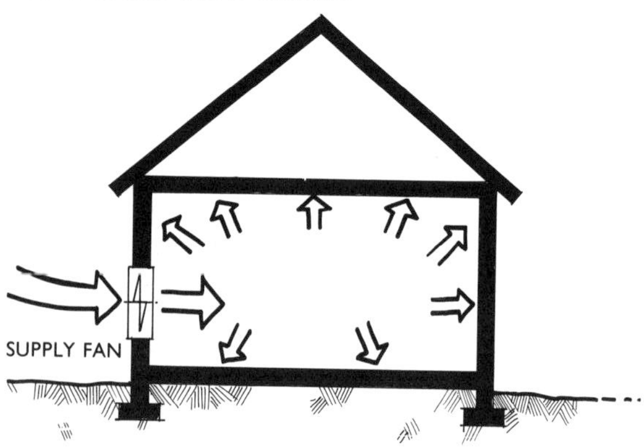

Fig. 18-9 Building Pressurizaton by Supply Fan. *A* Supply Fan *pressurizes the home, encouraging outward leakage through cracks and openings.*

Disadvantages

• Local contamination sources (eg. kitchen ranges) cannot be effectively exhausted.

• Large amounts of heat energy may be wasted in a leaky house.

• Cold drafts may result near the supply fan.

• House pressurization by supply fan can increase air leakage and cause hidden condensation damage.

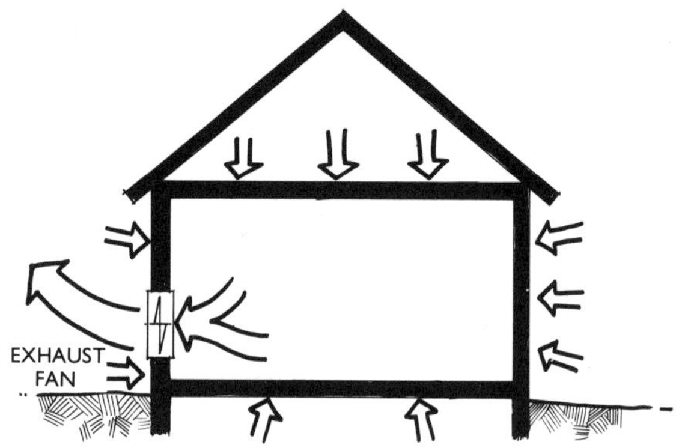

Fig. 18-10 Building Depressurization by Exhaust Fan. *An* Exhaust Fan *depressurizes the home, encouraging inward leakage through cracks and openings. This leakage can include chimney gases, and fumes from building materials.*

Exhaust fan: The exhaust fan removes air from the home, causing a slight negative indoor pressure. This negative pressure tends to bring air in through any available opening. The exhaust fan is particularly suited to removing, at their sources, such local contamination as cooking fumes, kitchen moisture, and water vapor in bathrooms. The kitchen range hood fan and bathroom ceiling fans are always exhaust fans. ***When using an exhaust fan it is essential to provide an opening somewhere in the house where outside air can enter to replace the air exhausted by the fan.*** This is particularly true for tightly sealed houses. If this is not done, effective exhausting will not take place and dangerous backdrafting from chimneys may also occur.

ADVANTAGES AND DISADVANTAGES OF EXHAUST FANS

Advantages

• They can remove local contamination (eg. cooking fumes), and prevent them contaminating the household air.

Disadvantages

• They tend to reduce the house's air pressure, bringing in air and possible contaminants through cracks, chimneys, and other openings.
• They increase uncomfortable cold drafts through cracks.
• They produce large heating and cooling energy losses. (See Air to Air Heat Exchangers, below, for solutions.)

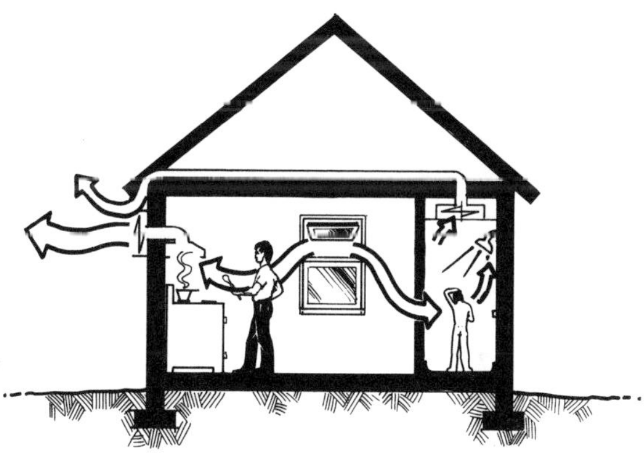

Fig. 18-11 Balanced Indoor Air Pressure. *Every large exhaust fan must be balanced by an air supply to prevent unwanted infiltration and chimney backdrafting.*

Recirculating fan: Installed in every central forced air heating/cooling system is a large fan which recirculates room air. These units draw room air in through ducts, pass it through a filter, then heat it or cool it, as required, and re-distribute it throughout the home. Such systems are for heating and cooling and are not primarily intended for ventilation. (See the Home Heating/Cooling chapter.)

Many recently installed central forced air systems add a simple fresh air connection to improve ventilation during the heating or cooling season when doors and windows are tightly closed. This is a small, 3″–6″ diameter metal pipe which brings outside air in to the furnace on the "return side." (The side where the room air returns to the unit.) This pipe is usually equipped with a damper valve, allowing control of the amount of air it delivers to the furnace. Its advantages are that it assures an adequate and controlled fresh air supply during the heating or cooling season, and it tends to slightly pressurize the house, reducing random leakage of air in through cracks. Outside air is also preheated in winter and combustion air sometimes supplied to the burner by this method.

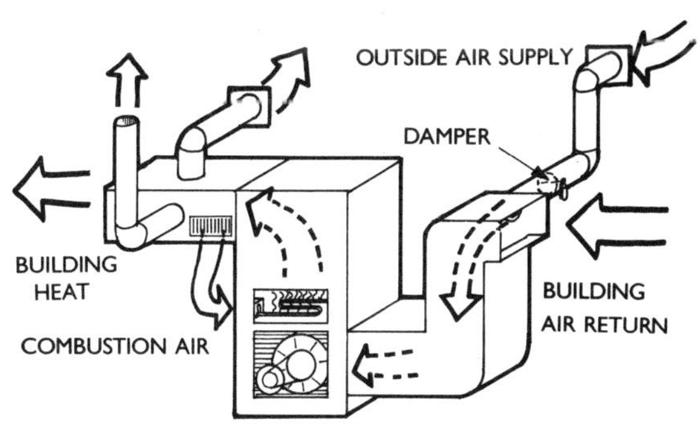

Fig. 18-12 Air Supply to the Furnace. *Every warm air furnace should be fitted with an* Outside Air Supply *connected to the return air duct. This will ensure adequate ventilation in winter, and reduce house depressurization due to exhaust fans.*

Cautions: Where an outside air supply is in use with a forced air system, ***make sure its intake pipe is located where uncontaminated air is available.*** It should be well away from garages, streets, household sewer vents (pipes which pass through the roof to vent the drains), soil, and allergenic plants. Be sure it is also equipped with a sturdy screen to keep out rodents, insects, and birds.

If you have a forced air furnace without an ***outside air supply,*** check with a heating contractor whether one can be installed. This is particularly important if you plan to tightly weatherseal your home to save energy. A *combustion air supply* is a small pipe leading to the burner bringing in outside air to provide oxygen for the flames of a furnace or water heater. (See the Home Heating/Cooling chapter.)

WHOLE HOUSE FAN SYSTEMS

Fan systems which ventilate the entire house are often used for controlled ventilation, particularly in tightly sealed homes. The most popular type in energy efficient homes is the air to air heat exchanger, also known as a heat recovery ventilator. Another type is the simple humidity fan.

Air to air heat exchanger: To maintain comfort during cold or hot seasons, ventilation air drawn into the home from outside must be either heated or cooled. At the same time, air that is being removed from the house by kitchen and bathroom fans is wasting the energy that was used to heat or cool it. The purpose of the heat exchanger is to provide controlled ventilation, while *transferring* the heat between outgoing and incoming air, in order to save energy.

A heat exchanger typically requires two small fans and a heat transfer unit. These are generally mounted in a box connected by metal ducts both to the rooms of the house and to the outside. During the heating season, one of the fans, the supply fan, draws cold outside air in to pass through a complex matrix before introducing it to the house. This matrix is a series of metal or plastic plates sandwiched together in alternate layers. (See Fig. 18–14.) Flowing through this matrix is the exhaust air, which is being extracted from the house (usually from the kitchen and bathroom) by the other fan. The heat from the exhaust air is absorbed by the matrix and transferred to the supply air, without the two air paths ever actually mixing.

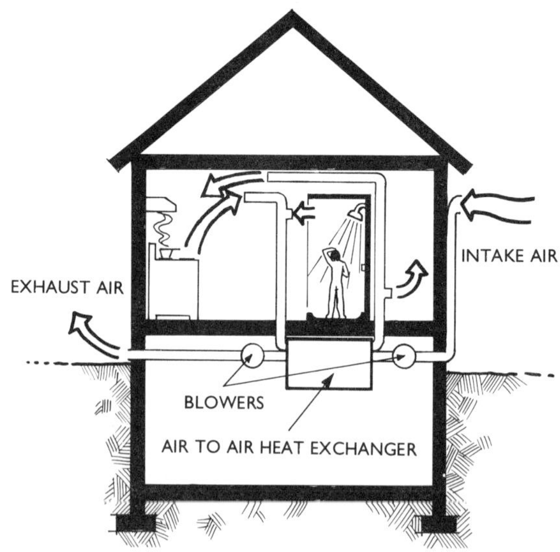

Fig. 18-13 Air to Air Heat Exchanger. *An* Air to Air Heat Exchanger *saves energy by transferring heat between exhaust air and intake air. Stale humid air is generally drawn from bathrooms and kitchens, and passed through the unit before exiting.* Intake Air *is provided to replace* Exhaust Air *and minimize pressure imbalance.*

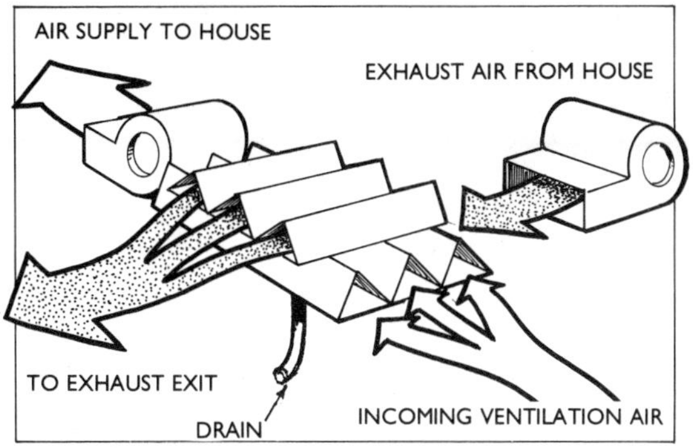

Fig. 18-14 Inside the Air to Air Heat Exchanger. Exhaust Air *passes over metal plates, which are also in contact with* Incoming Air. *Heat is transferred through the plates, and condensation is removed by the drain.*

ADVANTAGES AND DISADVANTAGES OF AIR TO AIR HEAT EXCHANGERS

Advantages

- They deliver controlled ventilation in tightly sealed houses.
- They reduce ventilation energy costs.
- They can increase ventilation in "imperfect" houses to reduce contamination problems.
- They constantly balance exhaust air with an equal amount of incoming air, so that the air pressure balance in the home is not upset.

Disadvantages

- They are not expected to perform well unless the home is built and sealed to current energy efficiency standards.
- They are costly ($600-$1,000), and require some maintenance.
- A number of health related problems can occur. (Described below.)

The transfer of heat through the matrix often causes condensation when the warm air comes into contact with the cool plates of the exchanger, releasing some of its moisture there. (This is the same process that occurs in the winter when windows become fogged by moisture.) This moisture may then freeze, blocking exhaust air, or it may collect and support the growth of bacteria and fungus which can then enter the air supply. Well made units are built with an automatic defroster and condensate drain, which prevent the accumulation of moisture hazards. ***Regular cleaning will still be necessary to reduce the risk of bacterial contamination.***

The material which makes up the matrix is also a concern. Plastics, paper, and metal types are all available. The paper types are questionable, due to their tendency to collect moisture and dirt, as well as to easily become perforated. The plastic types are doubtful due to their tendency to outgas fumes, particularly when heated by a defroster. This is of particular concern to the environmentally sensitive. The metal type are usually aluminum and expected to be safe.

(These devices are not necessary in mild climates, as long as ample ventilation openings are provided.)

Humidity fan: These rudimentary central ventilation systems are similar to the air to air heat exchangers but lack their air supply and energy saving heat recovery features. They are connected to the kitchen and bathroom by ducts, and they incorporate an exhaust fan which draws moisture laden air from the house. They include a humidistat, which is an automatic wall mounted switch that works like a furnace thermostat, but senses humidity instead of heat.

An automatic humidity fan may be appropriate if you have condensation problems, or live in a humid region. These systems are much simpler and less expensive than heat exchangers. They can serve a useful function, particularly in moderate climates where energy saving is not a main concern. If you plan to use a humidity fan, remember to include a source of supply air to prevent excessive depressurization of the home. This could be provided by an air duct through the wall or by a small supply fan.

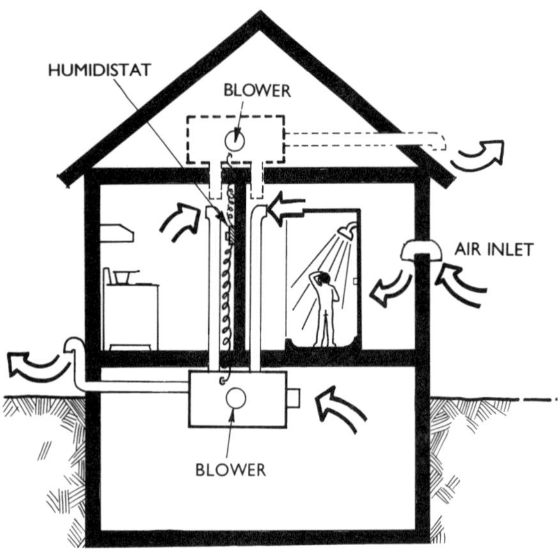

Fig. 18-15 A Central Humidity Fan *in the attic or basement automatically exhausts air from the bathroom and kitchen, preventing the buildup of indoor humidity. An* Air Inlet *must be provided.*

ADVANTAGES AND DISADVANTAGES OF HUMIDITY FANS

Advantages

- They are designed to control the excess moisture buildup in the home which can lead to discomfort, damage to the home, and health problems.
- They are relatively inexpensive.

Disadvantages:

- Supply air is not usually incorporated and must be provided for separately.
- A humidity fan is *not* a substitute for a proper exhaust fan for the kitchen range.
- Intake air may require preheating.

PREVENTING CONTAMINATED VENTILATION AIR

Outdoor air drawn into the home for ventilation may be contaminated with urban, industrial, agricultural, or pollen products. Where it is too contaminated for direct use, especially by the sensitive individual, it must be treated. Ventilation air can also become contaminated by the building itself and by its immediate surroundings.

The most common outdoor causes of contamination are auto exhaust, chimney emissions, airborne plant materials, pesticides and other yard and garden chemicals, fibers from building materials, and sewer gases. Some of these may come from streets or neighbors and be out of your control. However, the careful location of air inlets can alleviate some of these problems. Auto exhaust, yard and garden chemicals, and some plant materials, are usually most concentrated near the ground. Chimney discharges and sewer gases are generally highest near the roof. Consequently, when a supply fan is incorporated into the house or when an opening window is planned, use these suggested clearances from the sources of contamination:

- Locate the air inlet at least 8 feet above ground. Higher is often better.

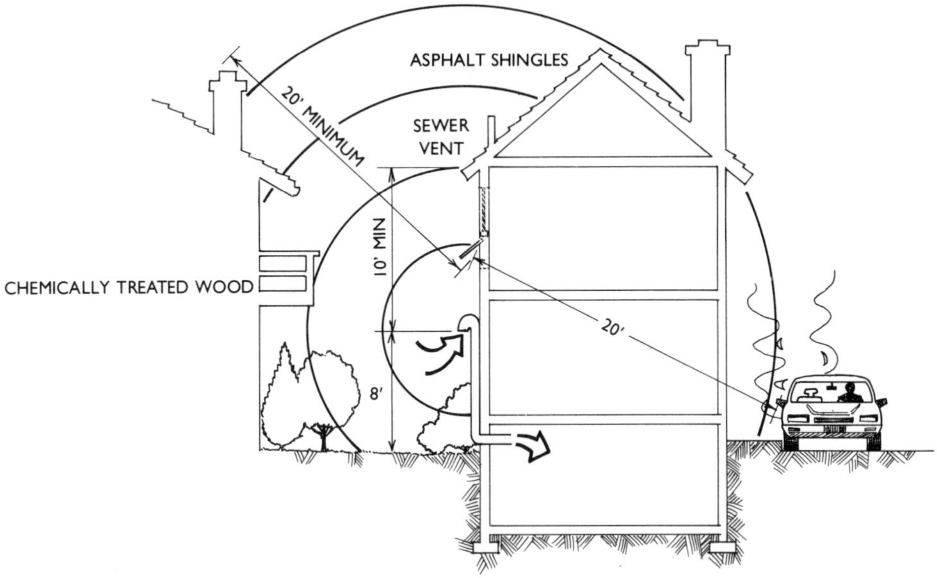

Fig. 18-16 Air Intake Clearances. *Maintain safe clearances between air inlets and such contamination sources as automobiles, chimneys, sewer vents, ground surface, and pollen producing plants.*

- Locate the inlet 20 feet away from any chimney, garage, or roadway.
- Locate the inlet 10 feet away from a sewer vent.
- Place the inlet to project 1 foot or more from the outside wall.
- Do not locate the inlet where it is exposed to materials containing asbestos. (This includes some types of shingles and factory made siding manufactured more than 10 years ago.)
- Where there is a sensitive individual in the house, be especially cautious about asphalt products, such as roof shingles and siding, as well as chemically preserved wood. These will release gases, particularly when heated, that can enter ventilation openings and affect people indoors.

AIR TREATMENT DEVICES

To prevent the buildup of indoor contamination due to unacceptable outdoor air, or pollutants from within the home, some form of air treatment will be necessary. There are two type of devices: the filtration systems which remove suspended particles from the air, and the chemical "scrubbers," which remove unwanted gases from air. The most complete and effective devices do both, and treat not only incoming supply air, but also the air inside the home. For successful indoor air treatment, these devices must treat recirculating air, because they will not remove all contaminants on the first time through.

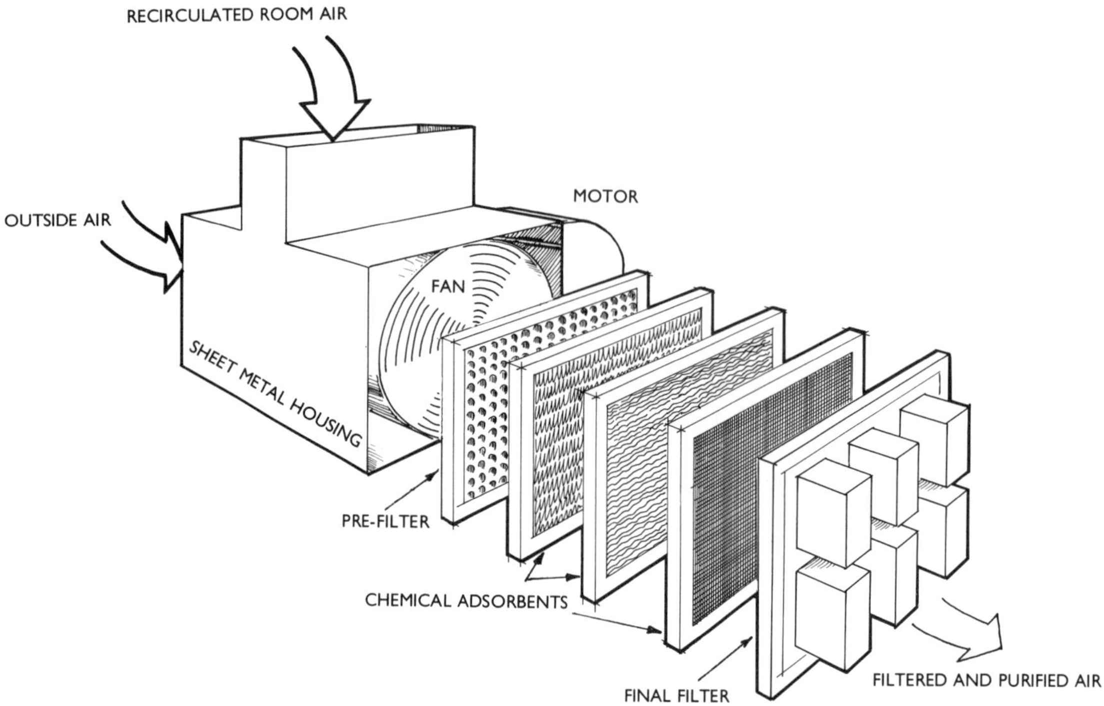

Fig. 18-17 Air Purification System. *Recirculated room air and outside air are mixed, and fan forced through a series of* Filters *and* Chemical Adsorbents *before returning to the room. The fan motor should be located outside the airflow, to reduce contamination.*

These devices may be single room units mounted in ceilings or below the floor, or they may be whole house air purification systems, centrally located and connected to the living spaces by ducts. Small portable units are also available. Though these are not as effective as the larger commercial units, they can be used to treat a small, closed room.

FILTERS

Common filters are either fibrous materials which trap particles as air passes through them, or electronic devices which remove particles by capturing them with an electric charge. Though these are usually part of a central heating system, in the health conscious home they can also be part of an independent air cleaning system.

The common fiberglass furnace filter is one of the least effective filtration devices available. It may also release dangerous glass fibers, gases from adhesives, scents, and disinfectant. (Filters may have been treated with oils, plastic resins, natural and artificial scents, and hexachlorophene, a potent disinfectant linked with chemical hypersensitivity reactions.) Even for their intended use in furnaces these filters are crude at best. The one good thing to be said about them is that they are very forgiving of neglect, and will still allow air to pass even when heavily loaded.

Fabric air filters: Among the higher performance filters is the pleated fabric type, made from layers of fabric fastened to a frame. These are far more effective than, and are also available as replacements for conventional filters in home furnaces. They must, however, be serviced more often than glass fiber filters. (In telephone directories they are listed under AIR CLEANING EQUIPMENT.)

A range of very high performance fabric filters is also available, which require special frames and stronger fans to force air through them. These resemble multiple vacuum cleaner bags, and must be discarded when a quantity of dirt is trapped inside. This type is generally not adaptable as a direct replacement for conventional furnace filters, but will require extra hardware.

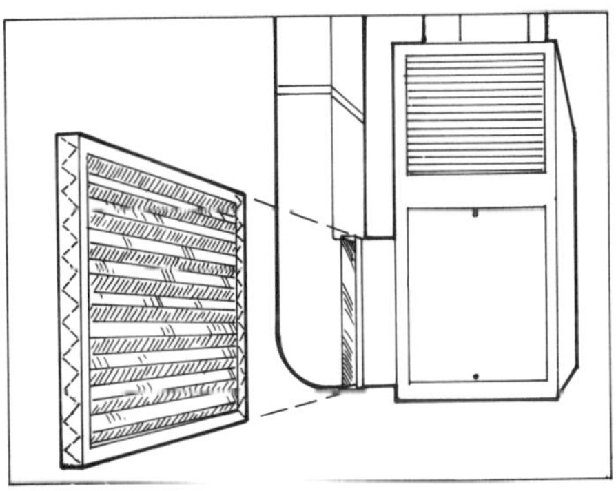

Fig. 18-18 A Medium Efficiency Filter *can be used to replace the standard, low efficiency furnace filter.*

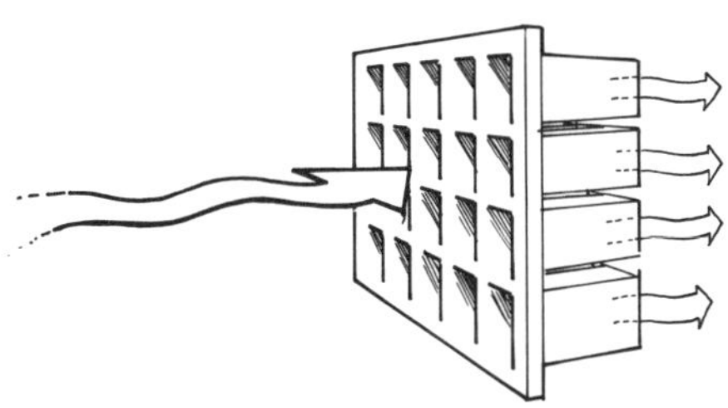

Fig. 18-19 A High Efficiency Filter *is very effective for reducing airborne dust. It requires a separate fan and housing, however, and cannot be used in place of a furnace filter.*

Electronic and electrostatic filters: Generally available as separate parts of central air cleaning systems, some models are available which fit into a furnace in place of the conventional filter. In these units a static electrical charge is generated by an electronic circuit. This change attracts dust particles to a collector plate from which they must be removed with regular cleaning. Though these devices are generally very effective in removing particles, they may produce ozone, a highly irritating contaminant.

Consumers' agencies have done extensive testing on the effectiveness of these units, but little information is available on the amount of ozone generated. Due to the possibility of respiratory irritation it would be wise to avoid the electronic type of filter if there is any sensitivity or chronic respiratory illness in the home. There are new electrostatic filters now available called the "electret" type. They use no electricity and produce no ozone, and are made from permanently charged static plates which attract dust. These plates must be regularly cleaned.

Chemical adsorption devices: These devices actually remove from the air unwanted gases that cannot be trapped by filters. They are made up of various chemicals which are held within a frame much like a filter frame. When air is passed through them, a reaction takes place which either physically traps the gas or changes it chemically so that it is no longer active. Adsorption chemicals are generally well contained within their frames, and are usually followed by a filter to trap any particles that escape.

Activated charcoal is the most common chemical adsorption medium. It is very inexpensive and highly effective for certain things, such as organic compounds with high molecular weight. This would include smoke, and the petroleum solvents used in paints, polishes, and waxes, as well as many odors produced by cooking. Charcoal must be discarded once it has adsorbed its capacity of contaminants, or else it will begin to release them again. It is not very effective, however, for filtering some lighter gases, such as formaldehyde, nitrogen dioxide, and ozone, all serious respiratory irritants.

Other media: The naturally occurring mineral alumina, combined with potassium permanganate or copper salts, is a common chemical absorption medium. It is known as the "catalyst", or "low temperature catalyst" type. It will actually cause chemical change to the offending gas, rendering it harmless or absorbing it. Though it is more costly than the others, it is generally longer lasting and can sometimes be regenerated. These materials are more effective for such gases as carbon monoxide and nitrogen dioxide, which are not trapped by charcoal. Ideally, these various adsorption materials will be combined in a system to achieve the benefits of all. A fully effective system will have a prefilter, followed by two or more stages of adsorption media, and then a final filter.

Where air purification systems are used for the environmentally sensitive, all filter media must be self tested for suitability. As mentioned above, treated paper and plastic filter fabrics are just two of the potential problem materials. If you are sensitive to the paper, and an alternative material is not available, an extra stage of charcoal adsorption may be required, for example, after the paper filter fabric.

Before buying a filtration and purification system, be certain that you know what the problems are in your home. Each system has some merits and weaknesses, and none is good for all situations. Some testing of your home and some consumer research will be necessary. (See the GETTING HELP section.)

ROOM AIR CLEANERS OR PURIFIERS

A great variety of portable air cleaners is available which can be effective for small areas. These circulate room air through various types of filtration and chemical adsorption media, and then return it to the room. *They are not a substitute for adequate ventilation, but will help reduce contamination and odors in small, enclosed spaces. Room air cleaners can be of some help to the environmentally sensitive in reducing unavoidable traces of contamination in the bedroom or sanctuary room, for example. Consumers' agencies have tested these units and can provide good information. Consult them before buying one, as manufacturers' literature may not be reliable. One small disadvantage of these units is that their filters require replacement as they become overloaded. If they are poorly maintained, micro-organisms will breed in the clogged filters, creating a health risk.*

Make sure to select a size with the right capacity for the room to be treated, and remember that these units are intended for enclosed rooms of moderate size. Do not expect them to be effective in large open plan houses, or to protect you from contamination at work if you work in a large office area.

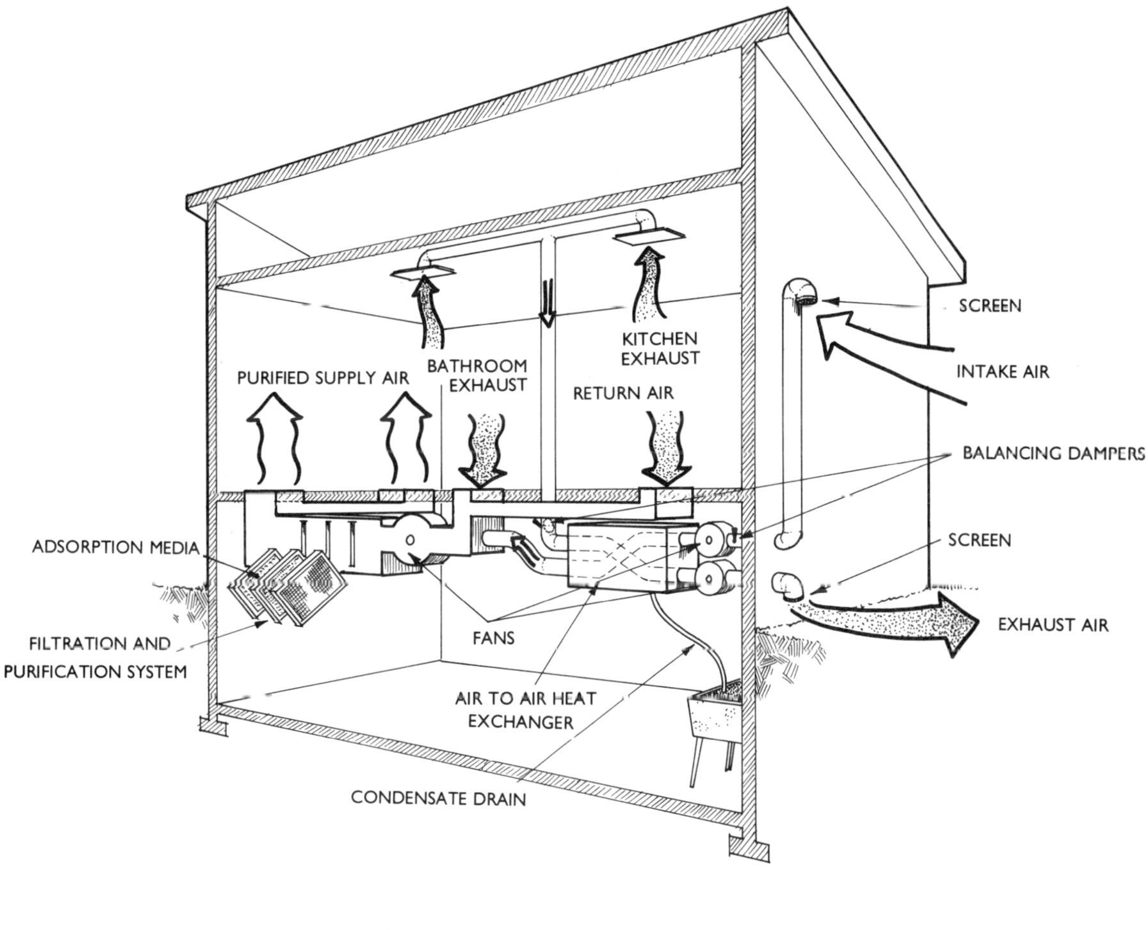

Fig. 18-20 An Energy Efficient Whole House Ventilation System. *House air is recirculated through a* Filtration and Purification System *and delivered to living areas. Outdoor* Intake Air *enters the system through an* Air to Air Heat Exchanger. Exhaust Air *is drawn from the kitchen and bathrooms to balance* Intake Air, *and passes through the* Air to Air Heat Exchanger *before exiting. Heating is provided by separate means, such as radiators or heated floors or ceilings.*

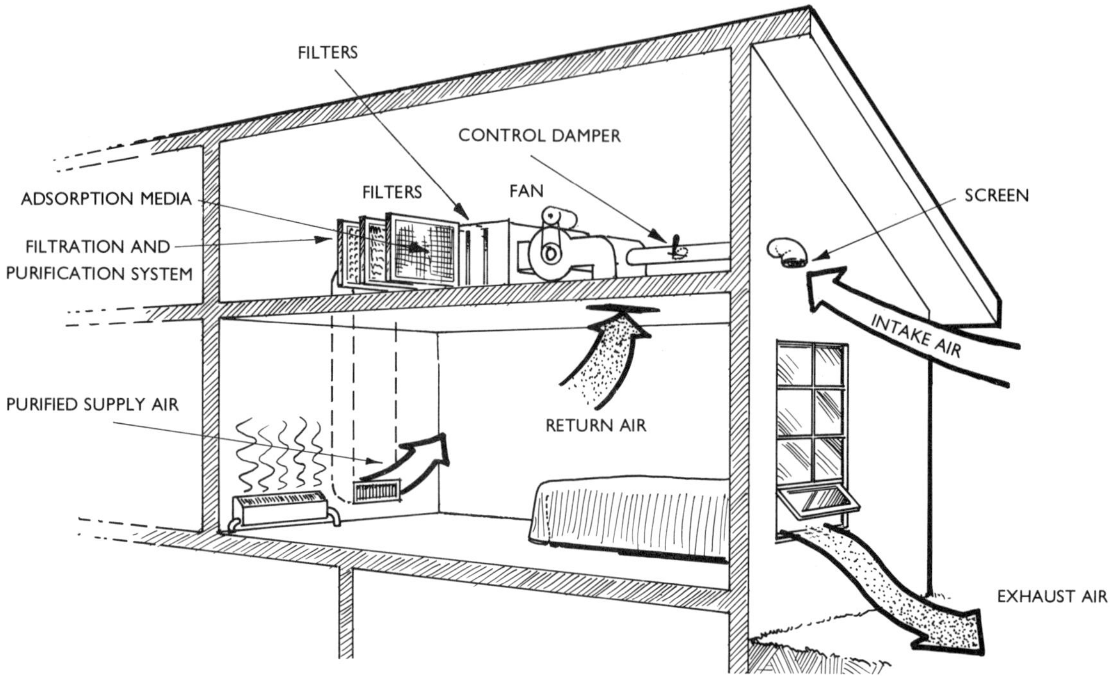

Fig. 18-21 A Single Room Air Purification System. *Room air is recirculated through a* Filtration and Purification System *and delivered to the room. Outdoor* Intake Air *is drawn into the* Return Air *stream and filtered and purified along with room air.* Exhaust Air *exits through a small window or other opening. This system is more effective than a portable unit, and can also treat intake air. Heating is provided by separate means.*

Homemade air filters: You can make a simple portable filter (Fig.18-22) to trap dust from the air in a closed room. Buy a medium efficiency pleated filter first, *then* have a sheet metal shop make a box sized to hold it on one end, and mount a furnace blower to discharge air from the other end. Place the unit on the floor and run it for two hours when the room is unoccupied. The powerful fan circulates the room's air, trapping dust in the filter (to be discarded months later when it appears soiled). For best results face it in a new direction each half hour. Anyone with dust allergy may use it twice a week or more. Filters are found at Filter suppliers (Yellow Pages). A 20″ × 25″ × 2″ or bigger filter is best. Heating contractors have new and used furnace blowers.

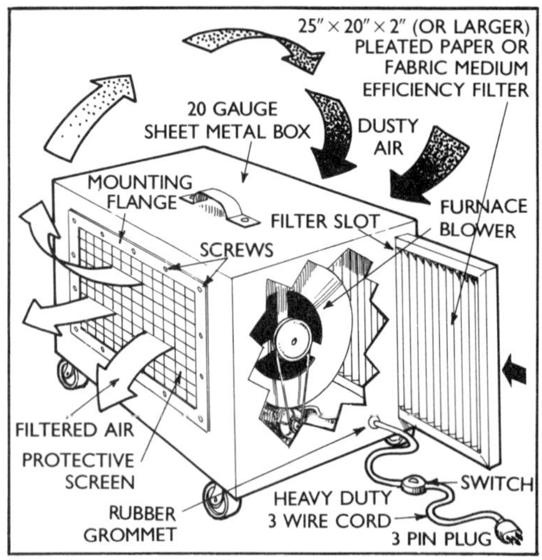

Fig. 18-22 A Simple Homemade Air Filter. *A heavy duty 3 wire cord is passed through a rubber grommet to a switch and a 3 pin plug. A ½″ mesh protective screen is placed over the fan. (For ease of handling casters and a handle can be attached.)*

19 HOME HEATING/COOLING

Home heating and cooling systems have improved dramatically in the past 20 years, and a wide range of sophisticated equipment now faces the homeowner or builder. The high cost of fuel has not only generated interest in energy efficient buildings, but has also created a demand for new systems. Solar heating, home heat pumps, high efficiency furnaces, and electronic controls have all become available. But though their safety has recently improved remarkably, there are still a number of health hazards associated with home heating and cooling systems.

Home Heating and Cooling Hazards

• Gas and oil fumes from fuel fired furnaces and appliances can enter the air in your home, causing discomfort, headaches, nausea, or severe reactions, in chemically sensitive persons. These fumes are known to be one of the most serious air contamination hazards. They should be avoided in the health conscious home. When renovating a house for someone who is hypersensitive, it may be necessary to remove all of the gas pipes as well as all the gas appliances.

• Leaking or backdrafting chimneys allow hazardous combustion gases to enter the home.

• Fuel burning appliances consume room air, causing negative pressurization leading to infiltration of contaminants.

• Wood heaters produce flue gases which may enter the home when opening the heater for loading, through faulty chimneys, and by returning through air inlets. These gases include irritants, toxins, and carcinogens, and are mixed with soot. They cause serious air pollution.

• High temperature surfaces of heaters and furnaces "fry" dust, contributing to air contamination.

• Boiler systems contain toxic glycol antifreeze, or other solutions, which can leak into the home or enter the water supply through faulty valves.

• Heat pumps or air conditioners can leak refrigerant gases. These are irritants and can cause serious reactions in sensitive people.

• Duct work will collect dust, debris, and often moisture. This can contaminate home air with allergens and pathogens.

• Solar heat "active" storage systems using rock beds or liquids can introduce dust, radon, and chemical contaminants into circulating air. They are often located where they cannot be cleaned.

CONTROLLING HUMIDITY

Your home may need humidification or dehumidification during the heating or the cooling season. (See the Thermal Comfort chapter for more about humidity.) If you do not have a relative humidity indicator, use this simple test to measure relative humidity.

MEASURING HUMIDITY

Place a thermometer in a suitable inside location away from drafts and heaters. Wait

5 minutes for the temperature to stabilize, and record the reading. Then wrap a small piece of cotton gauze or soft absorbent fabric that has been moistened with water over the thermometer bulb. (The bulb is the small chamber at the bottom of the glass tube that is filled with colored liquid.) There should be no more than one or two thin layers of fabric covering the bulb, and it should be wrapped around it if possible. Wait 10 minutes and record the reading. The temperature drop should be about 10° to 12°F for best conditions. See the Thermal Comfort chapter, Figs. 3-3 and 3-4, for humidity conversion.

Table 19-1

Advantages and Disadvantages of Home Heating and Cooling Systems

<table>
<tr><th>Type</th><th>Advantages</th><th>Disadvantages</th></tr>
<tr><td>PASSIVE SOLAR HEATING SYSTEM
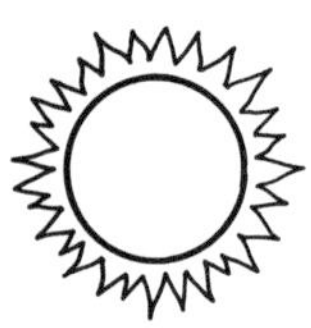</td><td>Free. Clean. No dust frying or stirring.</td><td>Poor control. Costly to install solar features. Heat losses in cold weather.</td></tr>
<tr><td colspan="3">Warning: Heat storage materials must be safe and accessible. Ceramic tile, concrete or brick walls and floors are preferred.</td></tr>
<tr><td>HOT WATER RADIANT
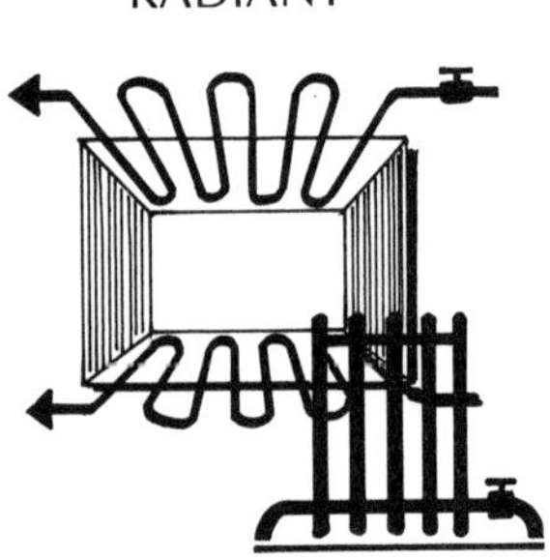</td><td>Gentle even heat. Clean. No dust frying or stirring. Can be individually controlled. Can be supplied by electric boiler, heat pump, or outdoor boiler. Will not transport contaminants.</td><td>Costly to install. May use toxic antifreeze solutions. Cannot be easily used for cooling. No air filtration.</td></tr>
<tr><td colspan="3">Warning: Heated surfaces may outgas contaminants.</td></tr>
</table>

HOME HEATING/COOLING

Type	Advantages	Disadvantages
ELECTRIC RADIANT low temperature and high temperature types 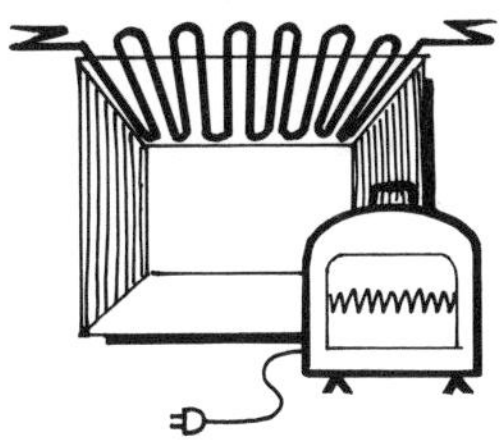	Low temperature ceiling panel types heat evenly. No dust frying or stirring. Easily individually controlled. Will not transport contaminants. High temperature types are inexpensive.	No air filtration. Low temperature units are costly to install. High temperature types will fry dust and become extremely hot.
Warning: Heated surfaces may outgas contaminants. Potential electromagnetic pollution.		
ELECTRIC CONVECTION HEATERS baseboard or wall type 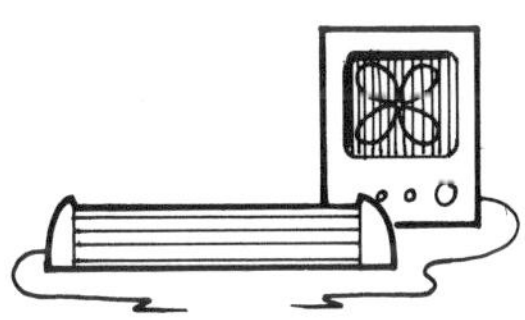	Inexpensive to install. Individual control.	Costly to operate. Will stir and fry dust. Surfaces become extremely hot. No air filtration.
Warning: Heated parts will outgas extremely. Potential electromagnetic pollution.		
INDIVIDUAL HEAT PUMPS 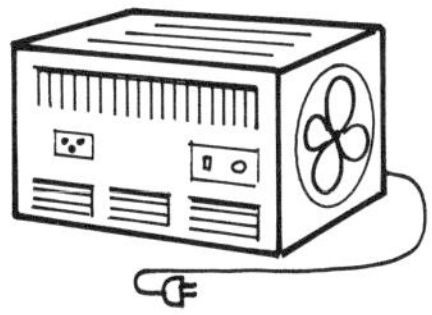	Can heat or cool. Inexpensive to operate. Can filter air. Individual control.	Units are costly. Noisy. Can become contaminated with microbes.
Warning: Refrigerant can escape. Plastic parts and filters will outgas.		

HOME HEATING/COOLING

Type	Advantages	Disadvantages
CENTRAL FORCED AIR 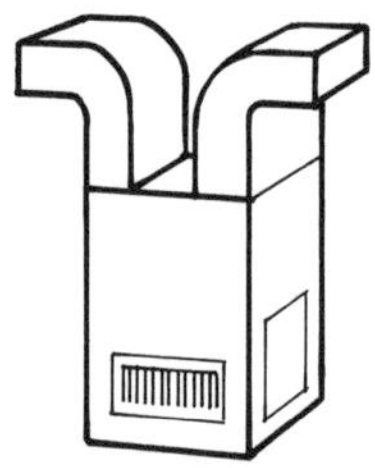	Units can be electric, fuel fired, or heat pump. Air is filtered. Can have cooling, air purification, and humidity control. Inexpensive to operate.	Oil and gas contamination. Flue gas contamination. Will stir and fry dust. Will transport contaminants. Noisy. Difficult to clean. Centrally controlled.
Warning: Fuel fumes and flue gases are serious hazards.		
WOOD, GAS, OR OIL HEATERS 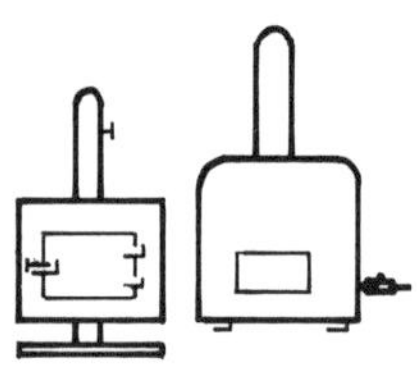	Inexpensive to install and operate.	Oil and gas contamination. Flue gas contamination. Fire and burn hazards. Will stir and fry dust. No air filtration. Poor control.
Warning: Serious fuel fumes and combustion gas hazards.		
PLENUM HEATERS 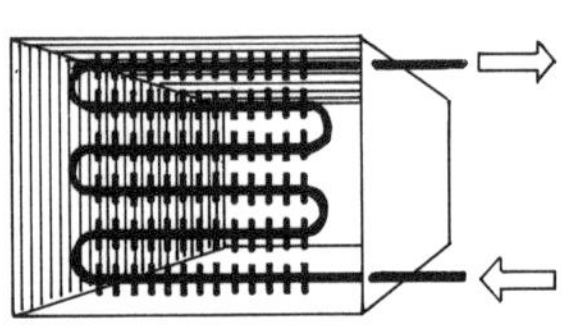 HEATED LIQUID FROM BOILER	Liquid heated loop fits in warm air duct. Boiler can be anywhere. Air is filtered and can be purified. For economical heating and cooling can be connected to heat pump. Will not fry dust. Can be added to existing forced air system.	Costly installation. Difficult to clean.
KEROSENE *Warning*: Extremely toxic flue gas. Fire hazards. Inadvisable for everyone.		

Healthful Heating and Cooling

SIMPLE PASSIVE SOLAR SYSTEMS

These systems simply take advantage of winter sunlight arriving through carefully placed windows. The heat is stored in walls or floors for overnight use.

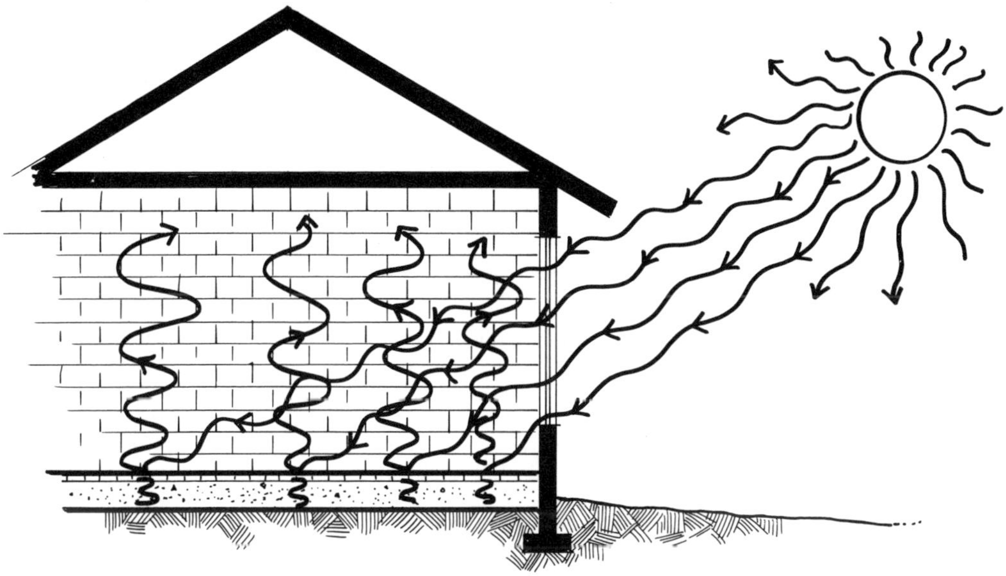

Fig. 19-1 A Simple Solar Storage System

LOW TEMPERATURE RADIANT SYSTEMS

These systems all use heated liquid coils which do not exceed approximately 240°F.

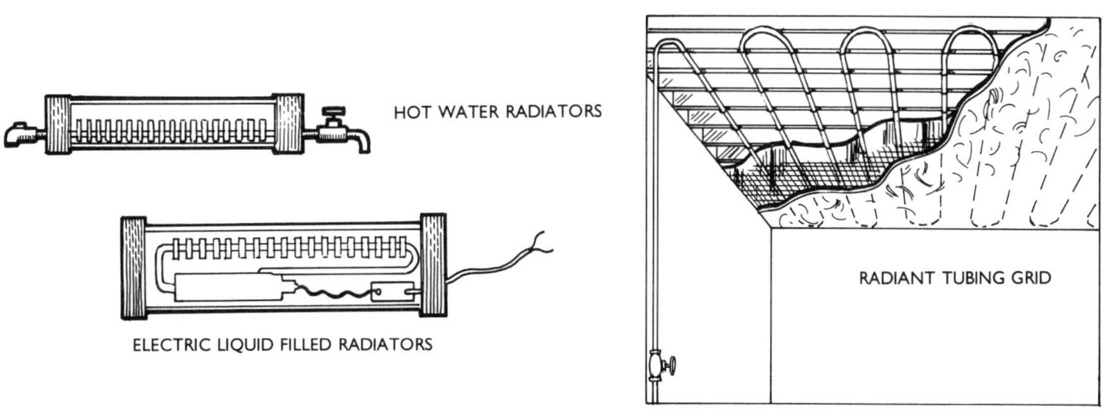

Fig. 19-2 Radiant Heating System. *This system uses low temperature liquids (less than 240°F.). (See the Construction Notes chapter for details.)*

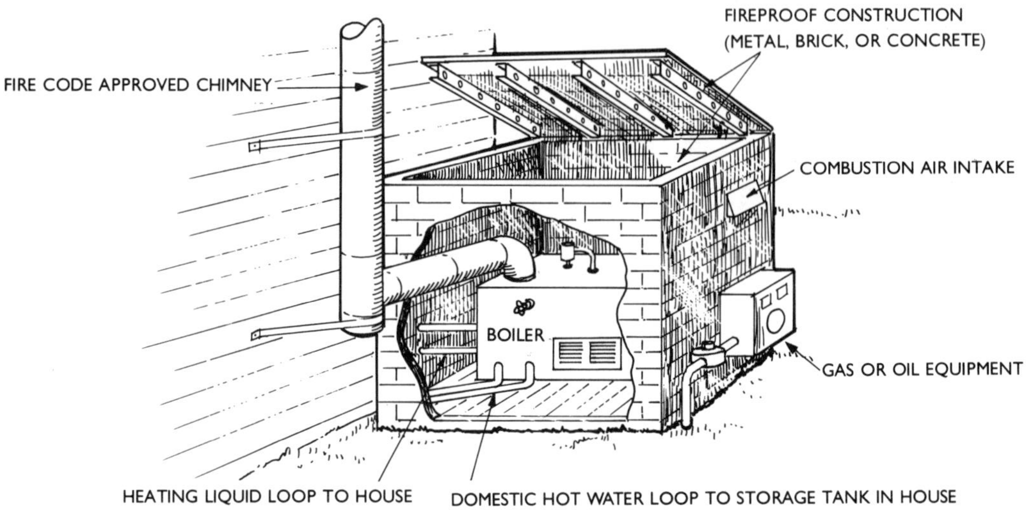

Fig. 19-3 Outside Furnace Room. *A gas or oil fired boiler can be located in a separate room to prevent fuel and combustion gas contamination of house air. The room must be of* Fireproof Construction *and equipped with an* Air Intake *and* Approved Chimney. *All* Gas or Oil Equipment *and piping must be located outside the home.*

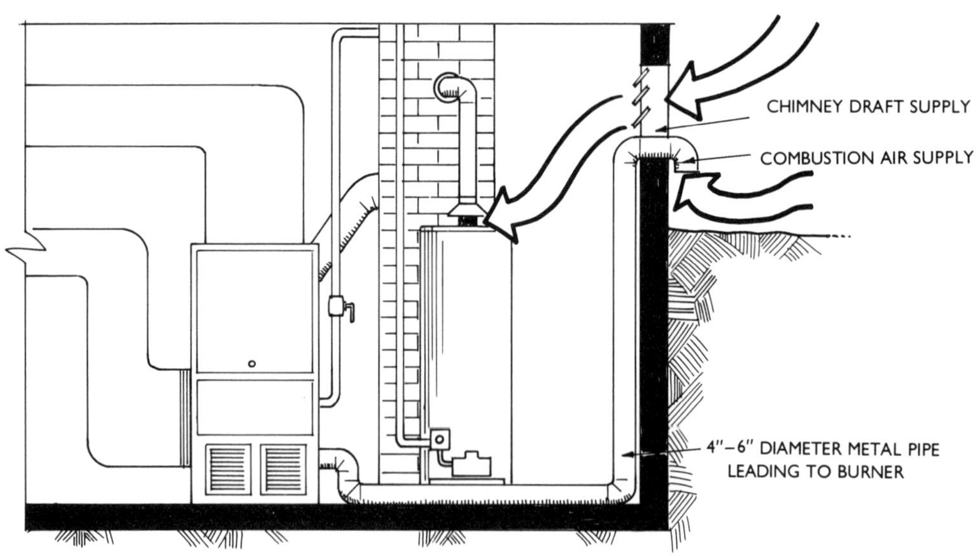

Fig. 19-4 Inside Furnace Room. *An inside furnace must be provided with a* Combustion Air Supply *and a* Chimney Draft Supply *to prevent air contamination. New forced draft type furnaces are equipped with a combustion air connection.*

OUTDOOR BOILER ROOM INSTALLATIONS

If fuel fired heating is the only affordable means in your region, a boiler can be installed in an outside furnace room. The boiler will supply heating liquid and domestic hot water through pipes to the house. This room must be of non-combustible construction, and all gas or oil piping must be outside of the house. If an electric heat pump is chosen for heating and cooling, it can be mounted in an outside room to reduce the hazard of refrigerant leaks, and to isolate noise.

INDOOR FURNACE ROOMS

All houses with indoor fuel burning furnaces must have a supply of outside air for combustion. If the house is built to energy efficiency standards there must also be adequate air intakes to allow draft air for the chimney. This should have an opening of at least 40 square inches in area, with a screen to prevent rodent and insect entry. *Induced draft furnaces are now available which considerably reduce the risk of flue gas contamination.* These use a small fan to feed a constant supply of air to the flame and maintain chimney draft. In these, the combustion air is piped directly to the burner.

SAFE DUCTWORK

If your heating system requires ductwork, be certain that it is *all* constructed of sheet metal, and is provided with cleaning and inspection openings. Cleaning should be performed yearly by a professional furnace cleaning service, with a large truck-mounted duct vacuum.

In many areas local codes allow floor cavities to be "boxed" with a sheet metal panel nailed to the bottom edge of the joists; these are then used to draw cool return air back to the furnace. This system allows dust to collect on rough wood surfaces where it cannot be readily cleaned, and floor grime to sift through cracks. This debris will contaminate heating systems and spread dust throughout the house.

SAFE HEATING SYSTEM MATERIALS

Remember that the materials used in a heating system are particularly critical to the environmentally sensitive. When heated, seemingly benign materials can become unacceptable sources of contamination. Sensitive persons must test heating equipment in operation to be certain of its acceptability.

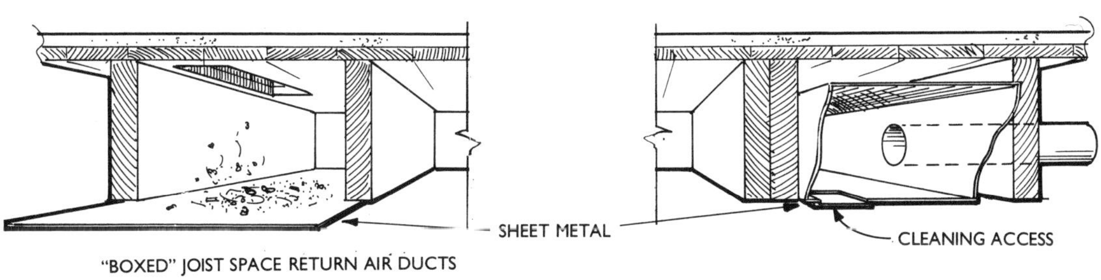

Fig. 19-5 Air Ducts. *All air ducts must be of* Sheet Metal, *without liners, and should be equipped with a* Cleaning Access. Boxed Joist Space *ducts collect dust and cannot be adequately cleaned.*

Table 19-2

Chimney Types and Uses

Type	Uses	Maintenance	Cautions
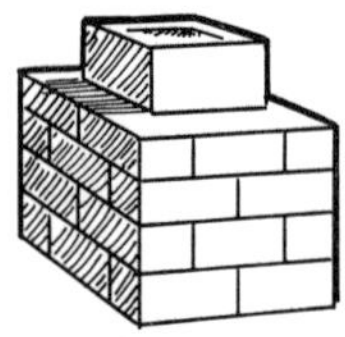 *Lined Masonry* (Standard flue sizes 8″×8″ to 16″×16″.)	Wood stoves Fireplaces Oil or gas furnaces	Clean and inspect yearly for wood stoves. Every two years for other uses. (Avoid handling, or inhaling soot.)	Check liners for cracks and deterioration. Check for loose bricks and cracked mortar. Check at roof for flashing damage. Maintain 2″ clearance to wood
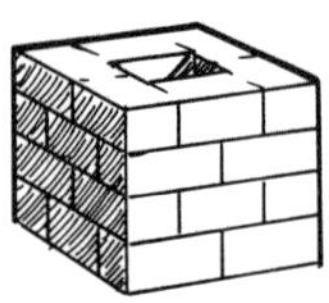 *Unlined Masonry*	NOT recommended		Unsafe for all uses due to leakage and poor heat resistance.
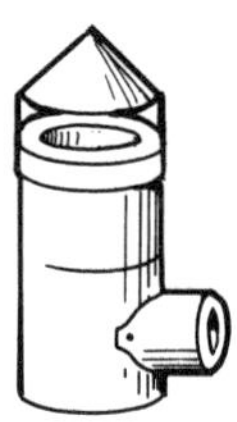 *Insulated Steel* (Standard flue sizes 6″ to 10″.)	Oil furnaces Gas appliances Factory made fireplaces (where approved by fire code).	Clean and inspect every two years, or annually if serving a heavily used fireplace. (Avoid handling or inhaling soot.)	No longer recommended for wood stoves in many areas. The outside of the chimney may overheat. (Maintain 2″ clearance to wood.)
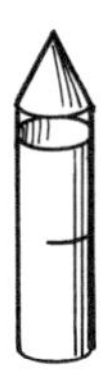 *Gas Vent* (Standard flue sizes 3″ to 6″.)	Venting of gas appliances.	Inspect every two years.	Watch for corrosion damage.

Type	Uses	Maintenance	Cautions
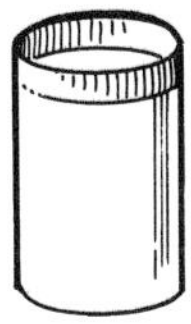 *Steel Stovepipe* (Standard flue sizes 5″ to 10″.)	Connecting stoves, furnaces, and water heaters (all types) to chimneys.	Inspect yearly. Clean and inspect monthly if used to connect wood stove to chimnney	Observe fire code clearances. (Usual minimum 12″ to wood surfaces.) Use stainless steel, or heavy plain steel for wood stoves, galvanized steel for oil and gas stoves.

20 HOME MAINTENANCE

Controlling contamination at its source is the first priority in a health conscious home. In previous sections, air quality and ventilation, heating systems, and selecting materials and furnishings were discussed. These fixed systems, structural elements, and furnishings, often all involve major decisions and sometimes large investments to change. We must also consider the non-fixed items brought into our homes for daily use, such as cleaning products and equipment. These are very important for maintaining a healthy home. Usually they require only simple decisions and small investments. In fact, changing maintenance methods and products can often simplify our lives and save money, while still improving the conditions around us.

Cleaning and maintenance with "convenience" products can introduce hundreds of chemical contaminants into indoor air and onto surfaces which contact our skin and food. Many are serious respiratory irritants, others are toxic to tissues, a few are known or suspected carcinogens.

Among the hazardous products found in the household are organochlorine pesticides, chlorine, phenols used in furniture polish, waxes, wood preservative; volatile petroleum solvents (acetone, benzene, mineral spirits, naphtha, toluene, xylene) used in paints, cleaners, glues; ethanes, ethylenes, alcohols, ketones, used in cleaning fluids; ammonia, formaldehyde, used in cleaners, glues, waxes, paints, disinfectants; and polymer resins, used in floor wax, paints, varnishes.

You will notice some of these hazards because of their strong odor. However, others have no odor at all, or their presence is masked by strong scents added to create an impression of "freshness." Air contamination is also caused by poor maintenance and cleaning of furnaces, heaters, and stoves. A food spill on a stove top or oven can produce carbon monoxide, toxic smoke containing benzo-pyrene (a potent carcinogen), and other pollutants when it becomes hot.

House cleaning and maintenance has changed dramatically in the past two generations, from a way of life occupying homemakers and weekend do-it-yourselfers, into a dreaded chore which robs busy people of what they consider their precious leisure time. However, the devices and products that have liberated us from drudgery do not come without a price, and part of that price is an added health risk. While it is not necessary to return to the ways of our grandparents, it is important to at least do the following things:

- ***Arrange your home and furniture to minimize maintenance.***
- ***Reject "convenience" products unless all contents are known and proven safe.***
- ***Try a few safe, simple, inexpensive substitutes for convenience products to discover the best combination for your needs.*** (See below.)

Design for Maintenance

Much household cleaning and maintenance is avoidable, or can be reduced by following a few simple principles when designing or arranging your home interior.

Durable Materials: Using durable materials in key locations is basic for reducing maintenance. A ceramic tile floor, for example, requires only occasional sweeping and light mopping to keep it shining.

• Consider covering heavy soil surfaces, such as splash areas behind stoves, with tile or hard plastic laminates to simplify cleaning.

• Try using glass or metals for shelving, table tops, and shelf liners.

• Use stone, brick, or concrete for some interior walls, especially in such heavy use areas as entries.

• Use hard plastic laminates for cabinet surfaces, edges, and splash areas.

• Choose durable fabrics which wear and fade least. They are also the most likely to be chemically stable and to outgas the least.

Appropriate Materials: Always select materials for their intended use.

• Do not use carpeting in bathrooms or kitchens, for example, because it will absorb and hold moisture and spills, and will support the growth of fungus.

• Rough textured wall and ceiling finishes will collect dust and are difficult to clean. Do not use them in kitchens, bathrooms, or playrooms.

• Fixed carpets in entries and halls are inadvisable because of heavy wear and dirt collection.

• In kitchens and bathrooms avoid porous countertop materials, such as wood, because they cannot be easily cleaned.

Design Simplicity: Reduce the number of materials used throughout the house. Doing more with less will mean fewer maintenance problems.

• Reduce the number of complicated joints and trims between various wall, ceiling, and floor surfaces.

• Consider using a few bold forms, such as deep window recesses, large trims and projections, rather than a multitude of fine details.

• Keep your house plan simple, reduce the number of corridors, turns, and dead ends.

• Keep the kitchen and bathrooms in easily accessible locations.

Reduce Traffic and Wear: Place traffic flows so that living rooms, bedrooms, and other light maintenance areas are away from heavily used paths.

• Consider a half-bathroom, and a storage area for childrens' outdoor toys, and other often used items, near a convenient entrance.

• If you use the outdoors a lot, have a telephone installed, and a clothes and shoes storage area built, near the entrance closest to your yard or garden. This will reduce the number of trips indoors.

• Have brick pavers, cement, or gravel paths leading to every entrance, and a rough doormat to reduce tracked in soil.

Reduce Cracks and Dirt Traps: Minimize narrow, unuseable spaces between furniture or cabinets and walls, unfilled cracks, and high shelves or ledges that are difficult to reach.

• Enclose upper kitchen cabinets to the ceiling, where possible. Have refrigerators installed with a cabinet above. Remember if there is a surface to collect grime and clutter, it will.

• Pay attention to edges, which are the high maintenance points where damage begins. Counter edges, table edges, and doorjambs should be durable and rounded where possible.

• When choosing ceramic tile, try to use the largest size appropriate for a particular use. Small mosaic tiles have large amounts of grout space which will require cleaning and repair.

• Open stairs collect large amounts of soil underneath in difficult to clean areas. Always use solid stairs indoors to keep the soil on top.

Buy Good Quality: If you do some simple cost calculations, over a 10–15 year period you may be surprised to discover something that a lot of shrewd investors already know. It often costs less over a long period to spend more now, as long as it is money spent wisely. Consider a ceramic tile floor in an entry, for example. This floor, installed, costs 50% more than a hardwood parquet floor, and over twice as much as a vinyl floor. Over a fifteen year period the parquet floor will require about thirty waxings, two sandings, and minor repairs. With heavy use it may be ready for replacement. Over the same period the vinyl floor will have been waxed sixty times and replaced once or twice, depending on use.

The initial installation of the parquet or vinyl will involve glue which outgases for a long period, the regular waxing will require a great deal of labor, costly wax, and add to the air pollution burden. The replacement alone of the vinyl will increase its cost to equal the cost of ceramic tile. By comparison, the ceramic will require only occasional sweeping and mopping over the fifteen years. It will still be in good condition and will probably last another fifteen years. Even if you borrowed the extra money for quality materials and had to pay interest on it for the fifteen year period, the total cost will still be the same or less, and you will have something lasting when it is paid for.

Surface Cleaning Equipment

The home vacuum is by far the largest investment that we make in cleaning equipment. Its effectiveness, and any possible undesirable side effects, are important to consider in the health conscious home, particularly where dust allergies are concerned. The typical cannister vacuum or upright portable not only removes dust from the soiled area, but it also disturbs dust from adjacent areas, releases trapped dust, produces ozone, objectionable noise, and oil and plastic vapors. It may also spread scents, and disinfectants, such as hexachlorophene, from treated filter bags into the room air.

Built-in Vacuums (Outside exhaust and motor type): These systems produce the least dust disturbance, the least air contamination, and the least noise because the motor and exhaust stream are located outside. There are air operated power head units available which increase their effectiveness on carpets yet do not produce fumes as electric motors do. However, built-in vacuums are costly, and may be difficult to install in some homes, such as those without basements. They are generally connected with P.V.C. plastic pipes, which will add to your home's air contamination. You can substitute these with metal pipes on request. (Ask your supplier or installer.) Consider installing an outlet near your furnace, air conditioner, and radiators, for regular dust removal from them.

Portable Vacuums: All portable vacuums discharge exhaust into the room. The exhaust tends to stir room air and raise dust. It also contains escaped dust, motor fumes, and other things which affect sensitive people. The best portable home vacuums are often the shop vacuum type, with the motor on top. They have large filter bag capacities, often with a second filter over the motor and exhaust, and they discharge their exhaust well above the floor. Low profile cannister vacuums discharge air horizontally at floor level and tend to raise dust. On any type of vacuum cleaner, power heads will be necessary for effective carpet cleaning.

Some machines use a water bath to filter dust from air. These are very effective and do not allow dust to escape, but they must be cleaned and rinsed regularly.

Hand-Held Vacuums: These "convenience" tools are not very effective for anything but the lightest soils. They have very weak suction, small capacities, poor filters, and are only appropriate for car interiors or other difficult to reach locations.

Using Vacuums: Vacuums are best suited to fabrics and carpets. A dampened dust cloth or mop is far more effective on hard surfaces, and will raise far less dust. ***Keep your vacuum working effectively by changing your bag when it is half full.*** When possible, change it outdoors, then clean the inside of the machine with a soft brush and damp cloth before replacing the bag. Before bringing it in, run the machine for 30 seconds to remove the loose dust that is always discharged after a bag change.

Brooms: Wherever possible, damp mopping is better than sweeping as it prevents raising dust. Finding and choosing good brooms and mops will present some problems, particularly for the environmentally sensitive. Most brooms today are fabricated from plastics, such as polypropylene and nylon, or from natural fibers such as corn straw. These may be irritating or allergenic for some people and must be selected with care.

Mops: Sponge mops are often made with cellulose sponge which contains no plastics. This is the type of sponge which becomes hard when dry. Mops which remain soft are made from foamed plastic resins, and should be avoided. Plain white string mops are made from cotton twine which is generally acceptable for most people. After using such a mop, rinse it thoroughly and then dip it in a final rinse of water containing a few teaspoons of white vinegar or borax. Wring it out and stand it up to dry. These steps will prevent mildew growth.

Safe Maintenance Products

There are a few safe and inexpensive common household products that are effective for many cleaning needs. They can replace most hazardous and costly formulated products. (See Safe, Effective Cleaning Methods, below.)

Baking Soda: Common baking soda is effective for light cleaning, removing odors, for cleaning teeth, as a polish, as well as many other uses. It is non-corrosive, slightly abrasive, and safe to ingest.

Washing Soda: Common sodium carbonate is effective for heavily soiled laundry and general purpose cleaning.

Borax: Common powdered borax is effective for light cleaning, removing odors, and for preventing the growth of mold. It is available in grocery stores in the laundry section.

Vinegar: Common white vinegar is effective for cutting grease, removing odors, and preventing the growth of mold.

Pure Soap: Bar or flake soap, if made without additives, is an effective and gentle cleaner for many uses.

T.S.P.: Trisodium phosphate is a heavy duty all-purpose cleaner for grease, soil, and stain removal, available at paint or hardware stores. It is, however, corrosive to skin, and must be used with care.

Chlorine Free Scouring Powders: Such products are effective for heavy duty cleaning of pots, tubs, sinks, etc. They have a mild chemical bleaching action without hazardous chlorine. (Products with chlorine are labeled as containing a chlorine compound.)

Chlorine Free Bleach: This is an effective laundry product where bleaching is necessary. It is safer and gentler than chlorine bleach.

Mineral Oil: This is a safe and odor free petroleum oil, available at pharmacies. It is useful for wood and furniture polishing and for cleaning greasy hands. It is also non-toxic if ingested in very small quantities.

Beeswax: Melted beeswax can be added to mineral oil to make a natural and durable furniture polish.

Safe, Effective Cleaning Methods

General Purpose Soap: For hands, dishes, laundry, and light cleaning, use pure bar or soap flakes without perfume additives. To make liquid soap, dissolve flakes or powder in warm water and store in a glass jar for use.

For Laundry: Pure soap flakes or unscented commercial detergent (if individually acceptable). Add ½ cup of borax or vinegar to the rinse water to remove soap residue and odors. To remove heavy soils, use 1 teaspoon of T.S.P. in the wash water.

Window Cleaning: 2–5 tablespoons of white vinegar in 2 cups of water. Apply with a pump sprayer, then wipe with an absorbent cloth.

Heavy Cleaning of Walls and Floors: 4 tablespoons T.S.P. to 1 gallon of hot water. Add more T.S.P. if necessary. *Caution: Wear rubber gloves when handling. T.S.P. is mildly toxic if ingested.*

Dishwasher Detergent: If commercial detergents are unacceptable, try ½ teaspoon pure soap powder (not much more, to prevent oversudsing) with 3 tablespoons baking soda. For heavy cleaning, try ¼ cup of sodium hexametaphosphate, a safer cousin of T.S.P. It is available from chemical supply houses.

Carpet Cleaner: Prevention is the best carpet cleaner. Do not use carpeting in heavy traffic or soil areas. Spot cleaning with a solution of ½ cup borax to 1 quart of water and a stiff bristle brush is the best method for maintaining carpeting. Vacuum well when dry. Odors from spills or smoking can be removed by sprinkling with baking soda, leaving it for a few hours, and then vacuuming. (A few pounds will usually cover an average living room area rug.) If commercial cleaning is necessary, consider removing non-fixed carpets outside the home for the cleaning. Steam process methods are best, and produce the least reside to attract further soil.

Caution: Commercial carpet cleaning solutions can leave chemical residues and odors. Ask to test a sample of all solutions to be used before hiring a carpet cleaner.

Hand Cleaner: Mineral oil rubbed into greasy hands will clean them gently. Wipe off on soft paper or cloth before washing.

Oven Cleaning: Prevent oven spills by baking in a covered dish whenever possible, or by using a cookie sheet or foil sheet below to catch overflow. For microwave ovens use a microwave safe large glass or ceramic dish. When heated, oven spills create serious air pollution and lingering odors. Self cleaning ovens deliver all of this pollutant burden to the air in your home during the self clean cycle.

To remove stubborn oven crust, apply a paste of chlorine free scouring powder and water to the warm surface. Allow to dry, then scrub with a fiber scouring pad. If necessary, use pumice powder or steel wool.

Tub and Tile Cleaner: Use equal parts of vinegar and warm water to remove soap films and spots. Regular use will prevent fungus growth. To remove fungus stains, try a chlorine free bleach or scouring powder.

Plugged Drains: Try a plunger, or a garden hose type drain cleaner. The inexpensive hose adapter for this type is available at hardware stores. Have a simple cleanout plug installed by a plumber so the trap can be cleaned periodically. Using 2 tablespoons of T.S.P. mixed into two cups of hot water from time to time will reduce grease accumulation. Allow it to stand for 1 hour before flushing.

Silver and Copper Cleaning: Place silver in an aluminum pan, or a sink or washtub with an aluminum pie plate in the bottom. Add hot water to cover the silver, a few teaspoons of baking soda, and a pinch of salt. Turn silver after 5 minutes. This treatment removes tarnish in 10–15 minutes by a gentle chemical reaction. Rinse silver well and dry thoroughly before storing.
Scrub tarnished copper or brass with a paste of lemon juice and baking soda. Rinse well.

Fruit Stains in Fabric: Rinse as soon as possible by pouring *boiling* water through stained area. Remove stubborn stains by applying lemon juice, and then placing in the sun for a few hours.

Fungus Retardant: Add 1 cup of powdered borax to each gallon of natural protein paint, or to homemade starch wallpaper paste, to resist fungus growth. In difficult areas or in damp climates, use calcium propionate (available from chemical supply stores). Wash mildew-affected areas with ½ cup borax per quart of warm water.

Floor Wax: Try a paste wax that requires buffing. Apply it with good ventilation, and then let the house air out well. It will last much longer than liquid "self-polishing" wax, and it is more chemically stable when dry.

Wood Furniture Polish: Use plain mineral oil applied with an absorbent cloth. Wipe dry after a few minutes. For a durable finish for new or finished wood, over a double boiler melt ½ pound of beeswax in 2 cups of mineral oil, and apply warm with an absorbent cloth.

Insect Control: Use window screens and flypaper to control flying insects. Consider herbal repellents for biting insects. Prevent entry of ants by plugging foundation holes and cracks with cement mortar, white glue, or a safe caulking compound. To prevent the entry of termites, shield all wood near foundations with sheet metal. Clean up food and kitchen spills immediately to reduce the spread of ants, mice, and cockroaches.

Remember that many safe products, such as herbal scents, will only repel insects, while poisons will destroy them. Whatever is poisonous to insects is likely to be poisonous to people and pets as well. For more information on pest control see Further Reading in the GETTING HELP section.

Hazardous Household Chemicals

The following household chemicals are either toxic or serious irritants. They should be avoided wherever possible. All of these are potentially serious health hazards to sensitive individuals, even in very small amounts.

Pesticides: These are hazardous for everyone, particularly the **organochlorine** families. (See the Indoor Hazards chapter.) Safer pesticides are rotenone, pyrethrin (extracted from the marigold flower), boric acid powder (toxic if ingested, but safe to handle and available from chemical supply houses); diatomaceous earth (fossilized tiny sea plants); and biological pesticides (such as the bacterium B.T., available from garden supply stores).

Organophosphate Pesticides: Diazinon, malathion, and parathion are also hazardous, though they do not remain in the environment like organochlorines. Organophosphates are serious nerve toxins causing nausea, headache, dizziness, and numbness. Children, the chronically ill, and pets are particularly affected by these, sometimes even when sprayed at some distance.

Chlorine Products: Bleach, scouring powders.

Ammonia Products: Household ammonia, window cleaner.

Oven Cleaners: All commercial varieties.

Drain Cleaners: All commercial varieties.

Mothballs: Made from toxic naphthalene.

Fungicides: All commercial varieties. (Many are formaldehyde based.)

Waxes, Polishes: Liquid or spray preparations, which contain potent solvents, acrylics, phenols, formaldehydes, etc.

Glues: All types, except animal product glues, and white glues.

Petroleum Solvents: B.B.Q. lighters, paints, thinners, and cleaning fluids.

Aerosol Products: They spread the product indiscriminately, and contain hazardous propellant gases.

Carpet Cleaner: All commercial varieties.

Household Deodorizers and Disinfectants: These products are irritating for sensitive people. Their main purpose is to mask the odors which result from problems which should be recognized and dealt with.

Scheduling Healthy Home Upkeep

In every health conscious home, a few important maintenance procedures should be marked on the calendar. Keeping to such a regular schedule for heating systems, kitchen appliances, and the water system, will be a great help for maintaining healthful conditions in your home.

Central Furnace/Air Conditioner Fans and Filters: Vacuum clean filter and housing every 30 days during use. Replace filters every 60 days. Also vacuum clean fan and housing yearly at the beginning of each heating/cooling season.

Note: Electrostatic filters should be cleaned every 30 days. The metal filter plates of some electronic models can be cleaned in the dishwasher.

Furnace and Air Conditioners: Vacuum clean heat exchanger or coils. Have burner/compressor serviced by a professional. Also have duct system vacuumed (by professional) yearly at beginning of heating/cooling season.

Heaters and Radiators: Vacuum clean the heat tubes and fins twice monthly during use.

• Chimneys: See the Home Heating/Cooling chapter.

• Air Conditioner: Clean the coils and the drip pan with a mixture of 1 cup vinegar to 1 gallon of water. Clean the drip pan drain weekly during the cooling season.

• House Fans: Disassemble and clean blades with a mixture of 4 tablespoons of T.S.P. to 1 quart of hot water yearly.

• Humidifier: Remove drum, or all moisture bearing parts, and water reservoir. Clean with soapy water, then soak in a mixture of 1 cup vinegar to 1 gallon of water weekly during use.

• Air Purifiers: Disassemble and clean collectors, filters, and fans monthly. Use a soft cloth moistened in vinegar-water mixture. Replace filters and adsorption media as recommended by the manufacturer.

The Kitchen:

• Stove: Clean burner pans, burners, and oven with 4 tablespoons T.S.P. to 1 quart hot water, or with a chlorine free scouring powder, as necessary.

• Range hood and fan: Soak the filter in a solution of hot water and 4 tablespoons T.S.P., or wash it in dishwasher. Wash inside hood monthly.

• Refrigerator and Freezer: Wash interiors with ½ cup baking soda to 1 gallon of warm water. Clean drain pan and drain holes and wash with soapy water once a month.

The Bathroom: Rinse tub and shower enclosures with a vinegar and water solution every month.

The Water System:

• Water filters: Backwash or replace filters as recommended by the manufacturer. Disassemble and wash housings in warm soapy water when replacing filter. Rinse well.

• Water heaters: Drain a few gallons from the sediment drain on the bottom of the tank once a year.

21 WATER TREATMENT

Clean water is fundamental to health, not only for drinking and cooking, but what is less well known, also for bathing and washing. The water that enters our homes, whether it comes from a clear spring, a deep well, or a city reservoir, is never "pure". It contains many minerals, salts, gases, and microorganisms, as well as man-made contaminants. Many of the natural components, such as the minerals, are quite harmless, or even beneficial to health, though some, such as selenium and nitrates, are harmful. Other components, such as gases, salts, and some microorganisms, will cause unacceptable taste or health risks. Our modern manmade contaminants are particularly unwelcome, and can be very serious health risks.

The most hazardous compounds found in water today are the inorganic substances, such as mercury, lead, and arsenic, industrial pollutants and agricultural chemicals, and the organochlorine compounds formed by the chlorine that is added to municipal water to reduce the level of microorganisms. In some areas water is dangerously contaminated with industrial chemicals, such as solvents, and pesticide and fertilizer runoff. *The absorption of some of these hazardous contaminants does not just occur through drinking water. Recent research shows that from 50% to 60% of the soluble contaminants that we absorb from water enter the body through the skin while bathing.*

If water tests indicate that significant levels of these contaminants are present in your water (see Water Testing, below), or if a member of your household is sensitive to the chlorine compounds in municipal water, home water treatment can be installed to remove a large proportion of the offending substance. For others, water treatment is a worthwhile effort for the improvement in the water's taste, odor, and appearance.

No water treatment system can remove 100% of any contaminant, and each type of system is only effective for certain types of contamination. If you decide after testing your water that you wish to treat it, choose the system carefully for the specific use. Beware of advertising claims and unscrupulous sales people when it comes to choosing a water treatment system. There are many unfounded claims for these units, high pressure sales tactics being used to sell them, and unjustifiably high prices. Many systems will not do what they are designed to do, while others are a $10 piece of hardware inside an impressive housing with a $300 price tag. (See Effective Treatment Methods, below.)

Types of Water Contamination

The type of contamination that may be present in your water, and the levels that are found there, are largely determined by the water's source, though small amounts of plastic compounds and metals are introduced by the piping system.

Table 21-1

Hazardous Substances Found in Ground Water

Substance	*Number of cities sampled*	*Percentage of cities with chemical present*
Trichloroethylene	25	36
Carbon tetrachloride	39	28.2
Tetrachloroethylene	36	22
1,1,1-Trichloroethane	23	21.7
1,1-Dichloroethane	13	23.1
1,2-Dichloroethane	25	4
Trans-dichloroethylene	13	15.4
Cis-dichloroethylene	13	30.8
1,1-Dichloroethylene	13	7.7
Methylene chloride	38	2.6
Vinyl chloride	25	4.0

Table 21-2

The Most Prevalent Dangerous Chemicals In Drinking Water

Chloroform (TCM)
Benzene
BCEE
Carbon tetrachloride
Nitrosamines
Polynuclear aromatic hydrocarbon (PAH)
Trichloroethylene (TCE)
Xylene
Selenium
Arsenic
Cyanide
DDT
PCBs
Toluene
Toxaphene (pesticide)
Methoxychlor (pesticide)
Endrine (pesticide)
Lindane (pesticide)
2, 4-D (herbicide)
2,4,5-T (herbicide)
Vinyl chloride
Mercury
Lead

City Versus Country Water

City water is closely regulated for some health hazards and is very unlikely to contain dangerous bacterial contamination. It is, however, almost always treated with chlorine to reduce the bacteria count. Chlorine combines with such organic compounds as natural methane gas (from decomposed material) in water, to form organochlorine compounds. The most common are the THM's (trihalomethanes), such as chloroform. These are suspected carcinogens. They also give water an unpleasant taste and odor.

Most important for those who receive water from a municipal system is the removal of chlorine compounds. This will not only reduce the risk of cancer, but will dramatically improve the flavor.

City water may well contain significant chemical contaminants from industrial discharge or hazardous waste disposal. For example, it may contain such residues as vinyl chloride (a potent carcinogen) from plastic pipe. Recent studies in the U.S. show that 4% of municipal water supplies carry vinyl chloride from P.V.C. plastic pipe. Contact your local water authority, and ask for a current report on the quality of your water. If your water district serves more than 20,000 people it is required to meet strict health standards.

If you do not receive municipal water, there is a much greater likelihood that your water may be contaminated by bacteria, parasites, or hazardous man-made chemicals. Lake or stream water is easily contaminated by surface runoff containing agricultural chemicals, airborne industrial fallout, and bacteriological activity. It is also vulnerable to leakage from chemical dumps, sewage, and industrial discharge. Lake or stream water is now unsafe in many areas because of these hazards. It must be monitored closely for bacteria, organic and inorganic chemicals, and toxic metals. (See Water Testing, below.)

Spring water, or shallow well water (less than 30 feet deep) is not as likely to be contaminated by surface activity. However, the source of this water is shallow groundwater, which is vulnerable to other types of hazards. Septic tanks and hazardous waste seepage can contaminate groundwater over large distances, particularly in limestone regions. Shallow wells and spring holding tanks are also susceptible to bacteria from poor maintenance or decaying vegetation. *A tank or well should be properly constructed with a complete concrete liner and a tight cover.* Spring or shallow well water should also be tested regularly for bacteria and organic compounds.

Deep well water from a properly constructed well is unlikely to be contaminated by bacteria or surface runoff. The deep water table is also less likely to be contaminated by hazardous waste seepage or sewage, though this has occurred in some places. However, two problems may arise with deep well water. One is the presence of radon gas if it is drilled in radioactive bedrock, such as some granite in New England, Pennsylvania, and Eastern Canada. (See the chapter Testing for Contamination, for radon testing.) Another may be the presence of dissolved minerals (hardness) if the well is in limestone formations. Hardness is generally harmless but can be a household nuisance.

One very serious health hazard from deep wells that has only recently been discovered, is the possibility of PCB contamination. This highly carcinogenic substance may be leaking from some deep well submersible pumps. Prior to the 1977–78 manufacturing year, some manufacturers of these pumps placed PCB's inside their oil filled, sealed motors, and these can leak onto the well water when the motor seals begin to wear out. Check with your supplier or the manufacturer if your submersible drinking water pump was manufactured before 1978. Or obtain a full list of the affected units from your local Environmental Protection Agency office, in the U.S., or from your local Ministry of Environment office, in Canada.

Water Testing

Always test water before deciding to treat it. Treatments are very specific for different types of contamination, and you must know what contaminants you are trying to remove. Use an independent test laboratory or a public health service. Do not accept the offers of testing by water treatment sales persons. (See the chapter Testing for Contamination.)

Understanding Water Treatment

There are several water treatment processes. No single one is the best for all problems, and each has its own particular maintenance needs and costs.

ACTIVATED CHARCOAL ADSORPTION

Activated charcoal grains are effective for removing many chemical contaminants, such as chlorine compounds, some organic chemicals (eg. solvents and oils), as well as some pesticides and dissolved gases. Charcoal filtering will remove most of the substances which cause odors. A good, large capacity charcoal filter can remove 80% or more of chlorine compounds when it is new, but it must be renewed regularly. Charcoal is not appropriate for removing bacteria or suspended solids, and can become a dangerous breeding ground for microorganisms if not properly maintained and renewed.

FILTRATION

Ceramic or fabric filters are used to remove particles from water. They are effective for removing suspended solids and most microorganisms such as protozoan parasites and bacteria. They are not effective for removing chlorine compounds or other dissolved chemicals.

REVERSE OSMOSIS

Membranes made from cellulose, acetate, or nylon, are very effective for removing many contaminants when water is forced through them at high pressure. This process will effectively remove chlorine compounds but not chlorine, many organic chemicals, such as solvents and pesticide residues, and some dissolved minerals. Though reverse osmosis will also remove bacteria and suspended solids, it is not a recommended practice as it will clog the membrane. Where bacteria and solids are a problem, water should be treated for bacteria and prefiltered before using a reverse osmosis unit. However, the membrane will eventually clog with any sort of use, and will have to be replaced.

PASTEURIZATION

Heating water to 160°F. for 10 minutes will kill bacteria, and also reduce the concentration of many volatile organic compounds, such as chloroform from chlorine. Boiling is still more effective. Large pasteurization units are available for whole house treatment, but they are costly to install and operate.

DISTILLATION

Distilled water is usually considered pure, and it is certainly free of bacteria. Its taste, however, is also very insipid. Home distillers do not remove chlorine compounds and other volatile organics effectively, because these will boil off before the water does, and will then re-enter the distilled water as it cools. Distillers also use a great deal of electricity.

ULTRAVIOLET LIGHT

Bacteria removal can be accomplished in the home with an ultraviolet light treatment unit. This is a tank with a lamp inside which kills bacteria as the water passes. These are available as "whole house" treatment units, but they are expensive and require a lot of maintenance.

CHLORINE AND IODINE TREATMENT

Though these well known treatment chemicals are effective for reducing bacteria content, they themselves present health risks. Sometimes, where home chlorination or iodination is used for bacterial control, it is followed by a dechlorination unit, such as one with activated charcoal. Unfortunately, the dechlorination process is not as reliable as the chlorination process, and water may still have a high chemical content after treatment. These systems are not acceptable in the health conscious home.

WATER SOFTENERS

Water softeners are only effective for reducing the mineral content (hardness) of water. Resin granules in the softener attract dissolved minerals, such as calcium carbonate ($CaCO_3$) from limestone, and sulfates. Common salt is used to wash the attached minerals from the resin and periodically flush them to the drain.

Hard water problems are not a health risk, though they are a nuisance. On the other hand, water softeners can become a health risk if used in drinking and cooking water.

The salt used for flushing the resin will enter the water, and this is a serious risk for those on low sodium diets for medical reasons. Many hard water problems can be overcome by using different soaps to improve suds and reduce the residue from washing and bathing. If water softening is necessary, consider using it only for laundry, bathing, and dishwasher water. Many water treatment specialists recommend connecting the softener only to the water supply serving the water heater, so as to reduce the risk of salt absorption.

Table 21-3

Sources of Water Contamination

Type	Major Sources	Health Risks
Bacteria	Surface water contamination (sewage, agriculture, rotting vegetation) of shallow wells, creeks, lakes, and rivers.	Disease causing pathogens. Also unacceptable taste and odor.
Organochlorines	Chlorinated municipal water combining with natural organic compounds. (See City Versus Country Water, above.)	Potential carcinogens. Also unacceptable taste and odor.
Man-made organic chemicals	Industrial waste (solvents, pesticides, etc.), agriculture runoff, leaking waste dumps entering surface or ground water. Plastic water pipe.	Potential carcinogens. Can cause chronic illness when absorbed in large amounts.
Metals (lead, mercury, cadmium, etc.)	Solder from water pipes, surface runoff from roadways, industrial emissions.	These are all toxic, and will accumulate in the body.
Minerals (hardness)	Dissolved from deposits in the earth, such as limestone ($CaCO_3$)	No major health risks.
Sediments (cloudiness)	Suspended solids from various sources.	Cloudiness does not necessarily indicate a health risk. Test for bacteria, however.

Effective Treatment Methods

Contaminant	Removal Method	Notes
Bacteria and Parasites	Boiling, pasteurization, distillation, ultraviolet treatment.	Always treat for bacteria first if tests indicate bacterial contamination. Ultraviolet may be the best method for a "whole house" system.
Chlorine Compounds (chloroform etc.). Other Volatile Organic Chemicals.	Activated charcoal, reverse osmosis, boiling.	These compounds enter the air when boiling. Always ventilate well.
Pesticide and Herbicide Residue	Activated charcoal, reverse osmosis.	This is only partly effective.
Minerals (hardness — $CaCO_3$)	Water softeners.	Treat only washing water.
Cloudiness, Suspended Solids	Ceramic, or other high performance filters.	Sand or disposable prefilters are necessary.

Water Treatment Equipment

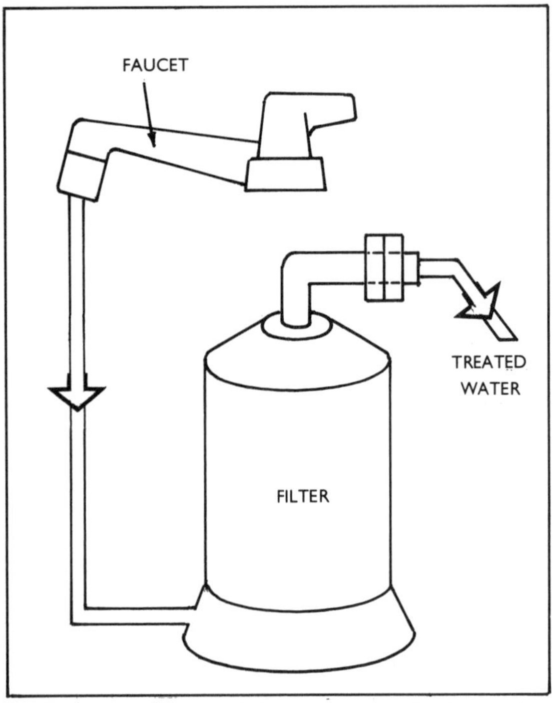

Fig. 21-1 A Typical Counter-top Activated Carbon Filter.

ACTIVATED CHARCOAL

These units are generally "flow through" types, which are connected to a cold water line. They will quickly treat fairly large amounts of water, but the disposable charcoal cartridge they contain must be changed regularly. Charcoal becomes contaminated with use, and if not renewed will begin releasing what it has trapped back into the water. Saturated charcoal is also a dangerous breeding ground for microorganisms. If the filter is used regularly, flushed for a period after standing unused, and renewed according to schedule, bacterial contamination will not be a problem unless your water is heavily contaminated with bacteria.

The general rule for charcoal is that more is better. The larger units, with a greater charcoal charge, are far more effective than small units, such as the type which screw onto a tap or shower head. These "convenience" units are probably not worth buying unless you are prepared to change them almost daily. The most effective of the larger cartridge types are those with a solid jacket casing. If the replacement cartridge has a screen or fabric casing it will not perform as well.

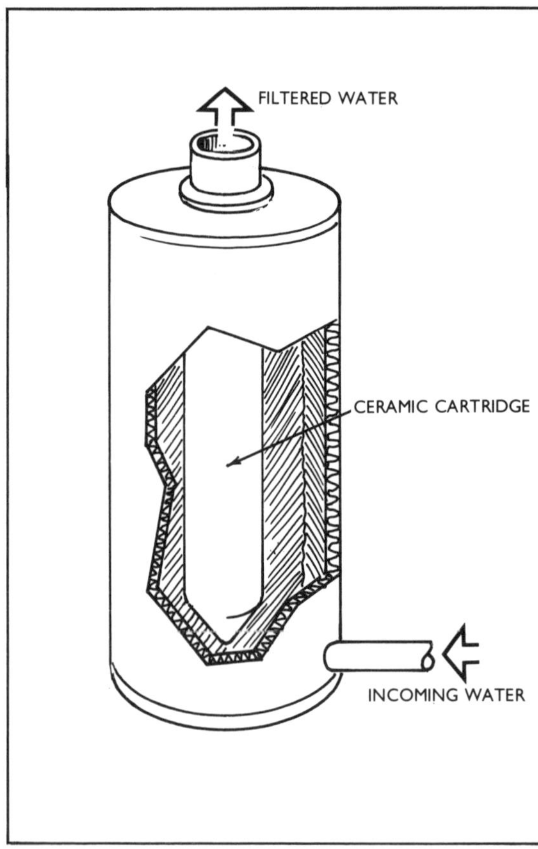

Fig. 21-2 A Typical Ceramic Cartridge Filter.

CERAMIC OR OTHER PERMANENT FILTERS

These units are slow, and are usually "by-pass" types which treat only a small amount of water for drinking or cooking. When the filter becomes clogged it is backwashed (used in reverse) for cleaning, and the back-wash water discarded. The filters are also periodically removed and washed. Ceramic filters are very fragile and must be handled with great care. A cracked filter is useless.

REVERSE OSMOSIS UNITS

These are very slow, and require a booster pump for best performance. The pumps are available in both hand operated and electric models. Reverse osmosis units are generally small "batch" type units, which are filled from a tap or pipe connection, pumped up, and left for a time until the treatment is complete. The filter membranes are periodically backwashed to reduce clogging, but will eventually become blocked and have to be replaced. These membranes are very sensitive to clogging with bacteria and small particles, and should be protected by pre-filtering and sterilizing the water. For small units water can be poured through a paper filter and boiled. For large units it can be passed through an inexpensive commercial disposable cartridge filter (available at plumbing supply stores.)

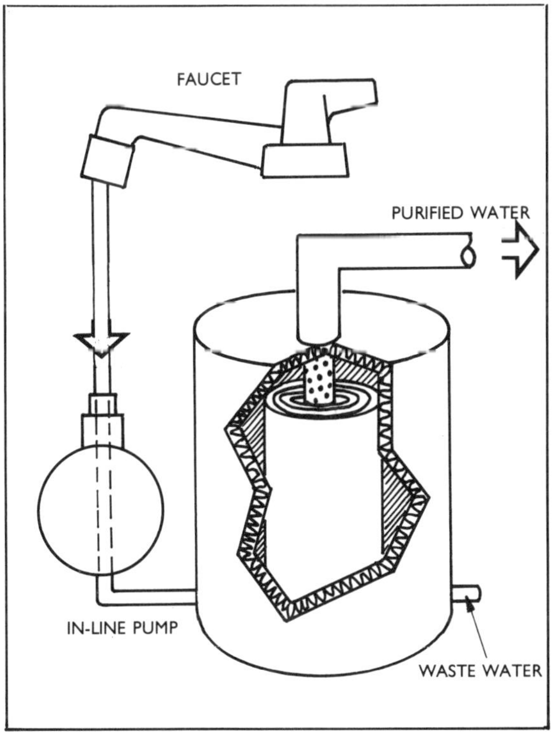

Fig. 21-3 A Reverse Osmosis (R.O.) Water Treatment System.

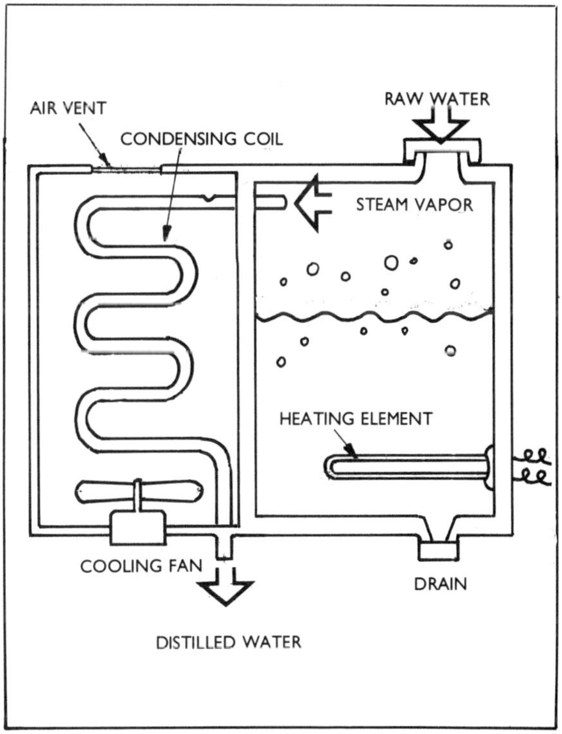

Fig. 21-4 A Typical Steam Distillation Unit.

DISTILLATION UNITS

These are generally small batch type, counter top units. They are very slow and use large amounts of electricity, but they are the most effective of all systems for removing bacteria and minerals.

ULTRAVIOLET STERILIZER

These are very complex and expensive, and will require permanent plumbing and wiring. They are generally whole house treatment systems, and should be chosen and installed by water treatment experts.

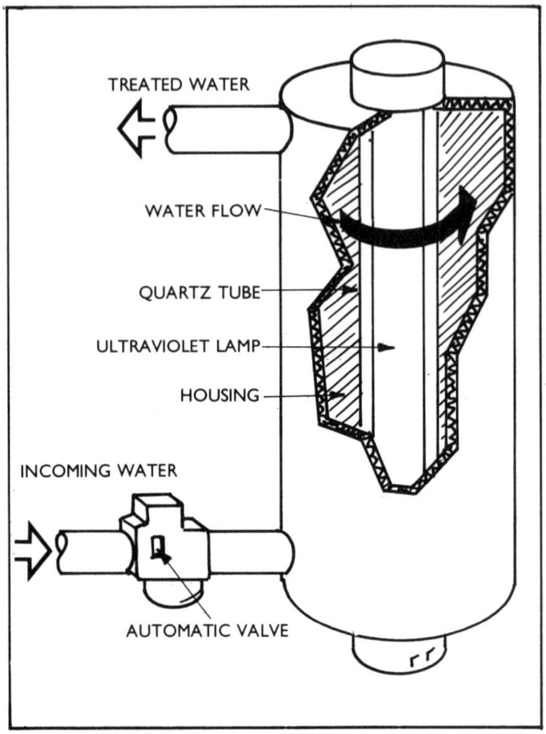

Fig. 21-5 A Typical Ultraviolet Sterilization System.

Sizing The System

Cooking and drinking water usually amounts to only about 2 to 4 gallons per day for a household. Bathing water is approximately 10 to 20 gallons per shower, and about 30 gallons per bath. The total water usage of an average household is about 200 to 300 gallons per day.

The smallest batch type charcoal or reverse osmosis units are counter top models, about the size of a toaster. These will only handle enough water for drinking and cooking. Treated water may be safely stored for up to two days in clean glass jars in the refrigerator. The filters in these units are capable of treating anywhere from 200 to 3,000 gallons of water before replacement, depending on the type of filter and contamination levels. Smaller units, such as those which screw onto taps or shower heads, are not recommended.

Larger, under counter units are the next size, and are connected directly to the plumbing. These are often connected to an extra sink tap which supplies only treated cold water. The filters in these units generally are capable of treating anywhere from 1,000 to 3,000 gallons of water before replacement.

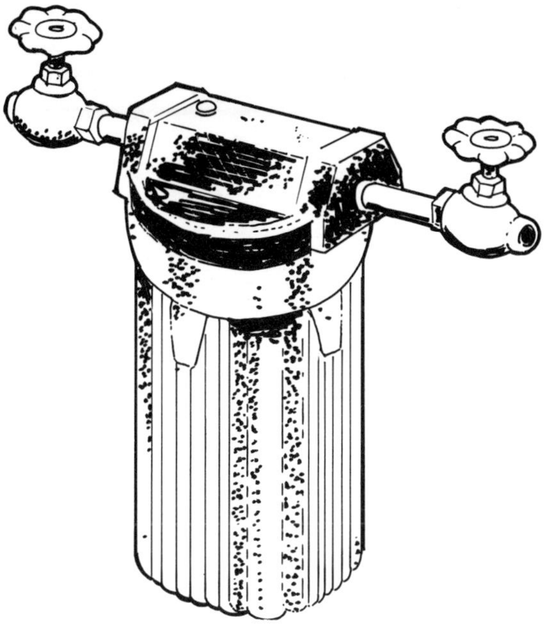

Fig. 21-6 A Typical In-line Charcoal Filter

The largest units available can be used to treat all of the water used in the house. Charcoal or reverse osmosis units of this size are available only from commercial suppliers and are very costly. They require permanent plumbing and electrical connections, and they must be installed and serviced by experts.

The safest approach to treating seriously contaminated water is with a whole house system, combining bacteria treatment and reverse osmosis or charcoal, as necessary. Though these are prohibitively expensive for most people, they may be necessary for the environmentally sensitive.

Note: For an excellent article on choosing a small water treatment unit, see "Consumer's Report," February, 1983.

Lead and Copper in Water

The copper pipes in your home release lead and copper into your water as it passes through them. This process is accelerated by the presence of chlorine or other chemicals. Though this is usually not considered a major health risk, some precautions should be taken. Research shows that much higher levels of lead accumulate in water when it is standing in pipes than when it is flowing through. Lead levels can reach 100 times normal after standing for 24 hours. Run your tap for 2 to 3 minutes before drawing drinking or cooking water if the tap has not been used for more than four hours. This will substantially reduce your lead dose, as well as improve the taste and appearance of the household's drinking water.

If you are building or renovating, consider having copper pipe with mechanical fittings installed, instead of soldered ones. This is more costly, but it can eliminate lead from your water. If you find you must use soldered pipe, ask for a special solder called 95/5. This is made for heating systems, and contains only ten percent of the lead that typical 50/50 solder contains. It has a higher melting point than typical solder, and is harder to work with, but the health benefits are worth the extra effort. "Lead free" solder is also available now in many regions.

SECTION V

Materials

22 MATERIALS AND SELECTION

One of the most difficult dilemmas facing anyone concerned with maintaining a health promoting home environment is the selection of safe materials. In many ways it is easier and less costly to make changes in our personal habits, diet, and exercise, than it is to restructure our surroundings. Personal change is certainly a good place to start, but once that is done the next step to consider is environmental change. One of the problems immediately encountered, in addition to cost, is the scarcity of good information about available materials and their alternatives. Of course, those fortunate enough to be designing a new home can better control materials and costs than those who are considering changing an existing one. However, when renovations are being considered, informing yourself will help you to make intelligent and economical choices about materials and methods. It will also enable you to choose and instruct your contractor or suppliers, or become more aware of health factors as a builder.

Food labeling with a full table of ingredients has been steadily progressing, as government agencies recognize the necessity of serving the health conscious and allergic sectors of the population, but *progress in listing the chemical properties of building materials has been moving more slowly.* Recent work by the United States Environmental Protection Agency has led to the classifying of some formaldehyde producing pressed wood products, but though work is progressing on a more complete listing system for a wider range of materials, we are still a long way from having adequate information and accountability.

The time has come to apply pressure upon manufacturers and government for better controls and public information. *Read product labels where available, and question your supplier or the manufacturer if the information is inadequate.* With large purchases, it is best to request information in writing, and keep copies of correspondence. Product information is legally regulated, and if you should have a claim against a supplier or manufacturer, you will need records.

Until more information becomes available, health conscious or sensitive people can make informed individual decisions based on their personal experience, obtaining professional help when necessary. (See the GETTING HELP section.)

The following table is a guide to building materials and finishing and furnishing materials, listed by generic type (by kind and not by trademark), with a rating-for-safety system based on the usual chemical properties of each material. Plumbing, electrical, and heating equipment is also included, as well as small appliances. Remember that manufacturing standards will vary widely from one producer to the next, and each item must be examined on its own merits. (See Testing Materials, below.)

MATERIALS RATINGS

A: These materials are generally stable (ie. they will not outgas or otherwise deteriorate), and are not expected to contribute significantly to indoor contamination. Except for the most sensitive individuals, and those already suffering from environmental illness, this group can be considered "safe".

B: These materials are potentially significant contaminants, and may be unacceptable to sensitive individuals. They should be self-tested for adverse reactions. (See Testing Materials, below.)

C: These materials have been clearly linked with serious contamination, and should be avoided by everyone whenever possible.

Table 22-I

BUILDING MATERIALS

The materials for each use are listed below in order of acceptability, starting with the most preferred. Individual acceptability, however, will vary with personal sensitivities and must be self-tested.

USE	MATERIAL	RATING	NOTES
Foundations	Concrete	A, B	If untreated, is usually acceptable for most people after curing. Concrete additives, however, may contain formaldehyde, petroleum oils, and detergents.

MATERIALS AND SELECTION

USE	MATERIAL	RATING	NOTES
Foundations (continued)	Glazed brick Concrete block Stone	A, B A, B A, B	If set with plain cement mortar masonry materials are usually free of contaminants. However, masonry foundations are more permeable than concrete to moisture and radon gas.
	Treated wood foundations	C	Contain wood preservatives which can introduce a large number of chemical offenders. In addition, they are difficult to seal against moisture.
Foundation coatings:	Cement based sealants	A, B	Contain no petroleum products. For most people usually acceptable for exterior use or interior patching. The acrylic additive often sold with this material should be used only if individual testing shows it to be acceptable. This has been found to be an effective and hypoallergenic sealant for concrete.
	5% silicone water repellent	B	Contains petroleum solvent. May be acceptable after curing or for exterior use.
	Asphalt emulsion	B	May be acceptable for exterior use underground, or where fully isolated from air intakes.
Building Frame	Reinforced concrete Masonry, brick, block, stone	A A	See the *Foundation notes.*

MATERIALS AND SELECTION

USE	MATERIAL	RATING	NOTES
Building Frame (continued)	Lightweight steel joist Lightweight steel stud Lightweight steel truss	A A A	May be coated with oily residue from factory which can be removed with detergent. Painted finishes should be self-tested for acceptability.
	Softwood lumber	B	Often contains preservatives. Tree resins are potential irritants. May be acceptable where fully isolated from the interior by a tight air barrier (See Construction Notes chapter.)
	Laminated lumber	C	Formaldehyde-based glues produce contamination.
Exterior Cladding (Siding)	Metal siding	A	Baked enamel finishes are usually quite stable.
	Stucco on metal lath	A	While plain stucco is usually acceptable to most people, some stucco mixes may contain acrylic additives and be placed on polystyrene foam outside insulation. Outgassed contamination from these products can enter through doors, windows, and cracks.
	Wood siding	B	Cedar, redwood, and pine are often acceptable when used outside. Be cautious as they do bother some. Avoid preserved wood siding which may contain PCP, mercury, or arsenic. Exterior paints and stains should be self-tested for acceptability.

MATERIALS AND SELECTION

USE	MATERIAL	RATING	NOTES
Exterior Cladding (continued)	Exterior plywood	B	Exterior-rated plywood is made with low formaldehyde-producing resins. It may be acceptable if confined to outside by a tight air/vapor barrier. (See Construction Notes chapter.)
	Chip board (Wafer board sheathing)	C	Contains large amounts of formaldehyde-based glue.
	Vinyl siding	C	Releases contaminating gases, such as vinyl chloride and plasticizers, particularly when heated.
	Asphalt shingles Asphalt sheathing paper Asphalt treated fiberboard	C C C	Release contaminating petroleum fumes, particularly when heated.
Exterior air barrier:	Untreated building paper Kraft paper	A A	Usually acceptable for this use. Such new materials as polyolefin have not yet been well tested for their chemical properties.
Roofing	Steel, galvanized Steel, painted Aluminum	A A A	Some may have oily residues from manufacturing which should be removed with detergent.
	Cement, clay, or metal tile	A	No reported problems.
	Wood shingles	B	While acceptable for many in their natural state, preservative treatments and fire retardants may render them unacceptable.

MATERIALS AND SELECTION

USE	MATERIAL	RATING	NOTES
Roofing (continued)	Asphalt shingles Tar and gravel Plastic or rubber membranes	C C C	Definitely release contaminants, particularly when heated.
Insulation	Foamed cement	B, C	This is a lightweight cement product that is foamed in place. The foaming agents in some formulations produce contaminants, however, and should be self-tested.
	Glass fiber batts Mineral fiber	B B	Usually acceptable when fully isolated from the interior. Fiber shedding, and formaldehyde or other compounds released from the binders produce contamination.
	Expanded mineral slag (vermiculite, etc.)	B	Though often acceptable, these are only suitable for horizontal surfaces. They also produce a fine dust which can enter the home if ceilings are not fully sealed.
	Cellulose fiber	C	Contains contaminating fire retardants, and produces fine dust
	Plastic resin foams (styrene, polyurethane, etc.)	C	May be acceptable only when buried as outside basement insulation.
	Urea Formaldehyde Foam	C	A very potent source of formaldehyde now banned for use in homes.

MATERIALS AND SELECTION

USE	MATERIAL	RATING	NOTES
Air/vapor barrier	Aluminum foil, paper backed foil	A	Adhesive backed foil tape is the least contaminating method of joining sheets. Do not use caulking compounds, if possible. Paper backed usually acceptable.
	Polyethylene sheet	B	May be acceptable to some if sealed behind an airtight inside finish. It will outgas, however, and may contain a large number of chemical additives for strength and durability.
	Vapor retarding paint	B	Latex paints are effective vapor barriers *as long as there is good coverage and very little air leakage through cracks.* Some find them acceptable once they have cured.
	Caulked systems (caulked polyethylene sheet, caulked drywall, etc.)	C	Large amounts of contaminating sealants used in these applications make them unadvisable.
Interior wall and ceiling covering	Plain plaster on metal lath Plain plaster on gypsum lath	A, B A, B	Gypsum lath may be unacceptable for some. Plaster additives and colorants can also introduce contamination.
	Brick, with plain, mortar joints	A	
	Solid hardwood paneling (maple, birch, alder, poplar, etc.)	A, B	A very costly option, but some hardwoods are acceptable for many. May be used unfinished or finished. (See *Paints* below.)

MATERIALS AND SELECTION

USE	MATERIAL	RATING	NOTES
Interior wall and ceiling covering (continued)	Gypsum board, taped and filled	B	Varies widely in composition from different manufacturers, and many unacceptable chemicals may be present in small quantities. Fillers may contain contaminating vinyl acetate and formaldehyde. (Special hypoallergenic fillers are available. See the section ENVIRONMENTAL ILLNESS AND YOU.)
	Solid softwood paneling (pine, cedar, spruce, fir)	B, C	These boards contain aromatic tree resins objectionable to some. Small amounts may be acceptable, particularly if well sealed with a finish, such as lacquer sealer.
	Brick veneer	B, C	Some are genuine brick. However, adhesives other than plain mortar can cause air contamination. Plastic brick is a source of air contamination.
	Interior plywoods	C	Glues in these are potent sources of formaldehyde, capable of producing 20 times as much contamination as exterior plywood glues.
	Prefinished interior paneling	C	Often vinyl coated, or treated with other objectionable plastics.
	Particle-board-based materials	C	Potent sources of formaldehyde contamination.
Floor systems Subfloor:	Reinforced concrete	A	See the *Foundations* notes, above.

MATERIALS AND SELECTION

USE	MATERIAL	RATING	NOTES
Subfloor: (continued)	Solid wood plank	B	Some woods may be acceptable, particularly if thoroughly covered. (Most hardwoods are.)
	Exterior plywood	B	Produces small amounts of formaldehyde. May be acceptable to many, particularly if sealed with an acceptable, self-tested finish, such as varnish.
Underlayment:			Underlayment will not be necessary if using the preferred floor finishes.
	Thin concrete, reinforced	A	This is an effective soundproof floor, and can be finished with tile or a cement finish. (See the Construction Notes chapter.)
	Exterior plywood	B	
	Exposure #1 particle board (showing stamp.)	B, C	Produce some formaldehyde but may be acceptable for some if used in small quantities. Edges and surfaces can be sealed with an acceptable, self-tested finish, such as varnish, to reduce out-gassing.
	Particle board (Other than Exposure #1 type.)	C	Potent sources of formaldehyde contamination.
Doors and windows Frames:	Metal	A	While acceptable for most
	Porcelain Steel	A	people, the gasket systems may
	Enamelled metal	B	produce contaminants and

MATERIALS AND SELECTION

USE	MATERIAL	RATING	NOTES
Frames: (continued)			offensive odors. These can be covered with foil tape (see *Air/vapor barrier,* above) or replaced with a more acceptable sealant, such as plain clear silicone. (See *Sealants,* above.)
	Solid hardwood	A	They may contain unacceptable glues, however.
	Solid softwood	B	May contain unacceptable glues and wood preservatives. Pine and other conifers not acceptable for the hypersensitive.
	Solid plastic	B, C	Made from fairly stable hard plastics which are relatively odor-free, but should be self-tested, particularly when warm.
Glass settings: (See *Sealants* above.)			
Adhesives, caulkings, and weatherstrip			
Adhesives:	White glue, yellow glue (water washable wood and paper glues)	A, B	Acceptable in small amounts for many. Contains acrylics, casein, and/or vinyl acetate, but no petroleum solvents.
	Hide glue (made from animal products)	A	From art supply stores. Has some limited uses for woodwork, but prone to mildew and moisture damage.
	Wallpaper glue	A, B	Starch-based wallpaper glue is widely acceptable; however, some commercial varieties contain unacceptable contaminating pesticides and fungus

USE	MATERIAL	RATING	NOTES
Adhesives: (continued)			retardants. Borax can be added to homemade starch glue to reduce mildew growth.
	Ceramic tile thin set mortar adhesive	A, B	A cement product acceptable to most. The acrylic additive sold with it should not be used.
	Ceramic wall tile adhesive (solvent-based)	B	Often acceptable, once cured, if thoroughly covered and sealed by the tile and grout. They contain toluene, benzene, naphtha, and other dangerous solvents, however, and must be handled with copious ventilation.
	Floor tile adhesive	B	See the Ceramic tile adhesive, above. (Water-based varieties are available from suppliers of hypoallergenic products. See the section ENVIRONMENTAL ILLNESS AND YOU.)
	Contact cement (solvent or latex based)	B	Acceptable for many when thoroughly cured and completely covered, as for applying hard plastic laminates to cabinets. Very dangerous to handle however; use outdoors where possible.
	Carpet adhesives	C	Similar to other solvent or latex adhesives, but because they are used over large surfaces and covered only by porous carpet they will outgas over long periods.

MATERIALS AND SELECTION

USE	MATERIAL	RATING	NOTES
Adhesives: (continued)	Construction adhesives Panel adhesives	C C	Sold in tubes and applied by a gun during construction. Virtually all will outgas for an extended period.
	Urea-based glues Plastic resin glue	C C	Potent sources of formaldehyde contamination in any application.
	Epoxy glue	C	Particularly hazardous and should be avoided. The hardeners are powerful oxidants, difficult to mix perfectly, and prolonged outgassing results.
	ABS solvent cement PVC solvent cement	C C	Glues for joining plastic pipe. Made from volatile solvents and plastic resins. Should not be used indoors, if possible. Small amounts may be acceptable where pipes are isolated from room air by a complete air/vapor barrier. (See Construction Notes chapter.)
Sealants:	Clear silicone (without additives)	A	Acceptable to most once curing is complete. The vapors from curing are temporarily troublesome but contain little or no petroleum solvent.
	Linseed oil putty Linseed oil caulking	A A	Contain oil of the flax seed, acceptable for many people. Not very durable, however, particularly for outdoor use.
	Silicone tub caulk	B, C	Contain mildew retardants, which are unacceptable to some people.

MATERIALS AND SELECTION

USE	MATERIAL	RATING	NOTES
Sealants: (continued)	Acoustic sealant	B, C	These common caulkings are petroleum-based, but may be acceptable to some people.
	Acrylic sealant	B	A latex type sealant, acceptable for some. Can be painted which may reduce outgassing.
	Butyl rubber sealant Polysulfide sealant	C C	Outgassing of petroleum solvents and lingering odors.
Weatherstrip:	Felt strip, metal bound	A	
	Hard vinyl strip	A	
	Soft plastic strip (vinyl or other)	B	
	Foamed plastic strip (white polyurethane or others)	B	Acceptable to some in small quantities, such as for door or window seals.
	Neoprene rubber strip (black sponge rubber)	C	Unacceptable due to lingering odors, and contains chlorinated hydrocarbons.

Table 22-2
FINISHING AND FURNISHING MATERIALS

USE	MATERIAL	RATING	NOTES
Paints, varnishes, polishes			These materials are described according only to paint *bases*. Paint *pigments* and other *additives* are also chemicals which vary widely between products. The suitability of each should be self-tested before selection.
	Baked enamels	B	Problematic for some when used in large amounts. Safe in small quantities.
	Casein paints Special Hypoallergenic paints	A A	Formulated from milk protein and other widely acceptable materials. (See the section, ENVIRONMENTAL ILLNESS AND YOU.) These may require addition of borax as a mildew retardant.
	Whitewash	A	Simply lime and water used as a paint, it is acceptable for most people, but is not durable.
	Natural walnut, natural olive oil	A	Safe wood finish for the hypersensitive, but may attract dust.
	Mineral oil	B	The petroleum product used in baby oil, it is acceptable for most people and makes a suitable finish for most woods and unfinished furniture. It requires periodic reapplication, however, as it is absorbed into the wood.

USE	MATERIAL	RATING	NOTES
Paints, varnishes, polishes (continued)	Natural shellac	B	A tree resin dissolved in alcohol that is acceptable for many people. Not very water or alcohol resistant, however, and unsuitable for wear surfaces, such as floors.
	Lacquer paints Lacquer wood sealer	B B	Acceptable for many after a brief curing period. Contain very volatile and toxic solvents and must be used with copious ventilation.
	Alkyd oil paint Linseed oil paint	B B	Acceptable for some after a lengthy curing period. Durable and suited to a wide range of uses, but contain petroleum solvents which outgas quite slowly. Extra heat and ventilation shorten curing time.
	Paste waxes	B	Many contain carnauba from palm trees, which is acceptable for most people. Also contain petroleum solvents which evaporate quickly, but may contain other unacceptable resins.
	Bees Wax	B	
	Urethane varnish	B	Some find this acceptable in small amounts once it is thoroughly cured. Its use on large surfaces, such as floors, should be avoided, however, due to long-term outgassing, especially when warmed. (See Solid hardwood flooring, below.)

USE	MATERIAL	RATING	NOTES
Paints, varnishes, polishes (continued)	Latex paints	B, C	A wide variety of formulations, all containing synthetic rubber and acrylics. These are the most common interior paints for all uses, and must be carefully self-tested. Outgassing of latex, colorants, mildew retardants, and other additives may continue indefinitely. Some reports note that adding 1½ cups of baking soda per gallon reduces objectionable odors.
	Furniture polish Danish oil finish	C C	Contain combinations of oils and solvents which can outgas for long periods.
	Liquid floor wax	C	Generally acrylic-based, and produce unacceptable outgassing for long periods.
	Epoxy paints Epoxy varnishes	C C	Produce large amounts of contamination for long periods.
Wall finishes			*Note:* See also interior wall and ceiling coverings.
	Some acceptable paints		See the *Paints,* above.
	Ceramic wall tile Wall tile grout	A A	See the *Adhesives,* above.
	Acceptable wallpaper Foil wallpaper (without Mylar)	B B	See the *Adhesives,* above.
	Vinyl wallpaper Self stick wallpaper	C C	Can produce vinyl and formaldehyde contamination,

USE	MATERIAL	RATING	NOTES
Wall finishes (continued)			plus various contaminants from the adhesive.
Floor coverings	Concrete Finishes	A, B	These dyes and waxes applied to the troweled concrete are maintained with colored paste wax. All should be carefully self-tested. Olive oil sealant safest for the hypersensitive.
	Ceramic tile in cement ("thin set") mortar (with cement type floor tile grout)	A	The most widely accepted and durable floor covering available. Acrylic additives sold with both the thin set type mortars and the grout should not be used by the chemically sensitive.
	Solid hardwood plank (maple, oak, beech, ash)	A	Widely accepted, durable. Urethane varnish, oil type or epoxy finishes are often unacceptable. A lacquer sealer, followed by a carnauba paste wax is durable and often acceptable. (Walnut oil best for the sensitive.)
	Wood parquet, wire bound	A	Parquet pieces come joined by staples or wire. Can be fastened with white or yellow wood glue (or other water soluble glue) if acceptable, and finished as hardwood plank floors. (See above.) Caution: May contain wood preservatives.
	Area rugs, untreated natural fibers	A	Cotton and wool rugs are acceptable for most people. Some may contain unacceptable chemical treatments, mothproofing, and dyes.

MATERIALS AND SELECTION

USE	MATERIAL	RATING	NOTES
Floor coverings (continued)	Area rugs, acetate or rayon fiber	A, B	Some of the synthetic fibers have been found acceptable, even for sensitive people.
	Ceramic tile fastened with adhesive	B	Some may be found acceptable, but they are not as durable as cement mortar settings.
	Parquet floors, pre-glued (or self-stick)	B	Adhesives used in these products will produce formaldehyde and other compounds. They may be partially sealed with paste wax to reduce outgassing.
	Synthetic carpets (nylon, polypropylene)	B, C	Sources of various contaminating gases, such as formaldehyde, toluene, xylene, and benzene. Glued or nailed down carpets also prevent necessary cleaning.
	Hard vinyl composition tile	B, C	Some of these materials are acceptable but should be carefully self-tested.
	Carpet pad, natural fiber	B	These may be allergenic for some people, They also collect dust.
	Carpet pad, foamed rubber, or plastic	C	Potent sources of air contamination.
	Soft vinyl tile Self-adhesive tile, no wax tile "Linoleum" sheet	C C C	Virtually all contain soft vinyl and other petroleum products which will outgas for long periods.

MATERIALS AND SELECTION

USE	MATERIAL	RATING	NOTES
Floor coverings (continued)	Simulated wood flooring	C	These prefinished sheets are made from particle board, a potent source of formaldehyde.
Cabinets	Metal frame and doors	A	Enamelled metal cabinets are durable, stable, washable, and relatively inexpensive.
	Ceramic tile tops and wall coverings	A	See *Interior wall and ceiling covering,* above.
	Solid wood frames and doors	A, B	Hardwoods and some finished (sealed) softwoods are acceptable for many people. Lacquer sealer followed by paste wax finishes are acceptable to many. Plain mineral oil can also be used.
	Hard plastic laminate tops ("Formica," "Arborite.")	B	Often acceptable, but only after the contact cement has cured.
	Exterior plywood frame and doors Exposure #1 rated particle board	B, C B, C	Produce small amounts of formaldehyde. They may be acceptable in small quantities, particularly if careful attention is paid to sealing all their surfaces and edges with hard plastic laminates or varnish, shellac or lacquer. (See *Paints,* above.)
	Interior grade plywood Hardwood veneered "cabinet stock" Standard particle board	C C C	Produce large amounts of formaldehyde. Particle board is by far the worst offender as it contains the most glue.
	Vinyl "Imitation wood" panels	C	Produce vinyl and formaldehyde contamination.

USE	MATERIAL	RATING	NOTES
Upholstery and furniture			
Frames:	Metal	A	Painted metals should be self-tested for acceptability.
	Hardwoods (maple, oak, birch, alder, ash, beech, mahogany, cherry, walnut, etc.)	A	The glues in solid wood furniture frames are unacceptable to a few people; they are present in only small quantities.
	Softwoods (pine, spruce, fir, cedar, cypress, larch, Philippine mahogany, etc.)	B, C	Contain tree resins which may make them unacceptable to some people. Some are acceptable if sealed with paint, varnish, or lacquer. (See *Paints*, above.)
	Exterior plywood	B	See the *Cabinets* notes, above.
	Exposure #1 type particle board	B	
	Standard particle board	C	See the *Cabinets* notes, above.
Fillings:	Natural fibers (untreated cotton, wool, jute, silk.)	A	Acceptable to most people.
	Metal springs	A	Acceptable when used in combination with natural fibers. But metal spring constructions are often padded with urethane foam or other plastic resin foams which are unacceptable, particularly in direct contact with the skin.

USE	MATERIAL	RATING	NOTES
Fillings: (continued)	Animal products, (feathers, down, hair.)	C	These are allergenic materials adversely affecting many people. Some find down products acceptable if covered with a suitable "barrier cloth". (See *Covers,* below.)
	Polyurethane foams Styrene foam chips Foamed rubber	C C C	These are all potent sources of contamination.
Covers:	Cotton "barrier" cloth	A	This is a specially woven cotton which allows some air and moisture to pass, while blocking allergenic materials, such as down, dust, feathers or mites.
	Untreated natural fiber fabric (cotton, wool, silk, linen.)	A	Acceptable to most people, even with direct skin contact.
	Acetate, rayon	B	Based on cellulose derived from natural fibers, such as cotton. They are acceptable to many people, though dyes and other treatments may make them unacceptable.
	Natural leather	B	Natural, undyed, hide covers are acceptable to many people, but tanning odors may contain hazardous formaldehyde.
	Nylon and polyester fibers	C	Made from plastic resins and may be irritating to skin. The outgassing of their plastic components, and their mildew, fire, stain, and crease resistant treatments make them unacceptable.

USE	MATERIAL	RATING	NOTES
Covers: (continued)	Vinyl fabrics, imitation leather	C	Potent sources of air contamination due to the outgassing of plastic products, particularly when exposed to sun and heat.
Bedding	Natural cotton filled futon Cotton and spring mattress	A A	The most widely available hypoallergenic mattresses. But check labels for possible fire or mildew resistant treatments which will make them unacceptable to some. Cotton batting must be washable and pre-washed.
	Silk covers Cotton "barrier cloth" covers Natural cotton, wool, or silk filling	A A A	See the *Upholstery* notes, above.
	Acetate, rayon fabrics	B	See the *Upholstery* notes, above.
	Animal products (feathers, down, hair.)	C	See the *Uphostery* notes, above.
	Vinyl mattress covers	C	Can be highly irritating and they reduce the capacity of fabrics to "breathe."
	Polyester fibers Polyurethane foam filling Foamed rubber or plastic	C C C	See the *Upholstery* notes, above.
Decorative materials	Metal, glass, ceramics	A	The safest types.
	Enamelled metals Porcelain enamelled metals Cotton, wool, silk	A B A	 May have objectionable odors. See *Furnishing* notes above.

MATERIALS AND SELECTION

USE	MATERIAL	RATING	NOTES
Decorative materials (continued)	Hardwoods	A	See the *Furnishing* notes, and *Paints,* above.
	Softwoods	B	See the *Furnishing* notes, and *Paints,* above.
	Wicker, reeds, grasses	B	Sometimes allergenic on contact but acceptable for many. May contain unacceptable fungicide, resins, or varnishes.
	Paper products	B	Often acceptable in small quantities. Books, newspapers, and art, however, may be unacceptable in quantity, or on contact. Ink and paint outgassing diminishes with time. (Also contribute to mold and dust allergy.)
	Hard plastics, plastic laminates ("Formica," "Arborite")	B	See the *Cabinets* notes.
	Hard nylon	B	Made from polyamide resin, and generally acceptable in small quantities.
	Soft plastics Thermoplastics	C C	Less stable than the hard plastics and will outgas chemical components.
	P.V.C. plastic A.B.S. plastic Polyester resin (fiberglass products, clear plastic castings)	C C C	Contain vinyl chloride, styrene, acrylonitrile, plasticizers, hardeners, and other chemicals known to be toxic or carcinogenic to humans.
	Acrylic resin ("Plexiglas," "Lucite")	C	Irritating to sensitive people even in minute quantities.

Table 22-3
PLUMBING, ELECTRICAL, HEATING, AND APPLIANCES

USE	MATERIAL	RATING	NOTES
Plumbing			
Supply piping:	Copper pipe with mechanical joints, such as "flared" type, or lead free solder	A	The most acceptable piping system and contains no lead.
	Copper pipe (lead soldered joints)	B	Most common piping. Contains lead solder, making it more prone to water contamination (due to electrochemical reactions with chlorine and minerals) than the mechanical joint or lead free system.
	Galvanized steel pipe	B	Is lined with zinc, which is toxic in large quantities. Zinc can enter the water via chemical reactions with chlorine and minerals carried in water. Also leaches cadmium.
	P.V.C. pipe (cold water use) C.P.V.C. pipe (hot water use)	C C	Contain vinyl chloride (a human carcinogen) which contaminates water in the pipes. Often used for public water supply. In some regions approved for indoor use by local codes.
	Polybutylene tubing	C	These flexible plastics are approved in many regions for inside piping. As their chemical properties are not well tested they should be avoided for both drinking and bathing water.

MATERIALS AND SELECTION

USE	MATERIAL	RATING	NOTES
Drains and vents:	Copper and brass pipe Iron pipe	A A	Stable materials, preferred for indoor use. However, they are costly, and require intensive labor to install.
	A.B.S. pipe	B	Contains acrylonitrile, vinylethylene, and styrene, which contaminate indoor air, particularly when it is heated. Usually acceptable if sealed inside walls and floors. (See the chapter Construction Notes.)
Fixtures:	Stainless steel Porcelain Enamelled steel Enamelled cast iron	A A A A	All highly stable materials.
	Fiberglass Cultured marble	C C	Both made with polyester resin and various hardeners and additives which outgas and contaminate air and water. Also less durable than steel fixtures.
Electrical System			
Wiring:	Steel conduit (E.M.T. or rigid type)	A	These isolate plastic-jacketed wire from room air. May also reduce electromagnetic fields in the home. Though a preferred wiring method, oily coatings on the tubing may be objectionable, and must be removed with detergent.
	Metallic sheated cable	A	Has a solid aluminum jacket and offers the advantages of steel conduit (above) at a lower cost.

MATERIALS AND SELECTION

USE	MATERIAL	RATING	NOTES
	Armored "flex" cable (BX type)	B	May be acceptable when sealed in walls, but contains oils and plastics which will easily penetrate its porous jacket and cause air contamination.
	Vinyl- and nylon-jacketed cable Mineral/asphalt-jacketed cable	B B	May be acceptable when sealed in walls, but contain vinyl, petroleum tar, and other products which outgas and contaminate air.
Boxes and cover plates:	Steel	A	The safest material, both for health and fire safety.
	P.V.C., A.B.S., and hard plastics	C	Electrical boxes cannot be effectively sealed in the wall and isolated from room air. Contain resins and other contaminating chemicals.
Lamps:	Metal and glass sealed fixtures (vapor-proof fixtures)	A	Designed airtight for damp locations, minimize fried dust, or plastic outgassing. Incandescent are best.
	Metal and glass recessed fixtures	A	Designed for recessed mounting in ceilings and should be ventilated to the outdoors.
	Compact fluorescents	A, B	Operate at low temperatures and will not fry dust. Some models are all metal construction.
	Conventional fluorescent fixtures	B	Can be acceptable for some uses, but often contain many plastic parts which will outgas.

MATERIALS AND SELECTION

USE	MATERIAL	RATING	NOTES
Lamps: (continued)	Bulbs enclosed in glass shades (incandescent types)	B	Widely acceptable if the lamp is isolated from room dust.
	Exposed light bulbs (incandescent types)	C	Likely to fry dust and aggravate allergy problems.
Heating/cooling systems	Radiant systems (hot water radiators, liquid filled electric radiators, ceiling mounted radiant electric, portable radiant electric)	A	Can provide excellent comfort while minimizing the stirring and frying of airborne dust.
	Central electric boilers	A	These compact devices can be located indoors to supply radiators.
	Electric water heaters	A, C	Glass-lined tanks are relatively hazard-free. A few have plastic-lined tanks, however, which are serious contaminants.
	Heat pumps, outside mounted	A	Can either heat or cool liquids circulated through the home. Locating them outside minimizes the possibility of leaking refrigerants (chlorofluorocarbons) entering the home. Be sure no insulation in heating chamber.
	Boilers, outside mounted (fuel burning boilers)	A	Fuel burning boilers can be fully isolated from the home to prevent fuels or combustion gases entering.

USE	MATERIAL	RATING	NOTES
Heating/Cooling systems (continued)	Electronic air filters	B	Acceptable for many when operating properly, but if poorly maintained can produce ozone and release trapped dust into air.
	Room air conditioners Heat pumps, indoors	B B	Acceptable for many, but can leak contaminating refrigerants into the home.
	Electric baseboard heaters (conventional type)	B	Acceptable for some people, though they stir and fry airborne dust. Oil coatings on new units produce highly irritating fumes when they are first used. Turn on new installations only with full ventilation.
	Electric furnaces (warm air type)	B	These forced air systems fry dust and spread contamination between rooms.
	Induced draft furnaces (gas or oil)	B	Designed for airtight, energy-efficient homes, with a small fan to ensure that combustion gases will not enter the home. More acceptable indoors if enclosed in an airtight furnace room to reduce the risk of fuel vapor entering living areas.
	Gas fired water heaters	B	Acceptable for many people if connected to a safe chimney on the outside.

USE	MATERIAL	RATING	NOTES
Heating/Cooling systems (continued)	Wood stoves, fireplaces	C	Release dangerous combustion gases, including carcinogenic benzopyrene, which pollute outside air and can enter the home. Wood stoves fry dust, and can overheat interior wall and floor surfaces, increasing fire hazards and outgassing of building materials.
	Oil or gas furnaces, indoor (forced air type)	C	Can leak fuel, release combustion gases, fry dust, and spread contamination between rooms.
	Humidifiers/dehumidifiers (See the *Heating* chapter.)	B, C	These can introduce mold and bacterial contamination into the home, or spread chlorine or minerals from water into the air.
	Heating and ventilation ducts	A, C	Sheet metal ducting with adequate cleaning access is the only acceptable system. (See the Home Heating chapter.) Fiberglass ducts and fibrous duct liners contaminate air with gases and fibers.
Appliances			
Kitchen:	Electric ranges	A	The safest type if vented outside with an exhaust fan.
	Steamers, slow cookers	A	

USE	MATERIAL	RATING	NOTES
Kitchen: (continued)	Microwave ovens	A, B	Produce minimal contamination, though there is a small risk of microwave radiation, particularly with older or damaged units.
	Refrigerators, outdoor pump	A	Commercial refrigerators have a separate motor and pump which can be located outdoors to reduce contamination from oils and refrigerants.
	Refrigerators (conventional type)	B	Metal- and glass-lined refrigerators are safest. Some sensitive people react to the plastic parts and oily fumes. There is also possibility of refrigerant leaks.
	Toaster, countertop ovens	B	Acceptable to some, but require the same ventilation as an electric range.
	Blenders, mixers, food processors	B	Contain brush type motors which produce irritating ozone and oil fumes. Though acceptable for some, should be used with ventilation.
	Gas ranges	C	Serious sources of air contamination and small gas leaks. If they must be used, operate them only with an exhaust fan and an open window. Electronic ignition types and ceramic burner insert types are slightly better.

MATERIALS AND SELECTION

USE	MATERIAL	RATING	NOTES
Laundry machines:	Electric dryers, outside vented	A	
	Electric dryers, inside vented	B	Inside venting is sometimes done for humidification and energy savings, but odors and fried dust will be unacceptable to some. Fabric softeners and anti-cling chemicals can be serious irritants to sensitive people and should not be used, particularly with inside vents.
	Automatic washers	B	Though acceptable to most, they produce oily fumes and detergent odors. Select laundry soaps carefully to reduce this hazard.
	Irons	B	Produce fumes from heated fabrics during use that are objectionable to some people.
Miscellaneous:	Induction type electric motors	A	Commonly found on fans, pumps, and other small machines. They produce little irritating ozone or oil fumes.
	Brush type electric motors	B	Commonly found on hand tools and other small machines, with vent slots on the side through which sparks can be seen while in operation. Produce ozone and irritating oil fumes which make them unacceptable for some. Also produce electromagnetic radiation.
	Hair dryers	C	Produce large amounts of fried dust, oily fumes, and ozone.

Materials Selection

A fundamental principle of the health conscious home is careful selection of all materials included in it, so as to minimize indoor contamination and the resulting health hazards. This is particularly critical for the environmentally sensitive, who may react dramatically to tiny amounts of specific contaminants.

After our diet, exercise, and health habits, the most important health influences encountered in the home are the materials that contact our bodies, and those found in the air we breathe. Contact items include underclothing, clothing, bedding, water, soaps, personal hygiene products, and, to some extent, furnishings. The major sources of air contamination within the home are smoking, combustion products of fireplaces, wood stoves, and gas appliances, including cookstoves, furnaces, and clothes dryers, building and finishing materials, household cleaning, maintenance, pest control materials, and natural radiation.

Once you have become aware of the need for environmental change, a useful strategy is to begin with intimate items, such as clothing and bedding. At the same time, it is wise to consider such obvious sources of air contamination as urea formaldehyde insulation, gas stoves, attached garages, and the presence of fungus. Many of these can be temporarily reduced by improved ventilation until the permanent changes can be made. By using this approach you may get some relief, rest better, and prepare yourself for the bigger changes.

Testing Materials

First read the label: If there is a label, and it lists any contents with which you are not familiar, or which you have doubts about, do some checking first. (See the GETTING HELP section for a list of resources and information.)

When selecting materials, it is important to understand the two distinct types of responses to environmental contaminants: First, the rapid reactions, such as eye, skin, or nasal/bronchial irritation, difficulty in breathing, faintness, nausea, and heart rhythm changes. Then, the latent reactions, such as long term weakness, increased common illnesses, sensitization, organ disorders, and cancer risks.

The first group of reactions is rapidly and relatively easily identified, and so can often be linked to specific contaminants in the environment. These reactions form the basis of personal challenge testing (see below). The second group consists of latent or subtle reactions, which are much harder to identify and link with environmental contaminants. Examples of these are undetected radiation, pesticides, asbestos, toxic metals, and other agents which pose long term threats to health and life without causing immediate symptoms. Identifying and eliminating these will require some preparation and research, and sometimes professional help, as well. (See the GETTING HELP section.)

PERSONAL CHALLENGE TESTING

For those healthy individuals who are concerned with prevention, a simple "sniff test" and some variations of it are all that is generally required to make intelligent choices about building and furnishing materials. If a sample of a tested material seems offensive in any way, then a bed made from it, or a room full of it, is clearly not acceptable. Remember also that you, or someone you live with, may become more sensitive or reactive to it with time.

For those experiencing environmental sensitivity, a much more complex procedure must be followed under the guidance of a trained professional, such as a clinical ecologist or general practitioner trained in clinical ecology. See the section ENVIRONMENTAL ILLNESS AND YOU.

The basic sniff test:

• First "clear" your senses by taking a walk outside or breathing deeply near an open window. It will, of course, be necessary to do this in a relatively unpolluted setting. Inside a fabric, furniture, or building supply store is generally not a good place to sample material, due to the presence of many conflicting odors.

• Briefly hold a sample of the material in question to your nose and sniff.

• Repeat the "clearing" procedure before sniffing each sample.

If there are peculiar or offensive odors, or symptoms of reactions, then this material should be considered very doubtful for use. If the material is a paint, adhesive, caulking compound, or any other product which is expected to cure or age rapidly, the following steps should identify any problem materials. Repeat the sniff test procedure with a sample which has cured for the period of time which you would consider reasonable to allow for its cure in your household. Remember that you may have to avoid the material during its curing period. Anywhere from five to thirty days, for example, might be an acceptable time to avoid a room in your house while paint dries. Remember, too, that the *conditions* under which a material cures must be appropriate for its intended use. Paint samples dried outdoors in the sun, or adhesives set in the oven, do not necessarily represent the state these materials will attain in actual use. If the material is a washable fabric, wash a sample of it a few times before sniff testing or testing it against your skin.

If the material fails the sniff test after curing or washing, reject it for indoor use.

Further sniff tests:

• Test a sample as above, but heat it first to the highest temperature that it might attain in service. This is particularly important for those paints, floor coverings, and finished materials which might be exposed to sunlight, heaters, or light fixtures during their actual use.

• Place a small sample of a bedding or clothing fabric which has been moistened with water in a clean glass jar with a tight fitting glass or metal lid. Place it in a warm place for a day or two, then open it and sniff. This is particularly effective for revealing fabric treatments, such as those containing formaldehyde, which can react with body moisture and become irritants. If the material fails this test, it is not appropriate for bedding or clothing.

Skin contact testing: Fabrics intended for clothing, bedding, or upholstery which have passed the "sniff" test can be tested further for skin contact. Place a sample of the material on your pillow at night and sleep on it, or "wear" it under your clothing against your skin for a few hours. If the material fails this further test, it is not appropriate for these uses.

WARNING: Persons experiencing symptoms of environmental sensitivity should not undertake any testing without the guidance of a health care professional. For these persons, a complex guided testing regime may be necessary, requiring a period of avoidance of contaminants and recovery before proceeding further.

Remember that the second category of environmental hazards produce no odors or symptoms. These will require time, skill, and sometimes professional advice to identify. For detailed information, refer to the chapter Testing for Contamination, in the GETTING HELP section.

SECTION VI

Environmental Illness and You

23 ENVIRONMENTAL ILLNESS

William J. Rea, M.D., F.A.C.S., F.A.A.E.M.

To understand illness, one must look at the environmental aspects of health and disease, since many things in our environment can trigger or influence them. Environmental illness is a disease process primarily triggered by environmental over-exposure. Classic examples would be asbestosis, black lung, mercury poisoning, and formaldehyde sensitivity. Three general categories of environmental factors can be triggers of ill health:

Physical Factors: These include heat, cold, weather cycles, positive and negative ions, electromagnetic radiation (including light), noise, and ionizing radiation (radioactivity).

Chemical Factors: These include (a) inorganic substances, such as lead, mercury, cadmium, aluminum, arsenic, asbestos, chlorine, nitrous oxides, sulfur dioxide, ozone, beryllium, nickel, copper, and many others; (b) organic substances, among which some of the more common toxic ones are formaldehyde, benzenes, toluene, xylene, and many other substances derived from gas and oil, chlorinated compounds, including organochlorine pesticides, chloroform, trihalomethane, pentachlorophenols, polychlorinated biphenyls (PCBs), and various herbicides; other substances like organophosphates, pesticides like malathion, parathion, carbamates and pyrethrins, and thousands of others.

Biological Factors: These include bacteria, viruses, fungi (molds), parasites, foods, animal dander, and some dusts and pollens.

WHAT IS CHEMICAL SENSITIVITY?

One prominent aspect of environmentally triggered disease is chemical sensitivity. This is defined as an adverse reaction to low levels of toxic chemicals which are generally believed to be subtoxic (i.e. not harmful) in air, food, and water. How these adverse reactions are manifested will depend on: (1) which tissues or organs of the body are involved, (2) the toxicity and pharmacologic nature of the substance(s) involved, (3) the exposed individual's susceptibility (i.e. his or her nutritional state, genetic makeup, and toxic load at the time of exposure), and (4) the length of time, and amount and variety of

Dr. Rea has been a specialist in both heart disease and environmental medicine for over twenty years. He and his research team use a specially designed, controlled environment that is considered the most advanced in the world. In his research and treatment center he works with a team of physicians and surgeons from many specialties, and research scientists in immunology, biochemistry, physics, psychology and pollutant chemistry. As well as helping the environmentally ill, they have found over the last twenty years that the average "normal" individual benefits markedly with the removal of pollutants from the person's environment. With an uncontaminated environment, they have seen improved brain function, increased vigor, improved resistance to viral infections, and retarding of the aging process.

other body stresses (total body pollutant burden). There can also be complications from reactions to combinations of exposures (synergism).

Chemical sensitivity or any environmental sensitivity can be triggered by three types of exposure:

Massive exposure: This occurs in cases of industrial catastrophe, such as the one that occurred in Bhopal, India. It may also occur in wartime, such as the nerve gas exposure during W.W. I, or the herbicide exposure during the Vietnam War.

Chronic exposure: This kind of exposure occurs where there is chronic accumulation of environmental incitants over a long period of time. (For example, exposure in the workplace or the home to formaldehyde.)

Exposure with infection or massive injury: This occurs after a viral or bacterial infection, or another non-related, massive injury.

SYMPTOMS OF ENVIRONMENTAL SENSITIVITY

Environmental sensitivity is usually manifested in the major organ systems, especially those related to the smooth muscle (respiratory, gastrointestinal, neuro-cardiovascular, genito-urinary) systems, and the skin. There are usually a variety of symptoms, depending on the specific toxicity of the substances, the severity of the exposure, the number of organs involved, and the patient's individual susceptibility. One can often experience early signs of environmental overload before the specific fixed named disease occurs.

There is a period of opportunity, between optimum health and identifiable end-organ diseases, when one can reverse or prevent end-organ failure. This time span can occur days, weeks, or years before a recognized disease occurs. Early symptoms and signs may be unexplained weakness, temperature intolerance (especially to cold), unexplained swelling of eyes, hands, feet, spontaneous bruising, "floaters" in the eyes, and little red spots in the skin that look like freckles (petechiae). One's judgment and perceptions may be subtly impaired, as indicated by clumsiness, recent memory loss, and inability to remember numbers. Yellowness of skin that is not jaundice, sudden passing out, sluggishness after eating, irritability, extreme fatigue, and intolerance to medication and alcohol may also occur.

Individuals with environmental sensitivity may experience aggravated problems after childbirth or surgery. Joint and muscle aches and pains, unexplained heart irregularities, bloating and gas, recurrent respiratory and throat infections, food intolerances, and many other symptoms may be present.

UNDERSTANDING ENVIRONMENTAL ASPECTS OF HEALTH AND DISEASE

There are four principles involved in understanding the effects of the environment on health and disease.

The first is the *total body burden or load.* This is the total number of incitants (i.e., environmental factors which contribute to disease) that the body has taken in at a given time. Total load not only consists of the previously stated physical, chemical, and biological contaminants in air, food, and water, but also the emotional, psychological, and spiritual state of the individual.

The fact that this load fluctutates on a daily basis explains why an individual can at times be very tolerant in his environment and at other times be almost totally intolerant.

The second principle is the *masking* (*acute toxicological tolerance*) or *adaptation* phenomenon. Masking is the situation occurring when a person gets so "used to" an incitant that he fails to make a connection between cause and effect. For example, when a dangerous contaminant with a foul odor enters and stays in one's environment, if nothing changes, after a period of time one gets used to it and does not smell the odor any more. The contaminant may then continue its toxic effects, increasing the total body burden without one's being aware of it. Masking appears to be a short term "trade-off" for survival, with an accompanying long term cost. This cost may occur soon after exposure, or 20–30 years later, as the body becomes overburdened with contaminants. One example is tobacco smoking, which eventually results in heart and blood vessel diseases, lung failure, and cancer, and/or skin diseases. Long term exposure to car exhausts causing kidney failure in auto mechanics, is another example. Exclusively eating refined, low fiber foods, resulting in hemorrhoids, constipation, and colon cancer, is yet another. Anyone suffering exposure to "masked" incitants can establish the cause by avoiding the suspected substance for 3–5 days. If this avoidance test is done, reexposure to the suspected offender, be it food, chemical, or electromagnetic exposure (e.g., high voltage power lines), will give a clearly defined reaction. This test can be reproduced as many times as needed to conclusively establish cause and effect. Care must be taken to distinguish between the initial *withdrawal symptoms*, which occur after avoidance, and the actual *reactions to the incitant itself*. The initial symptoms are similar to the well-known, classical withdrawal symptoms which occur after removing drugs from an addict, alcohol from an alcoholic, or food from a food addict.

The third principle of environmental exposure is *bipolarity*. Here the body's immune and non-immune detoxifying systems are activated after exposure to incitants. These body defense systems respond to combat substances that they identify as a threat by their chemical "fingerprint". The first phase of response is an active period of detoxification by both the immune and non-immune (enzyme) systems. This *stimulatory phase* may last for minutes, hours, months, or years, depending on the virulence or toxicity, length and volume of exposure to the substance(s) involved, and the quantity of nutrient fuels available to respond. However, once the response systems become depleted, a *depressed phase* follows, allowing first early symptoms, and then clearly identifiable diseases to occur.

This depressed phase should not be confused with withdrawal syptoms. Withdrawal symptoms probably occur as a result of the sudden removal of the incitant(s), which causes the slow turn-off of the detoxifying systems. The changes in the body during this period are recognizable as classic withdrawal. The depressive phase, on the other hand, is due to the depletion of the body's response system, and will result in organ dysfunction and organ failure. Withdrawal from alcohol, for example, may give headache, muscle pains, and all the syptoms of a hangover for the first few days. The depressive phase of alcohol exposure, on the other hand, results in psychosis and liver failure.

Often, a stimulatory phase of the brain occurs paralleling the stimulatory phase of the immune and non-immune systems. During this period, a person may develop a "high," and not recognize that the substance(s) that produce the reaction are harmful to him or her. Because the substance is not perceived as harmful, the person will allow repeated exposures to the substance, causing an increase in total body load. When an individual is first completely removed from the substance, he may get extremely uncomfortable and seek out more exposures to stave off further withdrawal symptoms. This is easy to recognize as the pattern occurring with all addictive phenomena. People may also seek out other addictive (termed "cross-reacting") substances in order to stave off their addiction withdrawal symptoms. They may begin drinking soft drinks, eating junk foods, or specific foods to which they are sensitive and which often exaggerate their reactive responses.

The final principle necessary to the understanding of the environmental aspects of health and disease is *biochemical individuality.* Biochemical individuality is our uniqueness and accounts for our individual susceptibility. No two individuals are exactly alike. We have individually differing quantities of carbohydrates, fats, proteins, enzymes, vitamins, minerals, and immune parameters with which to respond to environmental factors. This individuality either allows us to clear the body of noxious substances or contributes to our body burden.

The biochemical individuality of each of us is dependent on at least three factors: genetic makeup; the state of the fetus's nutritional health and toxic body burden during pregnancy; and the individual's toxic body burden in relation to his or her nutritional state at the time of exposure. For example, due to these variable some individuals are born with significantly smaller quantities than normal of a specific enzyme (ranging from 25% to 75%). While he or she may be able to respond to an environmental stimulant, this response is often considerably less adequate than that of the individual who was born with 100% of the specific enzyme and immune defenses. There are over 2,000 genetic metabolic defects already described in the research literature that appear to be "time bombs," awaiting environmental triggers to elicit their expression. The odds are high that any given individual may have one or more of these genetic defects. A common example of the "time bomb" effect is provided by children with phenylketonuria (P.K.U.) who appear to be healthy only if they do not take in phenylalanines, but due to genetic causes are unable to effectively cope with the common phenylalanines group of amino acids. If they take in too much food containing phenylalanine (e.g., milk, egg proteins), their overloaded systems allow brain damage to occur.

HOW BODY MECHANISMS RESPOND TO POLLUTANTS

The body mechanisms which respond to pollutant overload are the immune system and the enzyme detoxification system. The immune system involves the gamma globulins, such as the immunoglobins IgE, IgG, IgA, IgM, and IgD. It also includes both T & B lymphocytes, phagocytes, macrophages, eosinophils, mast cells, and basophils. These are all specific immune devices carried in the blood system. Any or all of them can be involved in the body's response to environmental exposure. The enzyme detoxification system is a chemical reaction which can occur within any cell, and which generally fits into four categories. The first three are oxidation, reduction, and degradation. These are chemical processes which affect foreign substances, and which are also involved in food breakdown, while the last general category, conjugation, appears to be almost exclusively for eliminating foreign substances. The fact that three of these mechanisms respond to both foreign substances and foods, partially explains why an individual who is exposed to toxic chemicals may also become sensitive and intolerant to foods.

One needs nutrients to keep these systems running efficiently. Once nutrients become depleted, these systems cease to function effectively, and toxic buildup will increase total body load, causing dysfunction and disease. Environmental pollutants may damage these detoxification systems in several ways:

1) They may sensitize one's immune system, causing excessive reaction to minor exposures.

2) They may cause malfunction of one's immune system due to nutrient depletion. Such depletion may occur in the following ways:

– By *over-utilizing the available nutrients* when the immune system is kept active by increased load.

– By *competitive absorption,* occurring when the incitant is selectively absorbed, instead of the necessary nutrient.

– By *selective malabsorption,* occurring when the incitant has caused damage to the enzyme system, reducing its ability to absorb certain necessary nutrients.

– By *selective nutrient depletion,* occurring when the diet does not contain adequate amounts of certain nutrients as a result of food addictions, or of monotonous or highly selective diets.

CONTAMINATION OF AIR, FOOD, AND WATER

By virtue of the increased population and technology of the 20th century, we all are severely exposed to environmental contamination in our air, food, and water.

Air Pollution: Studies done by the U.S. Environmental Protection Agency (EPA) show that there has been no fresh air in the U.S. for 20 years. Today, the best air available is found at certain sea shores, mountain tops, and in unpopulated areas, such as deserts. Using this air as a reference, the pollution gradient increases sometimes by thousands of times in cities, depending upon weather conditions, polluting industries, number of automobiles, and surrounding agricultural practices (spraying, fertilizing).

The major environmental inorganic chemical outdoor air contaminants are *car-*

bon monoxide (mostly from car exhausts); *ozone* generated from the action of sunlight on air pollution caused by burning of fossil fuels (coal, gas and oil); *nitrous oxides* occurring from burning of fossil fuels (coal, gas, oil); *sulfur dioxides* coming from refineries, cars, sour gas fields, catalytic converters; *particulates* coming from silicon compounds, pollen, molds, hydrocarbon particles; and *lead* coming from leaded gas, paint, and factory emissions. Electromagnetic pollution from radar, radios, and T.V. stations, power plants, and power lines, is also present. Organic chemical pollutants come from car exhausts, industries releasing pesticides, and other chemicals, fertilizers, cattle, and the natural biologic production of gases such as methane.

Indoor pollution has been discussed in several chapters of this book. The main health offenders are as follows: fossil fuel heat (gas, oil, coal, wood); pesticides, formaldehydes, synthetic materials (carpet, mattresses, foam rubber, plastics); T.V. sets, electric blankets, incoming power cables and electric power outlets, and other electric devices.

Food: Food can cause problems due to the natural toxicity of the food itself, such as potato skins; inadequate nutrient value and contamination, due to widespread farming with the use of pesticides on unbalanced, artificially fertilized soils; the addition of preservatives and additives, which, according to EPA studies, are contained in 100% of commercial foods; and food sensitivity.

Water: U.S. drinking water is probably now as contaminated with toxic chemicals, as it was 75 years ago with bacteria and viruses. This is partially due to chlorination and other treatments, but it is also due to contamination of its sources. Most drinking water is recycled in some way, coming from sources already contaminated by industry or agriculture. If it comes from rivers, one gets all the wastes from upstream. If it comes from reservoirs, one will have the agricultural runoff of pesticides, herbicides, defoliants, and fertilizers. If the water comes from wells, they may contain runoff from toxic waste dumps (of which there are over 60,000 in the U.S.), or factory dumps, or agricultural runoff. Some waters also contain a small amount of radiation from natural sources.

PREVENTION AND TREATMENT

Once one understands the facts and principles in evaluating the effects of the environment on the individual, one can proceed with prevention and treatment. *Avoidance of as many pollutants as possible is the first step in prevention and treatment.* This can be done by controlling, as much as possible, the indoor environment, the air, and food contaminants. For example, as has been discussed in this book, avoidance of combustion heating or cooking (with oil, gas, coal, wood) in the house is important. Thousands of patients suffering from environmental exposure have found that gas heat was keeping them ill. It is better to avoid these devices or keep them outside, using a boiler with piped-in water for central and local heat. The routine spraying of pesticides and herbicides is another factor that can cause severe problems. Most of these are nerve toxins which can make people anxious, depressed, or hyperactive. They can also cause headaches, instability, and mood surges. Household cleanliness, steam cleaning, and local cleaning treatment with borax and other safe techniques will often control the problems and minimize the need for chemicals. The presence of *formaldehyde and other chemicals in pressboard, plywood, foam rubber synthetic carpets, and other items is a major problem*. Environmentally sensitive people suffer heart irregularities, transient strokes, recurrent bladder problems, premenstrual syndrome, asthma, bronchitis, and diarrhea, with exposure to these. Metal and hardwood furniture and floors will often solve these problems. Mattresses which are made of foam or have foam for fire proofing can cause severe problems. If one wakes up in the morning feeling tired, stuffed up, "headachy," and swollen, it might be due to the mattress. Dyes in the rugs, drapes, and furniture may be a severe problem, especially the darker azotic chemical dyes. Pastels and white colors tend to be less toxic. Natural fibers are recommended as long as they are not moth proofed, permanent press, or otherwise chemically treated.

One's food should be as little chemically contaminated as possible, as fresh as possible, and grown on soils that are highly nutritive. As large a variety as possible should be eaten. A rotating diet, eating the same food no more than one day out of every four, is necessary for treatment, but it is also a good measure for preventing new sensitivities. Variety will put less strain on the specific immune and enzyme detoxification system elements, allowing them to be at their optimum at all times. We have seen thousands of patients who are sensitive to the additives and preservatives in foods, as well as being specifically sensitive to some of the foods themselves. *Not only drinking, but bathing water should be treated to be less polluted*, as some studies are showing a high skin absorption of toxic volatile chemicals. Water treatment by reverse osmosis and charcoal filtering of the whole water supply to the building is the best approach. All filtering parts should be of stainless steel and glass. Charcoal should be used after the reverse osmosis membrane in order to remove the plasticizers that it may have introduced. Distilled water and spring water are also good drinking water supplies. However, all containers should be of glass or stainless steel because of the high contaminant potential of plastics. Some studies show that 50% of the chemicals in the containers will eventually leach into the water. *Sweating by sauna, or along with any exercise*, if done in a non-polluted area, will also help eliminate body pollutants and maintain a better preventative life style.

Replacement of depleted vitamins and minerals appears to be essential for good health. This is often necessary, because most available foods are grown with pesticides, herbicides, and fertilizers on depleted soils which are less than optimum for plant nutrition, so that their nutritional quality is not as high as it should be. In addition, food processing often destroys nutrients. Contaminated foods also require more unnecessary response of the body's detoxification systems. If ingested along with water and air pollutants, they may put a strain on these systems, causing vitamin and mineral deficiencies.

Pollutants also cause direct depletion effects on vitamins and minerals. In addition there may at times be selective absorption of the toxic chemical over the vitamin and mineral. Levels of pollutants can now be measured in homes, and in the blood samples of people living in them. (See Tables 23-1 to 23-6, below.)

The day is upon us where the maintenance of health and the treatment of disease is entirely possible through less toxic living.

Tables 23-1 to 23-4, below, show the presence of pollutants in an average home in a residential area. The homemaker living here was made ill by these levels of toxic chemicals. Tables 23-5 and 23-6, below, show the levels of pesticides and volatile organic chemicals in the blood of two large sample groups of chemically sensitive patients.

Table 23-1

CONTAMINATION IN AIR SAMPLES FROM PATIENT X'S HOME

	Breakfast Nook	*Living Room*	*Carport Steps*	*Bedroom*	*Backyard*
Diazinon	0.527	0.709	0.056	0.603	ND
Dursban	0.259	0.369	Trace	0.237	ND
Trifluralin	0.004	0.011	ND	0.017	0.030
beta-BHC	0.007	0.004	0.004	0.004	ND
Heptachlor	0.033	0.024	0.029	0.024	ND

Concentrations are given in micrograms of the compound per cubic meter of air.
ND = None Detected

Table 23-2

CONTAMINATION IN WATER SAMPLES FROM PATIENT X'S HOME

Compounds	*Home Water*	*Office Water*
Dieldrin	0.014	0.008
Trifluralin	0.014	ND
p,p,'DDE	0.008	ND
trans-Chlordane	0.004	ND
cis-Chlordane	0.002	ND

Concentrations are given in micrograms of compound per kilogram of water.
ND = None Detected

Table 23-3

CONTAMINATION IN WALLPAPER AND CLOSET SAMPLES FROM PATIENT X'S HOME

Compounds	*Wallpaper*	*Carpet*
Diazinon	99.4	374.4
Dursban	24.1	30.7
Heptachlor	0.7	0.3
Trifluralin	1.5	ND
trans-Chlordane	0.1	ND
cis-Chlordane	0.1	ND
Endrin	0.1	ND
Mirex	1.6	ND

Concentrations are given in micrograms of compound per gram of sample.
ND = None Detected

Table 23-4

CONTAMINATION IN SOIL SAMPLES FROM PATIENT X'S HOME

	Pillar Beneath Bedroom	*Pecan Orchard*	*Kitchen Steps*	*Pond*
trans-Chlordane	6459	14	5112	8
cis-Chlordane	3681	8	2745	5
trans-Novachlor	3899	8	2756	4
cis-Novachlor	813	3	714	1
Oxychlordane	56	ND	ND	ND
1-Hydroxychlordene	321	ND	107	ND
Heptachlor	1971	·4	1465	3
Heptachlor Epoxide	1415	4	303	2
Diazinon	Trace	ND	ND	ND
Dursban	ND	ND	Trace	ND
p,p'DDE	ND	2	ND	2
p,p'DDT	ND	3	ND	2
Mirex	ND	7	ND	7
Trifluralin	ND	1	ND	ND
Dieldrin	ND	1	ND	ND

Concentrations are in micrograms of compound per kilogram of soil.
ND = None Detected

Table 23-5

PESTICIDES PRESENT IN THE BLOOD OF CHEMICALLY SENSITIVE PATIENTS

Pesticide in blood	*% Distribution in 200 chemically sensitive patients*
DDT and DDE	62.0
Hexachlorobenzene	57.5
Heptachlor Epoxide	54.0
beta-BHC	34.0
Endosulfan I	34.0
Dieldrin	24.0
gamma-Chlordane	20.0
Heptachlor	12.5
gamma-BHC (Lindane)	9.0
Endrin	5.5
delta-BHC	4.0
alpha-BHE	3.5
Mirex	2.5
Endosulfan II	1.5

Note: These toxic chemicals should not be in the blood in any amount.

Table 23-6

VOLATILE ORGANIC CHEMICALS IN THE BLOOD OF CHEMICALLY SENSITIVE PATIENTS

Volatile organic chemicals in blood	*% Distribution in 114 chemically sensitive patients*
Tetrachloroethylene	83.1
Toluene	63.2
Xylene	59.7
1,1,1-Trichloroethane	50.5
Dichloromethane	49.7
Ethylbenzene	39.2
Chloroform	36.9
Benzene	23.4
Styrene	22.0
Dichlorobenzene	10.5
Trichloroethylene	8.6
Trimethylbenzene	3.2

Note: These toxic chemicals should not be in the blood in any amount.

24 LIVING WITH ENVIRONMENTAL ILLNESS

Jean Enwright

I am one of those people allergists now describe as "sensitive," who must be very careful of what they eat and wear, with what they wash themselves, their clothes and their home, what is in their home, what environments they expose themselves to, whether or not they can meet with people (depending on how many are involved, and what toxins, if any, they are wearing), and where they will be meeting. For a time I had to give up all jobs at least temporarily, including motherhood, and I will never be able to work full time in my chosen profession of teaching again. I have been diagnosed as having multiple allergies and sensitivities. When asked to answer the question on a medical form, "Will this patient recover?" my physician could only write, "We hope so." In other words I have a chronic illness with which I must learn to cope.

Many times I have been asked when I thought the illness began, and at what point did I become sick. After considering the complexities of the disease I realize I have had symptoms since early childhood. When I observe other members of my family I see that they also display symptoms. I can not attempt to answer this question as my knowl-

Jean Enwright, author of this candid account of the numerous problems resulting from allergies and chemical sensitivities, lives in Alberta, Canada. She has compared herself to a miner's canary—the caged bird once taken down into the mines whose death would serve as an early warning to the miners against the undetected poison gases which could also kill them as long as they remained unaware of their presence.

Though we are all at risk in the continued presence of certain chemicals in our modern environment, and many people already suffer unpleasant reactions, as yet only a minority has been medically diagnosed.

Jean Enwright has written this account in the hope that sharing her experiences will serve as a timely warning to us all. Her resolute struggle to overcome the enormous obstacles with which she has been faced cannot help but inspire anyone with similar problems. Just as important, it encourages all of us to inform ourselves and come to grips with this little known threat to our well-being.

The medical specialty in which doctors work with patients to uncover the relationship between their environment and their ill health, and to help them avoid inciting factors, is known as clinical ecology or environmental medicine.

The terms allergy and hypersensitivity describe an abnormal reaction to substances that your system recognizes as foreign which do not cause reactions in most people. Things which cause such reactions include pollens, danders, mold, dust, foods, drugs, air pollution, perfumes, and a host of chemicals. These things are called allergens, or incitants. The symptoms they produce can occur in almost every organ of the body and often masquerade as other illnesses. They can affect the skin, eyes, ears, nose, throat, lungs, stomach, bladder, vagina, muscles, joints, and the entire nervous system, including the brain.

edge is too incomplete, but there was a point at which I wish medical science had intervened on my behalf. Of course, a time arrived when I realized and accepted the fact that I had the illness and began to deal with it. I will go into further detail about dealing with it subsequently, but will first give a brief, semi-medical life history.

In 1943 I was born in London, Ontario, Canada, where I received my basic education and teacher training. At 19 I moved to central Canada, teaching there, in southern Ontario, and in Alberta. There I married, lived in or near small towns, and had two sons. Eventually we settled in Calgary, where I taught part-time. I became divorced, and then attempted to complete a Bachelor of Arts degree at the University of Calgary, planning to return to full time teaching. However, at that point this illness began to dictate my future.

Looking back, the first symptoms I can recall were irregular heart palpitations starting at age 4 or 5, increasing aches and pains in extremities and tummy by 10, strep throats and severe acne during puberty, headaches by midteens, and by the time I began to teach, virtually all symptoms I detail later were appearing infrequently in very mild form.

I had been to a number of doctors who did not recognize the nature of my illness, before I eventually went to see a general practitioner trained in clinical ecology, who understood the cause of all my symptoms. His main concern was with the potentially fatal symptom of depression. Now that I, too, understand the processes involved in environmental illness, I am able to see the state of my emotions as a guideline in charting my progress towards health. Depression itself was so distinctive a feature in my life (and in the lives of a large percentage of my relatives), that it has left a clear pathway in my past. At 11 I abruptly went into a depression, the controlling kind that dominates all one's experience. Even when I felt well it grabbed me, and no matter how hard I fought my mood sank, and I felt helpless to change it. This problem continued, only varying in degree until at 31, after having a general anesthetic, it seemed to lessen, and almost to vanish. But, as I became progressively more ill with environmental reactions, it returned. It was not until quite recently, when *I learned how to change my diet and environment* that I became *much healthier — and the depression appears to be gone*. I feel I am in control.

If the general medical practitioners I have seen over the years had been trained to identify environmental illness, I wonder if I would be as ill as I have become. For instance, correct medical intervention during a bout of reactions in 1983 might have changed the course of my life. At that time, I was hired to teach English for three and one half months in a junior high school. It was a dream coming true, and I enjoyed the aliveness of kids at the junior high school age. But I was able to work for only five weeks before I became ill. My health, my pleasure in teaching, my enjoyment of the children all vanished. I was diagnosed by two doctors as having a viral infection, but the symptoms lasted six months. Hoping to be helped, I went to another doctor who specialized in prevention. As I became sicker and sicker on his prescribed remedies, he became more impatient with me, and so I stopped going to doctors.

In 1984 I finally became a converted believer in environmental illness, when a psychologist friend pointed out that I had begun feeling more depressed at exactly the time I started driving a VW Rabbit (I think it was the upholstery fabrics which caused the problem.) No other diagnosis and related treatments had worked in the least. In fact, any treatment I had tried before this had just made me more and more discouraged, because with every attempt at first I felt hope, and then, with incorrect treatment, desperation. I felt terrible all the time. Also I did not understand the emotional links between poor health, chemical sensitivities, and psychological problems. I was starting to give up on myself, and though I had a greater desire to be doing many things, I felt a growing frustration at my increasing debility.

I also had many, many symptoms. There was such a mass of them, that it was difficult even to start to recognize a direct cause and effect between toxin and reaction. I am going to describe all the debilitating ones, as this may help those who suspect they have the illness, and would like to know more about it.

For example, my feet hurt and I had arthritic-like symptoms in various parts of my body at various times. I could not wear high heels without immediate and lasting discomfort. It was hard to buy shoes at all, because the fourth toe on my left foot needed a great deal of room and always seemed to curl up and then hurt if anything pressed on it. I was unable to run—indeed had to be careful walking—because my ankles were very unsteady. They twisted and were easily hurt. Sometimes, when I put on shoes, I got a headache. At the time I thought this was because the heels were probably ill-fitting and threw my back and neck out slightly. Invariably my legs ached except when I was asleep. I was developing varicose veins.

Gastrointestinal problems were constant. I was constipated almost always, except when I had diarrhea. Hemorrhoids began to be a problem. I was always painfully and embarrassingly gassy. There were usually stomach pains, and after some meals they were very sharp. At times, after eating, there seemed to be a bar horizontally across my stomach. An ache frequently developed somewhere back of my appendix. Sometimes I thought it was because I ate fat, sometimes I wondered if it was because I did not eat often enough. The left ovary and uterus always seemed to be painfully swollen. The discomfort was so pronounced, the ovary seemed to be in a constant state of ovulation. At times it felt as though spikes were being driven up into the right side of the floor of the abdomen. Periods were an almost crippling agony of pain and swelling. Sometimes the flow was practically impossible to contain, and I felt very shaky and exhausted for several days.

I was constantly "carrying my shoulders," and it was not possible to relax enough to let my shoulders rest in the normal position. I frequently tried to relax myself enough to drop them, but could never do so for more than a few seconds. (I am still able to use my shoulders as a guide to how chemically overloaded I am.) My entire body was constantly very tense, and I now understand how this tension caused my ankles and feet to hurt so much, and why I could not run, and had to be conscious of where and how I walked. When I risked all and wore a pair of high-heeled boots, I balanced only on the balls of my feet. I teetered precariously around as though the boots had no heels. Try as I did, I could not relax enough to let my feet rest on the heels of the boots, and I had to avoid stairs, and uneven or slippery surfaces.

Sometimes my throat was sore, like "instant" strep throat. Sometimes it hurt just at the voice box, at the front of the throat. My neck was stiff and sore. It was hard to turn my head to check in the rear window of the car. My right shoulder was so sore and stiff it was difficult to raise my arm to shoulder height, and the pain was starting to keep me awake at night. My hands and arms ached frequently, usually in one or both elbows, in my left fifth finger, my right hand, and one forearm.

Among this collection of pains one caused me real anxiety. It was the sporadic ache which occurred just below my right armpit. I feared it might be cancer, although I could never locate any swelling. The glands running along the bottom of the jaw were almost always uncomfortably swollen, sometimes hurting right up into the gums and teeth on the right side. When I started to experience face pains, I finally thought I was totally nuts, and must be a hypochondriac. Nobody ever gets face pains! They began along the base of the right jaw and stabbed upward into the eye. It was similar to the abdominal pain, and felt like a spike being driven into the eye. Although they could occur anywhere in the body, tiny muscle spasms occurred mostly around my eyes, usually off and on for a couple of days, or even up to a couple of weeks. The symptoms I felt most concerned about were the irregular heart rhythms.

I am extremely near-sighted and have been so since childhood, but my vision just seemed to get worse. At times it was improved, then it would be mixed, with one eye having clear vision, and one eye having blurred vision. It was quixotic. Though either eye could be clear, the imbalance became very noticeable when I was driving. At times my ears would suddenly seem to click, and afterwards I seemed to have two hearing systems, one internal, one external. External sounds remained quite clear, but I was simultaneously hearing my own voice, my breathing, swallowing, eating as though they were performed in a hollow cave. It interfered with my ability to hear what was going on around me. At times I experienced extremely painful Eustachian tube aches when exercising, or with even the slightest wind, or when swimming. Periodically, I would hear sounds in one ear, like whistling.

My face became sun- or wind-burned to the point of peeling within 10 minutes of exposure. My weight was 25 to 30 pounds beyond what it should be. It was steadily increasing, yet dieting caused major problems. I dieted for two weeks—ate slightly less but still ate a balanced diet—and had serious memory problems for a month. I lost no weight. Parts of my body were frequently swollen, particularly my eyelids, which almost looked transparent. Wearing a waistband was unbearable. My sense of taste had almost completely vanished, and I felt sick, ravenous, or unbearably sleepy after eating. I had to force myself to prepare and eat food, or even to be interested in it.

There were two constant symptoms which only changed in intensity, nothing eliminated them. I always had a headache. This was frequently accompanied by dizziness and the inability to tell what plane I was on. Was I standing up? Had I fallen over? Only by feeling what was against my face or looking around to decide where I was (in bed, outdoors) could I tell. The other was tiredness. I can remember standing in front of my class going over a reading selection and thinking I could not raise my right arm to point out the phrasing on the blackboard and stay standing up. I just did not have the energy. Lying in bed several hours a day was slight relief. I was too tense to sleep much or deeply. I had trouble falling asleep and staying asleep at night.

Though I know that my psychological problems stemmed partly from concern over my increasing debility, I learned they were also chemically based. My brain just could not function properly. It became impossible to follow any conversation, and I had trouble even remembering words. University classes were a nightmare, and I frequently could not finish a course. Over a 3 year period my results went from a term average of A– and B+ to first term test marks of D. After three weeks of classes in the fall of 1984, I realized that in order to pass any exam with my memory the way it was, I would have to read all texts and notes within 2 hours of writing. But this was impossible as I now was unable to read even more than half a page without falling into a doze.

I could not cope with life. Any occurrence, no matter how insignificant, was a major crisis. I was always dazed, and I could not make decisions. I had even become dangerous. My son Tim saved both our lives once when he alerted me to the fact that I was driving straight at another car. It was a clear day with no other traffic—I simply did not see the other car. In October I dropped some courses and re-registered one for January 1985, thinking that 3 months would be plenty of time to work at getting over these problems.

First, I reasoned that removing the toxins that were physically closest to me would have more effect than removing ones at a greater distance. I started with things that went *on* me or *in* me. I got rid of all makeup, soaps, toothpaste, deodorant, shampoo, detergents, fabric softener, and any synthetic clothing, except coats. I attempted to eat only organically grown food, and to drink tap water boiled for 45 minutes, or bottled water. Unfortunately there were a lot of factors which made these changes extremely difficult to put into place.

First of all, there was me. I was very ill (although I still did not realize it). I was confused, exhausted, in pain, and could not read. My psychologist friend had a friend with the illness. I talked with her friend a few times, and learned of some helpful books to read, namely Natalie Golos' *Coping with Your Allergies,* Theron Randolph's *An Alternative Approach to Allergies,* and William G. Crook's *The Yeast Connection.* She also introduced me to several other sick people, one of whom has become a dear friend. She herself was frighteningly ill, subject to such serious symptoms as collapse and convulsions. She and her husband were just beginning to look into the complexities of environmental illness. Being more sensitive than I, she reacted extremely quickly and specifically. She almost always knew what was "getting to her," and she had an acute sense of smell. I have absolutely none. (When our cat met a skunk I easily treated her.) For two and one-half years, almost every day, we called each other to share hopes, fears, laughter, pain, recipes, any new sources of organic food, encouragement, and symptoms. I would have been at a great loss without this partnership. Many of us feel guilty when we seem to be getting sicker, but if I called her and she had the same symptoms I had, then we knew it was not due to our own mismanagement, but possibly a southeast wind bringing pollution, or a temperature inversion, or the city adding some chemical to the drinking water. As well, her husband worked in the medical library of the University and kept us abreast of developments in the field.

Another restriction, which even now limits my choice of activities, was that I simply could not go out and wander through stores because of the toxins in them. In our local co-op grocery store, I could not go near sprayed produce, cleansers or detergents, clothing, plants, garden chemicals, automotive chemicals, or the bread display, because it was new and freshly varnished. Yet we needed food. I hated the place. I wanted to warn everyone about the toxins in that store, and the toxins in most of the food they were buying. Fortunately, there were lifesaving places in town—a farmer's market where some organic meat, eggs, chicken, and, in season, vegetables and fruit were available, and two health food stores where some organic grains, pure face soaps, biodegradable detergents, natural shampoos, tooth-brushes, and, occasionally, organic herb tea were available.

I was discovering how expensive organic food, or for that matter anything from a health food store, was. My first large expense was for cotton futons and futon covers for each of us. With my modest financial resources that seemed immense. I felt deeply discouraged about money. I learned of a woman who spent over $200,000 because of the illness. My income and savings seemed less than modest by comparison—they seemed non-existent. I had been divorced, a single parent, a university student and part-time teacher for several years. I had reached the stage where I was beginning to think I would be able to stop holding my breath financially speaking, because I would be teaching full-time in six months, or at most a year. My income would almost quadruple then. Now I had to start deciding whether to risk everything I had to get well. It took a year, but when I began to understand how sick I was, my first priority became getting well, so I risked everything I had on it.

There were concrete reasons for hope. *Within only two months of my very slowly and only gradually beginning this upheaval, two unexpected positive changes occurred.* Very abruptly my sense of taste returned. (I discovered how flavorful organic food is!) And by the end of November I had lost thirty pounds. It had come off quite reasonably, as I understand it now, but at the time this seemed bizarre. I would drop five and shoot up eight pounds, then drop two, five, three pounds, and rocket upwards again. Of course, it was primarily my reaction to the chemicals in non-organic food that caused this, but it seemed rather comical to me at the time. I was elated to be able to slip easily into a size ten jumpsuit, and I enjoyed the compliments from my co-workers. I had heard, read, and seen horror stories of people who had dropped too much weight too fast, and that was my only concern. Happily, I gained back a few pounds, and now I stay at this comfortable, sensible weight.

These very hopeful signs were tempered by the fact that I was still utterly exhausted and felt awful. By November I could enjoy about half an hour a week when I did not feel quite so ill. As a friend terms it, I was "less worse." By December it was half a day. Then during Christmas I began to feel worse, and by January I was not even thinking of returning to University. [This period coincides with increased exposure to the contaminants from the house's gas fired forced air heating system.—Editor.] I was just barely able to get to work, and feeling desperately ill. It was then I made an extremely difficult decision which was completely out of character for me.

I (and many other parents I'm sure), at least when the children are young or threatened, experience what I call the "Mother Mouse Syndrome." That is, if a mother mouse is separated from her offspring she will be very courageous, inventive, and persistent in order to be reunited with them. But though I had always been like the mother mouse, I chose to have my children move out to stay with their father, and felt no guilt pangs at all. I was so ill I only felt relief. They came for an hour or so after school every day, but I no longer had to deal with all the issues involved with child rearing: laundry, meals (those confusing, utterly frustrating, exhausting happenings, which involved two menus, two sets of preparations and cooking, and two kinds of shopping, for our two very different diets), homework, housework, hassles before bedtime, parent-teacher interviews, and getting up early in the morning. With my confusion, exhaustion, and poor memory I was often in tears of frustration, and could not cope. When they left I thought it would be for three weeks at the most, because I expected to be feeling better by then. In the end, the separation lasted ten months.

I began to lose hope, the key to survival. We humans are a tough lot, and we know how to endure. Over the ages individuals have survived immense hardship, and yet others who appear to be living very fortunate lives kill themselves. If one has hope, if there is some acceptable future, one endures. I, on the other hand, felt I had no future. All there was for me was illness and poverty. In all my imaginings when I was growing up these had not been part of my future. It seemed that unfortunate others had things like that happen to them, and in this marvelous modern world it was less common than in the old days. The poverty of the Bible, and the Great Depression were just something to read about. But reality for me, as I began to see it then, was illness and poverty, and this devastating necessity for isolation. I felt greatly betrayed, because not only was there no road leading into the future for me, but I also had no positive past to look back on, because everything I had done had made me ill. I had worked so hard to succeed, to become independent, strong, and financially secure. Now I would never be able to teach full-time again. The profession I had worked diligently in and for was gone. This was when I learned how to cry.

That winter was long and dreary. There were short periods when I still felt "less worse," and sometimes they did lengthen out to a few days' duration. I felt quite cheered by those times, but I had given myself a time limit for complete recovery, and I expected each "up" period to continue. Each time I slammed back into illness I felt guilty that I myself had caused the return. But I did not know what I had done wrong. I did not have control, the disease controlled me. My body rigidly ruled my life.

Despite all this, I continued my attempts to do the right things. *Our furnace was forced air fueled by gas, and every time it came on I felt dizzy.* Even though some days I awoke with ambition after "airing out" in my unheated bedroom at night, as soon as I turned on the heat, my immediate reaction was dizziness. This was soon followed by slipping into depression and feeling no desire to do anything except go back to bed. I had the heat vent turned off in my bedroom, and kept the window open at night. However, at −20°C I had to shut it. Since I was feeling the cold, and still struggling financially to be able to acquire natural fibre bedding, I was very uncomfortable. At times I awoke with frost from my breath on the covers. Needless to say all of me was huddled underneath. I did not even stick my nose out from under whatever I had piled on to stay warm. In the absence of a quilt I used extra sheets, doubled blankets, and topped off this strange but practical arrangement with pillows. In an attempt to be less affected by the furnace I kept the temperature low even in the daytime. Many cold days I spent most of the time in bed, just to be warmer.

Of course, I was rotating foods as advised by allergists to give the body regular rests from potentially negative foods. But since I live in an area where reliable organic foods are difficult to come by, and varieties of available fruits and vegetables are minimal, I could not follow a strictly rotated diet. I did not rotate foods by family, but simply by the food itself. Some foods I learned I reacted badly to, such as beef or milk, I never ate (unless it was to experiment to see if I was still allergic). Because beef was such a problem to me, I was very particular to eat separately any foods related to it. At first it was every two weeks for goat's meat or moose. Now I can eat beef as often as once a week. But when I first started to eat it regularly, it was once a month, and I have only been eating it regularly now for about ten months, and cannot be sure I will not react negatively again.

My diet that winter consisted of a single grain porridge or pancakes for breakfast. Lunch was a legume, or eggs and vegetables, and supper was four foods: a protein source (fish, legumes, poultry, meat), oil, and two vegetables. When I could get fruit I usually ate it with breakfast. This limited number and kind of foods was certainly not nutritionally complete, so I did take a supplement specially designed for very sensitive people. At this point I was even rotating the kinds of water I drank.

Since January I had been feeling increasingly depressed at my situation. In March the cat [A potential allergen.] was finally given to a good home. The same week I quit my job. A couple of weeks later I had a birthday and got another year older. I had modest means, was facing heavy financial needs, had no job, no pension, I was living a very solitary existence, my children were growing away from me.

For several months suicide was something I thought a great deal about. It seemed a reasonable choice. There I was on that pinnacle with no past, no future, and a miserable present. I had paid my dues. The boys were young, but tough and resilient. They had weathered rough times before, and they were strong enough to go on without me. I had our picture taken. I figured it was the last time for me.

Then my situation worsened still more when, in early July, I drove past a city work crew spraying herbicide, and started to get sicker. I was so ill I even envied Aids victims. They lived through 2 years of hell but they got to die, and were allowed release from suffering. I had to stay in hell here. And then, because I had been so ill so long, my backyard developed a large crop of weeds. Abruptly one morning a weed notice appeared on my front door, threatening that the city would come and spray. All I could do was cry. I sat on my futon and wept without being able to stop.

It was at this point that my outlook began to change. I found myself looking at a picture that had hung in the bedroom of my favorite grandmother, and, as I looked, I felt I would survive this crisis, and even lots more. From this point onward, despite setbacks, discouragements, and lots of tears, I knew I would survive somehow and eventually thrive.

It may seem that I proceeded through these hard times virtually alone, but that would have been impossible. It is true that I had to remain as isolated as possible, but the telephone was utterly vital to my survival. I talked for hours with my environmentally ill friend, and although a lot of these talks were very practical, often their greatest value was the human contact. The new doctor I went to also became a friend. I had become quite wary of the medical profession, as I became sicker and sicker without being correctly diagnosed. So I treated myself for approximately five months before I dared go to another doctor. This doctor was a general practitioner who had been helping his wife, who herself suffered from environmental illness. He had become familiar with the symptoms and ways to deal with them, and fortunately, he considered patients to be his equals. And he was a realist. When I bargained and begged to go back to University by September 1985, he said, "You're too ambitious". When I asked if there was a cure, he said that cure was a relative term. However, he did give me something concrete to go on: a time frame of two years, not for a cure, but for having most symptoms greatly reduced and to finally having renewed energy. It may sound strange, but in his office it felt safe to be a sick person. Here I was not stigmatized as a hypochondriac or considered slightly deranged. Instead, my symptoms were understood and carefully monitored. His nurse observed reactions of which I was not even aware. However, since I had to travel a couple of hours to get to his office, I only went when I was feeling well enough, and I ventured forth only two or three times a year.

The most important people in my life are my sons Timothy and Christopher, who were 12 and 10 respectively when this upheaval started. Just as the family problems created by the divorce were being resolved, this new onslaught hit us. In a way I was fortunate, because I had just learned how to go through a stressful life process. Though divorce is not environmental illness, the having to deal with great uncertainties and upheaval is the same. The choices one is forced to make are different, but I had gained experience in making momentous choices. In the present situation, however, I was alone in control, both of the family, and of how to deal with this illness.

At first, the boys were somewhat stunned as I explained what had to be done, adding naively that all would be fine within three or four months. They wanted to be supportive, but became very unhappy when I explained that our cat must go as a possible allergen. Because of their feelings the cat stayed, and I kept her until their father could take her, and she remained their cat.

Eating in our household was an immense problem. Many were the times I was just not interested and/or did not have the mental capacity to prepare very much. I was also terribly concerned about the boys' health. They both show early signs of the illness and as I never want them to become as ill as I am, I tried to make them eat in much the same way as I was eating. They are typical kids, with various likes and dislikes, and these "weird" new foods I served were often unappealing to them. It was not until much later, when I started eating more complex meals, and using recipes from a natural foods cookbook that they (and I) started to enjoy food again. When they were living away from me for ten months with their father, I had serious misgivings about their diet there, but at least they were not hungry as they were at times with me.

The boys were, and still are, forced to live a schizophrenic existence, because their father and I have different views of environmental illness. At times, he has wavered towards believing in its existence, but for the most part he does not understand it, and is even impatient with the whole idea. In my home the boys have absorbed a great deal about such things as unsprayed, organically grown food, the effect of eating refined sugar, natural fibre clothing, and toxic substances around the house. At their father's house they are exposed to the opposite view. They seemed to adapt to both perspectives, but they beg for sweet foods at my place. To them it seems that I alone have a problem, and I still am very uneasy about their weekend exposures, and worry about the lifestyles they live, with increasing illness and decreasing quality of life. Will they simply accept it as inevitable?

By far the most difficult time for the boys was when I became suicidal. Like most sick people, I was unpredictable, cranky, demanding, just plain hard to live with, and would sometimes cry a lot, and seem to scream at others for no reason at all. Recently we saw a movie about a boy close to my younger son's age. His mother has a terminal illness, and as much as she adores her son and shows it, she screams at him and throws things in her pain and frustration. I had acted like this, and I was glad my boys had a chance to see this as a shared human condition.

Today, our relationship is the best it has ever been. That is not to say there are no problems, but since I am so much healthier, when a problem arises I do not feel as though it is insurmountable.

The changes I had made in foods and clothing were helping, my weight stayed off, and I continued to be able to taste food. These were permanent improvements in my health, *but I was by no means well and major changes had to be contemplated in the house itself.* Facing this was difficult. It was like stepping off a flat rock in a thick fog. You hope you are walking off only a flat rock and not off a cliff. Controlling the other allergens was easier. If I touched, ate, or wore anything and then reacted negatively I knew those things were toxic to me. But if I had to spend hundreds or thousands of dollars on changing the house, I wanted to know beforehand that this would work. There was no way of knowing for sure. All I could do was follow the advice of others (those who could read and absorb technical information) and to some extent my own reactions within the house.

The house is a bi-level with approximately 840 square feet on each floor. The kitchen, living room, two bedrooms, and full bath room are upstairs. Downstairs there are 2 bedrooms, a half bathroom, the family room, and the furnace room. *My main thrust was and continues to be to get rid of obvious toxins,* like chemically produced synthetics. If I cannot give it away, throw it out, or sell it, it goes downstairs into the back bedroom. What I accomplished at first was minimal, and I grew wildly frustrated over my slowness. If only I was well enough to make all these changes I could be healthier! Now that I am feeling so much more secure in my health, I realize that what I did accomplish helped me, regardless of how slowly I did it. *Each item discarded was lessening the chemical load that I had to endure.* A partial list includes all my clothes, except shoes and boots (I still do not own a winter coat because I cannot tolerate one yet). I also discarded some furniture, some curtains and drapes, sheets, blankets, mattresses, all detergents (for clothes and dishes), all chemical cleaners, fabric softeners, nail polish, all cosmetics, our plants and, of course, our cat.

I would like to be able to say that when I got rid of a specific item I lost a specific symptom or at least that my overall health immediately improved. With a few exceptions, nothing quite so dramatic or helpful happened. But the few dramatic ones were very exciting! *The greatest of these was getting a new furnace. It was my most expensive gamble, and quite possibly the ensuing improvement in health has been the greatest.*

In the spring of 1985 a symptom, which had bothered me periodically, flared up so seriously that I was frightened. This was the soreness at the front of my throat, by the voice box, which seemed to be caused by a swelling after eating. But it was an erratic reaction, hard to pin down to a specific food. Finally, it began to occur when I drank water, becoming so intense that I was having difficulty swallowing. I first dealt with it by only drinking water when I was eating, so that the presence of foods would dilute the effect of the water's apparent toxicity. I had water from three different sources to rotate, and I drank one until the reaction became too strong, usually after two meals, and then switched to another. I was getting quite thirsty, but after a couple of very unpleasant weeks, the reaction began to diminish. Probably this was not because of the water alone, but because, as the weather warmed, I had the windows open more and the furnace on less, and so was decreasing the chemical load.

In the fall, I finally decided to install a furnace outside with a heated glycol (antifreeze) line running into the old furnace where there is a fan to force the heat upward. The glycol line also heats the water heater. *The advantage is that all gas is outside. The furnace is on a side of the house without windows, otherwise the fumes would enter the house.* Originally, I did not connect the throat swelling with natural gas. It was a reaction like many others which vanished and reappeared, and changed in intensity. I finally discovered the relationship while driving. Because I had "aired out" (been away from prolonged exposure to gas), when I got in the car within an hour after eating my throat swelled and hurt. I realized that it was not simply a reaction to food, but a reaction to the combination of ingesting food and exposure to strong concentrations of airborne petroleum products. For a while I stopped driving after eating.

Other major changes were a built-in vacuum system, and a water line filter which removes chlorine from all the water in the house. Now I can vacuum for an hour quite comfortably. With the regular vacuum, I became so irritable and furious, that only its loud engine could obliterate the sound of my voice saying words my mother did not teach me. I suspect I was reacting to the exhaust, and possibly also to the electrical current. I still have no idea whether the chlorine filter has helped or not.

Our house is by no means perfect, and probably never will be. I debate with myself whether to make any more major changes on a house situated in a city which is becoming increasingly polluted. Why invest in removing as many toxins as possible from a house when, in ten years if one opens the windows, brown air will frequently ooze in? The major changes I have made are the ones which I feel are absolutely necessary at this stage of my recovery.

The two rooms which I altered the most were the rooms I am in most often, the bedroom and kitchen. My main aim was to "air out" as much as possible at night, and to have a relatively safe refuge during the day, so I started with the bedroom. The furniture consists of a cotton futon and a box spring. The sheets, pillow cases, and some blankets are 100% cotton. One blanket is 100% wool, the pillows are cotton-filled and cotton covered. There is a small chair with a crystal lamp at the head of the bed, and a clock radio. I keep my clothes in the closet, or in an oak chest, and use an antique sewing machine to display a few treasures. On the wall above the bed are framed pictures and a brass oil lamp which has never been used. Pictures the boys made are on the wall above the oak chest. The hot air vent is always open now, so it is possible to keep the window open at night, even at minus 25°C. There are no curtains at the moment. The great problem of the room is its carpeting. If I could, I would have the floor tiled, and use wool or cotton mats. Since I have never been without the carpet (i.e., I have never withdrawn from it), I do not know what effect it has on my health. I speculate that without it, at this stage I might be able to sleep through the night and/or find myself with more energy.

The kitchen appliances are electric, although standing over the stove while cooking can be quite uncomfortable. At the beginning of my program, I did not use the dishwasher [because of the contaminating detergents], except to rinse dishes I had washed in pure soap. Now, for the last eight months, I can open a window and use dishwasher detergent, stopping the machine before the drying cycle, resetting it to rinse again, and putting in vinegar for a better rinsing job. The cooking pots and pans are either glass or enamelled steel. I keep soap and borax in the kitchen, while the dishwasher detergent is kept outside, in the milk chute. All plastic storage containers went, and I now use glass jars, aluminum foil, or for freezing, plastic bags. The table and chairs are varathaned oak (I use cotton pads on my chair), and the dry sink is unfinished pine. Happily, there are plants again in my kitchen! They are the ones said to help ameliorate indoor toxins—spider plants and golden pothos, and just for sheer beauty and youthful vigor, a baby jade plant. As clay pots always seemed to get moldy, all pots are plastic or ceramic. The real cat has been replaced by a painted cat plate, and pictures the boys drew on unbleached cotton material. They are framed in light, wooden, inexpensive embroidery hoops which hang on the wall. The boys have cotton futons and linoleum floors in their bedrooms. We try to adhere to the philosophy that less is better.

From an allergic's point of view, the living room is a disaster. It is carpeted and has overstuffed furniture. It would have been best to have thrown out the furniture, but with already discarding so much, and my feeling like a misfit on this planet, I just could not face an unfurnished living room. Now I simply stay out of there as much as possible. Unfortunately, the family room is not much better, but it has no carpeting and since the windows are above ground, there is good ventilation, though it can be rather nippy down there. The bathrooms were easy to strip of chemicals. The towels, bathmat, and toilet seat cover are all cotton. I wash the tub and toilet with pure soap, the walls, sink, and fixtures with baking soda, and the mirror with hot water and vinegar.

Overall, the house could still be a lot more comfortable. If I could have installed a fresh air exchanger, along with the furnace, we would be warmer. However, the alterations I have made have definitely been helping.

I will end with a brief chronology of the progress in my quest for improved health. For at least half the period I have described I was angry and impatient. I wanted THE solution. Which button do I push to make it happen? Gradually, I learned to be more patient, understanding, and accepting. I was better able to be accepting as I saw greater improvement in my health. At first, during a period of feeling well I would look back to compare the level of my health only over short periods of weeks or months. Now I can count the gains over years. Progress was extremely slow at first, then quicker, though there have always been times when I abruptly returned to earlier symptoms. I have included gains, therefore, not when they first appeared but when they seemed to be permanent.

Now, in January 1987, I feel full of optimism. Maybe my present gains are temporary, maybe not. It seems to me that the most recent health improvement has come from being able to work at delivering flyers, which involves healthy outdoor exercise. But it is considered a child's job, and, at first, beside being very tired (I delivered a while, came home and slept, then went out again), I had difficulty dealing with the fact that I was a teacher, a professional, and this was not my work. When it finally dawned on me what pleasures there are to be found in it (outdoors, seasons, exercise and people, people of all ages!) I realized how much it beat being in bed for two years.

Here is a brief summary of my progress over the past three years:

End November '84—Sense of taste returns. Thirty pound weight loss.

January '85—My sons leave to permit my further recovery.

March '85—I leave my teaching job. The cat goes.

Summer '85—Strong negative reaction to sun. Exhaustion, feeling "pressed down."

August '85—Despite being very ill, realized I could endure and have a future. Plastic glasses go. Bought glass and metal ones. Extremely painful reactions to synthetics; all clothes painful.

October '85—Central vacuum system installed. New outside furnace.

November '85—My sons return, and I feel human again.

January '86—Started to walk friend's dog—some days easy some days impossible. Beginning to trust memory. Sense of humour returns. Light reading becomes a pleasure.

Spring '86—Able to do more work in yard and garden.

August '86—Got up after six days in bed from exhaustion (but not feeling ill!), and got job delivering flyers. (Found it very difficult applying for jobs in summer heat.)

September '86—Still reacting negatively to clothes.

October–November '86—Flu. Kept delivering flyers, but slower and slower. Still not confident of the future.

January '87—Easily able to walk routes. Can even walk quickly. Able to wear clothes, even new ones, with minimal reaction. Only two kinds of fatigue instead of countless kinds. (Chemical and healthy tired.) Only need rest once a day, if that. Feeling more confident about what is in my future.

There have been many positive aspects to this quest. The boys and I have learned a great deal. We have been allowed to see and begin to understand more about ourselves individually, as a family, and as beings who inhabit this earth. We are far more questioning than before, but also more accepting of the traditional old ways that cause far less violation of the earth. All of us are very thankful that I am so much healthier, and we are looking forward to a healthier future. We enjoy my happier, more patient personality. I am greatly relieved now to understand why depression became a tradition in my own and earlier generations of my family. I am deeply grateful to be able to enjoy life and look forward to the future.

I was also much encouraged when I realized how sick I had been, and how much better I was becoming, though I was still living on this poisoned planet. I have had signs of illness for almost my entire life, yet I am healing. *My health improves constantly because I am removing toxins from my environment. Despite the fact that it is impossible to avoid toxins completely, I get healthier.* Surely the earth's situation can be bettered in the same way. What if each of us, planetwide, said "No more pollution for my family"? The implications are immense. The economic, social, and environmental upheaval would be incredible, but the final outcome could be as positive as it has been for our family. I feel much more hopeful for us all, and see this book as a step on the road to a safer world.

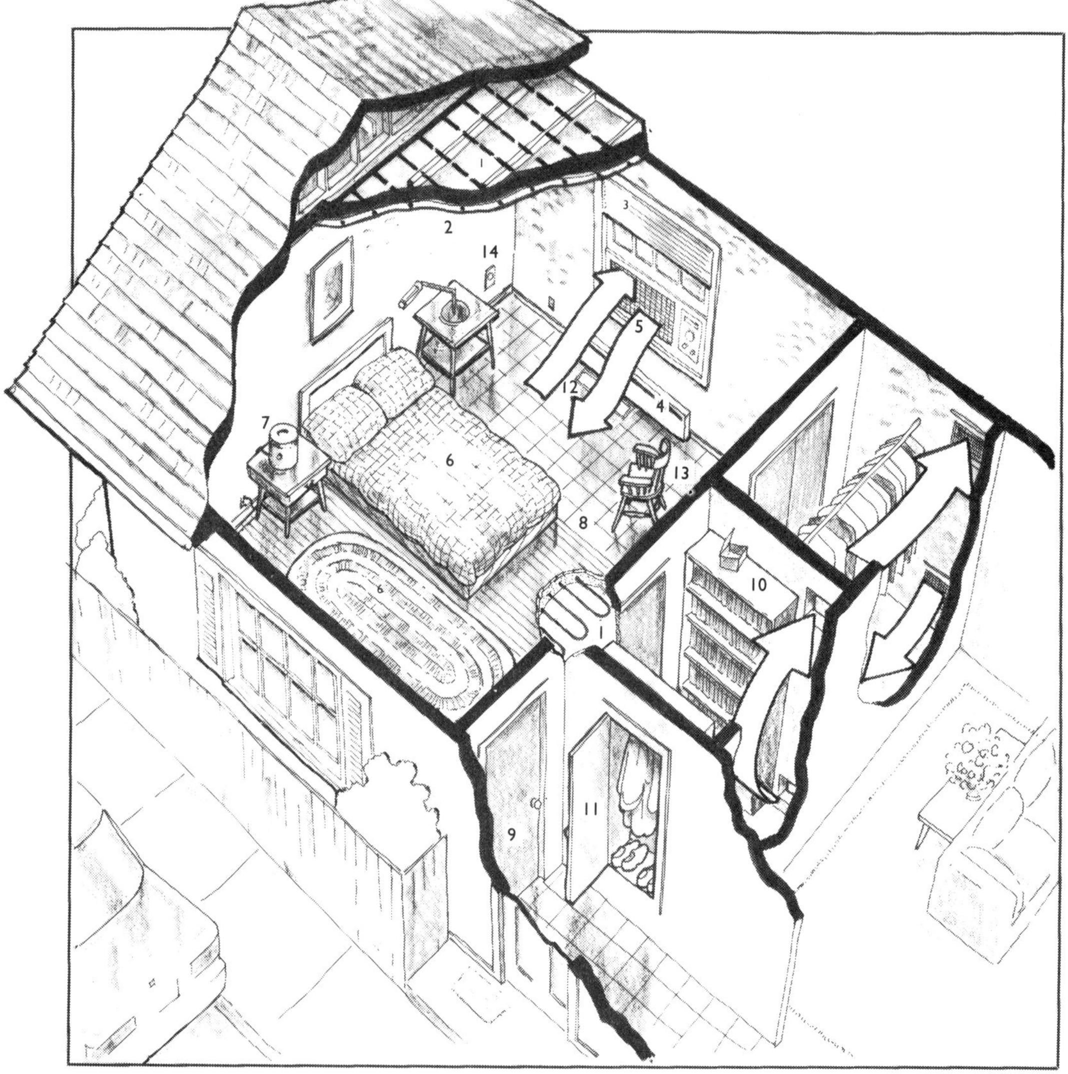

Fig. 25-1 A Sanctuary

1 HEATING PIPES IN CEILING OR FLOOR
2 UNTREATED PLASTER ON METAL LATH
3 METAL BLINDS
4 LIQUID FILLED HEATER
5 WINDOW FILTRATION/AIR CONDITIONER
6 UNTREATED COTTON BEDDING AND RUG
7 AIR PURIFIER
8 HARDWOOD AND CERAMIC TILE
9 SEALED DOOR
10 SEPARATELY VENTILATED STORAGE
11 ALCOVE WITH SHOES, ROBE
12 SEALED FURNACE DUCTS
13 HARDWOOD CHAIR
14 BUILT-IN VACUUM

25 THE SANCTUARY

A room in the home can be set aside as a special place of relief for the individual with environmental sensitivity. Converting a bedroom in a conventional home into a sanctuary, as free as possible from irritating conditions, is often an affordable means of providing a "healing place" when converting the entire home is impractical.

The sanctuary room is a retreat for:

- Relief during the hours of rest and sleep.
- Living with others whose habits may not be entirely compatible with the environmentally sensitive person.
- Living in an imperfect home.
- Preparing for forays into workplaces, or other public places with stressful conditions.
- Preventing illness due to exposure.

A sanctuary room will provide relief from conditions which are known to be irritating to the individual.

The sanctuary will generally require:

- An outside air supply as free as possible from chemical and biological contaminants. (See the Home Ventilation chapter.)
- Building materials and systems which do not contribute either to air contamination or contact exposure. (See the Materials and Selection chapter.)
- Furniture and fixtures which do not contribute to contamination and irritation. (See the Materials and Selection chapter.)
- Isolation from storage of problem clothing and household articles.
- A pleasant visual, thermal, acoustic, and tactile environment.
- Good maintenance practices to maintain these conditions. (See the Home Maintenance chapter.)

Necessary Conditions for a Sanctuary

Note: Individual requirements will vary, and those with severe environmental hypersensitivity must carefully sample and test each material before making a choice. (See Personal Challenge Testing, page 203.) The following guidelines, however, apply to most situations.

AIR QUALITY

Complete separation of the room air from the air in the rest of the house, and the installation of an individual air supply, is essential to controlling air quality in the sanctuary.

ISOLATION

- Tightly seal all heating vents or other openings with sheet metal or other non allergenic and fireproof material. (For safety reasons you *must* consult a heating contractor before doing so.)
- Plug all cracks in floors, walls, and ceilings. (Untreated plaster patching compounds are best.)
- Ensure that a tight air/vapour barrier is in place on all outside walls and ceilings. (Metal foil with metal tape seams is the preferred material. See the Construction Notes chapter.)

• Ensure that doors and windows fit tightly and are equipped with weatherstrip. (Fabric type strips which nail or staple on are acceptable for most people.)

AIR SUPPLY

(For detailed information on choosing ventilation equipment, see the Home Ventilation chapter.)

• Where clean outdoor air is available, simple cross ventilation through vents or windows will be sufficient.

• Where filtration of pollens or dust is necessary, install a high efficiency fan-driven filter, or an air conditioner with high efficiency filters. These are available as window mounted units. *Do not* connect central air conditioning or air filtration systems that serve the whole house to the sanctuary, unless the whole house is a carefully controlled environment.

• Where removal of gaseous contamination from outdoor air is necessary, install a chemical adsorption air purifier at the air intake. (See the Home Ventilation chapter.)

• Provide an exhaust outlet to relieve the pressure of incoming air.

• Use a high capacity room air cleaner where necessary to help reduce odors and air contamination in the sanctuary.

NOISE CONTROL

• Where outside noise is objectionable, use double or triple glazed windows to reduce incoming noise.

• Ventilation openings and air conditioners will admit noise, and are difficult to effectively baffle. Minimize noise by making sure that these face away from streets and other sources of noise and air contamination.

• Sanctuary rooms are likely to have a lot of sound reflection inside because they are uncarpeted and contain mainly hard surfaces. (See the Sound chapter.) To help reduce the resulting "empty room echo", which can be annoying, the wall and ceiling plaster finishes can be textured and acceptable area rugs and fabric wall hangings can be used. (For sound control methods see the Construction Notes chapter.)

Table 25-1

The Sanctuary's Building Systems

Component	Material	Alternatives (If individually acceptable)
Framing System	Lightweight steel	Softwood lumber
Insulation	Untreated mineral wool or glass fiber (sealed by tight air/vapor barrier)	
Air/Vapor Barrier	Metal foil, taped joints with foil tape	

The Sanctuary's Building Systems (continued)

Component	Material	Alternatives (If individually acceptable)
Walls, Ceiling	Untreated plaster, expanded metal lath; brick or concrete;	Untreated plaster on gypsum lath; hardwoods
Floors	Ceramic tile set in cement mortar	Hardwood strip or plank
Windows	Bare metal sash with well cured plain silicone glass settings	Enamelled metal
Doors	Hollow core metal	Hardwood
Finishes (Paints & varnishes)	Bare plaster; casein (milk) based paint	Other non-petroleum based finishes, or self tested and acceptable paints sealers and varnishes

Table 25-2

The Sanctuary's Furniture and Fixtures

Component	Material	Alternatives (If individually acceptable)
Bedding	Untreated cotton mattress, cover, blankets	Untreated wool or acetate material
Area Rugs, Hangings, Curtains	Untreated cotton (light colors)	Untreated wool, acetate, or linen
Furniture Frames	Metal, or solid hardwoods	
Window Coverings	Metal blinds	Untreated cotton, linen
Lamps	Certified, totally enclosed fixtures (glass and metal only)	Ventilated, recessed ceiling fixtures, conventional fixtures of metal or glass, compact fluorescents
Fixtures, Trims	Metals, solid hardwoods	

The Sanctuary Storage

Clothing that has been worn outside the home will adsorb smoke, perfumes, and other odors that are objectionable to the environmentally sensitive. Provide separately ventilated storage for such clothing, books, and other items that are not tolerated well in the room.

• Allow a small, outside air intake and exhaust opening for each closet.

• Provide a tight fitting closet door.

• Provide a small storage alcove outside the sanctuary room for shoes and overclothes which are used elsewhere in the home or outdoors.

Decorating the Sanctuary

Apply color using self-tested, appropriate paints, such as the casein based variety. Untreated cotton, linen, or wool fabrics, art prints, and watercolors on paper, are often tolerated by the sensitive, as well as metal, glass, or ceramic ornaments.

Hard plastic laminates, such as those used for kitchen counter tops, can also usually be used after the adhesive has cured. Do not use particle board or any plywoods as a base for these laminates in the sanctuary.

Heating and Humidity

Heating the sanctuary from a central heating system will be possible where a hot water type system is in use. *Do not* use warm air furnaces or conventional electric heaters, as they will introduce contamination from other parts of the house, and dust problems.

• In climates where heating, cooling, and dehumidification are necessary, a window mounted heat pump/air conditioner is a preferred system. This system must be self tested, however, as some acutely sensitive people react to the refrigerants and other materials used in these units.

• Humidification will not be necessary in most cases if the room is fitted with a tight air/vapor barrier. In extremely dry climates, however, or to treat illness, extra humidity is sometimes required. A portable steam humidifier operating with distilled water is the preferred method.

• A preferred heating system is radiant ceiling or floor heating, using a heated liquid. They must be installed with a tile or stone floor. These systems provide a gentle, even heat without introducing dust problems. Liquid filled electric baseboard heaters are also a good source of gentle heat that will not "fry" or stir up dust as much as conventional electric heaters. (See the Home Heating/ Cooling and Construction Notes chapters.)

• Portable liquid filled electric radiators can be an acceptable alternative. These are usually oil filled, however, and must be carefully watched for leaks. Some older units were also manufactured with highly toxic PCB's and must be avoided at all costs.

Maintenance of the Sanctuary

(For further details see the Home Maintenance chapter.)

Keeping the sanctuary free of dust, dampness, and other contamination, is the primary concern once clean conditions have been established.

• Installing a smooth cove base of ceramic tile or hardwood that is sealed to the wall and floor will reduce cleaning problems. Trims and mouldings without deep grooves can also be more readily dusted. (See the Construction Notes chapter.)

• A built-in vacuum cleaner will clean better than a portable one, without stirring up dust. For cleaning the walls, furniture, and other surfaces, damp cloth and damp mop dusting methods are best.

• Use no cleaners, waxes, disinfectants, or other products without careful testing by the sensitive person. Launder bedding and other fabrics only with soaps known to be acceptable. (See the Home Maintenance chapter.)

• Clean heating, cooling, and air cleaning equipment, and replace air filters, regularly.

• Check air conditioners and humidity equipment regularly for standing water. Dehumidifiers and air conditioners must either be drained continuously by a tube leading outside, or be drained and cleaned daily. Humidifiers must be drained and cleaned when not in use, and should be stored outside the room.

• Clothing, shoes, and other items which may introduce contamination should be stored for use outside the room. In acute circumstances, visitors to the sanctuary may be required to exchange street clothes for fresh garments before entering.

For further information for the hypersensitive, see the chapter Resources for the Environmentally Ill, and the GETTING HELP section.

26 RESOURCES FOR THE ENVIRONMENTALLY ILL

The following organizations and publications are specifically helpful for those wanting further information on environmental sensitivity and illness. They are also very useful for those concerned with prevention who wish to improve their diet and living conditions for better health. Most of these are volunteer organizations or non-profit societies, where memberships and donations are welcome, and there is often a need for volunteer help as well.

MEDICAL HELP

American Academy of Environmental Medicine
P.O. Box 16106
Denver, Colorado 80216

This is the U.S. organization of clinical ecologists. They publish a quarterly medical journal, "The Clinical Ecologist," and can provide a list of member physicians by region. This organization also accepts memberships from non-medical professionals and organizations interested in clinical ecology. H.E.A.L. (see Support Groups, below) can also provide information on A.A.E.M. member physicians in your region.

Canadian Society for Clinical Ecology
and Environmental Medicine
479 Roncesvalles Ave.
Toronto, Ontario M6R 2N4 (416) 536-9903
This organization offers educational seminars and services to physicians and other interested professionals.

ENVIRONMENTAL ILLNESS SUPPORT GROUPS

Human Ecology Action League
2421 W. Pratt, Suite 1112
Chicago Ill. 60645 (312) 665-6575

This is the parent organization for many regional environmental illness support groups. They publish "The Human Ecologist," a quarterly journal of information on E.I., and provide a wide range of support to members. H.E.A.L. can provide a list of regional organizations, clinical ecologists, product directories, travel directories, building consultants, and book lists. Membership is $20 U.S. per year ($25 U.S. for Canada), and includes a subscription to "The Human Ecologist".

Note: Local allergy associations can often provide information on local products and services.

In Canada:
Allergy Information Association
25 Poynter Drive, Suite 7
Weston, Ontario, M9R 1K8 (416) 244-8585

This self-help organization publishes a quarterly newsletter, and has local branches throughout the country.

PRODUCTS

Below is a partial list of suppliers of hypo-allergenic products. It is by no means complete, nor will everything supplied necessarily be acceptable to you. Remember that everything you buy must be self tested. Further product information is available in "The Human Ecologist" (see Support Groups, above), or by consultation with the information services listed above.

Most suppliers provide a free catalog on request.

The Human Ecology Research Foundation of the Southwest
8345 Walnut Hill Lane, Ste. 205
Dallas, Texas 75231-4262 (214) 361-9515

Along with its patient information and support services, this non-profit foundation sells selected products for the environmentally ill. All profits go to support services for E.I. patients. Write for a safe product list including building materials.

The Allergy and Health Emporium
5636 E. Mockingbird Lane
Dallas, Texas 75206 (800) 233-2606
(214) 828-4500 (Texas residents)

The Allergy Store
7345 Healdsburg
Sebastopol, California 95472 (800) 824-7163
(800) 222-9090 (California residents)

National Ecological and Environmental Delivery System (N.E.E.D.S.)
602 Nottingham Rd.
Syracuse N.Y. 13224 (315) 446-1122

Nigra Enterprises
5699 Kanan Rd. HE
Agoura, California 91301 (818) 889-6877

HOUSING CONSULTANTS

Below is a partial list of consultants who provide design and materials selection services for the environmentally ill. Other consultants can be located through H.E.A.L. or your local allergy association.

Mary Oetzel, Environmental Health Services
3202 W. Anderson Lane, #208-249
Austin, Texas 78757 (512) 288-2369

Dona Shrier, Designer
825 Northlake
Richardson, Texas 75080 (214) 235-0485

In Canada:
Bruce Small and Associates
Sunnyhill Research Centre
RR #1
Goodwood, Ontario L0C 1A0 (416) 294-3531

FURTHER READING

Clinical ecology topics:

Clinical Ecology, Iris Bell. Common Knowledge Press, Bolinas, Calif. 1982.

An excellent brief monograph on environmental illness. A good introduction for the medical practictioner who is unfamiliar with the problem.

Clinical Ecology, L. D. Dickey (ed.). C. C. Thomas, Springfield, Ill. 1976.

This is a comprehensive medical text containing 80 articles on environmental illness topics.

Human Ecology and Susceptibility to the Chemical Environment, Theron Randolph. C. C. Thomas, Springfield, Ill. 1962.

This is a major text on clinical ecology, written by a pioneer in the field.

The Mirage of Safety, Food Additives and Federal Policy, B. T. Hunter. Available from Wellington Books, Department THE, Rfd. #1, Box 223, Hillsboro, N.H., 03244.

This is an authoritative text on food additives and their health hazards.

The Clinical Ecologist, Journal of the American Academy of Environmental Medicine. (See Medical Help, above.)

This journal, available to A.A.E.M. members, is the major source for information on current research and practice in environmental medicine.

Environmental illness topics for the lay reader:

Sunnyhill, Bruce and Barbara Small, 1980. Sunnyhill Foundation, RR #1, Goodwood, Ontario, Canada, L0C 1A0

A very readable personal account of a family seeking alternative housing to deal with their environmental illness. Available from the authors.

Allergies and Your Family, D. J. Rapp. Sterling Publishers, N.Y., 1981.

A step by step approach to diet, personal care, and home maintenance.

An Alternative Approach to Allergies, T. G. Randolph, R. W. Moss. Lippincott and Crowell, N.Y., 1980.

An excellent discussion of the causes and symptoms of environmental illness, emphasizing diet, air pollution, and addictions. Includes case histories.

Coping With Your Allergies, N. Golos, F. G. Bulbitz, F. S. Leighton. Simon and Schuster, N.Y., 1979.

A practical guide to avoidance of harmful exposure in diet, and home and personal management.

The Experience, Ecologic Illness From the Viewpoint of the Patient, Iris Bell. X-Press, North Bend, Washington, 1982.

An account, for the lay reader or clinician, of the phases and symptoms of environmental illness.

How to Control Your Allergies, R. Formar. Larchmont Books, N.Y., 1979.

Practical suggestions for management of environmental illness.

The Allergy Self-Help Book, S. Faelten. Rodale Press, 1983.

A guide to detecting and identifying allergies; provides nondrug methods of treatment.

Allergy Relief, Rodale Press, 33 East Minor St., Emmaus, PA, 18049.

A monthly newsletter by subscription for the general reader.

Allergies and the Hyperactive Child, D. J. Rapp. Cornerstone, N.Y., 1980.

A practical, non-technical book on how to alleviate problems associated with allergies and hyperactivity.

SECTION VII

Getting Help

27 TESTING FOR CONTAMINATION

This chapter explains testing for household hazards, and lists test suppliers and information sources. Further sections cover selecting contractors for health conscious homebuilding or renovations, protecting yourself from demolition and construction hazards, and a list of further reading. All are intended for the reader with known or suspected health hazards in their homes, or for those who plan to build or renovate in a health conscious manner. Health related services for those with known or suspected environmental sensitivity are described in the section, ENVIRONMENTAL ILLNESS AND YOU.

TESTING

A number of simple laboratory tests may be necessary to determine if there are problems which need attention in your home. Some can be purchased by the householder and self administered, others will require the assistance of health care professionals and professional home testing services.

Radon

There are simple home tests that you can do for radon. These are pre-packaged air samplers which you place in the home for a period of time and then return to a lab for analysis. Making a few preliminary tests will help you determine if you have a radon problem which requires action. Further testing is usually required to determine the kind of remedy that is needed. These preliminary tests cost from $15 to $40 each. *Some consumers' agencies and health authorities are recommending that EVERYONE living in homes or apartments (below the sixth floor) with basements do a preliminary test.* Though some argue that this would be overly cautious, this is probably a good idea. *Test your home if you live with any of the following conditions:*

• If you live in a high radon area. (See Radon in the Controlling Indoor Air Quality chapter.) If you are buying a lot and planning to build, test the site before starting construction.

• If any neighbour has discovered radon problems.

• If your house has a cracked basement wall or floor, an earth basement floor, or any form of indoor groundwater sump. (This is a small well recessed into the floor containing a pump or valve.)

• If your home has a basement, and was built, insulated, and sealed to current energy efficiency standards.

• If your water comes from a drilled well located in bedrock.

• If your home contains large amounts of brick, stone, or concrete exposed to the interior.

PRELIMINARY TESTING

Two types of tests are available for preliminary screening to determine if you need further action.

The charcoal adsorption test: These inexpensive ($10–$20 including analysis) devices can provide rapid results and are preferred for initial testing. They are simply activated charcoal granules in a cannister which will adsorb radon gas. They require 3–7 days in your home and two to six weeks for mailed laboratory results. They are, however, adversely sensitive to moisture and cannot be used in such humid places as bathrooms. They are also limited to a 7 day maximum sampling period and cannot be used for long term testing.

Alpha track tests: These more costly ($20–$40 including analysis) devices are suited to long term measurements. They are preferred for detailed analysis of problem houses, and for such humid locations as bathrooms. They are small strips of photographic paper in cannisters which record the alpha particle tracks emitted by the radioactive decay products of radon. They require at least 1 month in place, but can be left in the home for a year or more to accumulate data.

USING RADON TESTS

Preliminary testing is best done with two or three devices at different locations in your home. Carefully follow the manufacturer's instructions. Testing during heating or cooling seasons, when the house is closed and ventilation is reduced, and sampling the most likely areas of radon concentration, will determine the "worst case" conditions for your home.

The basement (ground floor if you have no basement) is the best place to test first. Place the device 2 to 4 feet off the floor and away from windows, sumps, air grilles, sources of dampness (if it is a charcoal type), and basement cracks. First test playrooms or bedrooms in basements, children's bedrooms, and lower floors.

If you have a drilled well in bedrock, test the bathroom to determine the contribution of radon from well water. (Use an alpha track device.) Bathing with the window closed and fan off during the test period will help establish the "worst case" conditions.

Note: If you live in an area served by the Bonneville Power Administration (Washington State, Oregon, Idaho, and Montana), you may be eligible for a free radon test. Contact your regional BPA office. If you live in Pennsylvania, you may be eligible for state assistance for both testing and remedial action. Call the state toll-free radon line, (800) 237-2366.

INTERPRETING RESULTS

The laboratory will send back a report indicating radon levels in units of pCi/L (Pico Curies per Liter).

• If measured levels are under 2 pCi/L there is no cause for concern or for further tests.

• If measured levels are between 2pCi/L and 4pCi/L further tests should be done over an extended period, and in other areas of the home.

• If tests exceed 4pCi/L (the United States Environmental Protection Agency's recommended maximum for homes), professional help should be called in for further testing, followed by remedial action. (See Resources below, and the Controlling Indoor Air Quality chapter.)

• If tests exceed 20 pCi/L rapid action should be taken, using professional help.

Relocation in a safe building until the remedial work can be done is recommended if levels are very high (above 200 pCi/L).

- If the bathroom tests very high and the rest of the house does not, water samples should be lab tested and professional help sought. If water is the major source of radon, a filter will be necessary. (See Resources, below.)

RESOURCES

Suppliers of Charcoal Cannister Radon Tests:

The Radon Project
University of Pittsburgh
Pittsburgh, Pa. 15260
(Profits from sales support radon research.)

Environmental Measurements Lab.,
U.S. Dept. of Energy
376 Hudson St.
New York, N.Y. 10014
(Approx. $20 each.)

Alpha Nuclear
1125 Derry Rd. E.
Mississauga, Ontario
Canada L5T 1P3

Suppliers of Alpha Track Radon Tests:

Track-Etch Monitor
Terradex Corporation
460 N. Wiget Lane
Walnut Creek, Calif. 94598

Radtrak Radon Monitor
Glenwood Labs.
3 Science Rd.
Glenwood, Ill. 60425

Barringer Labs
5735 McAdam Rd.
Mississauga, Ont.
Canada L4Z 1N9

($16.50 to $66 each, depending on sensitivity. Analysis by Terradex included in price.)

Further information on approved suppliers of radon tests and recommended professional radon investigators is available from your local public health service, regional office of the United States Environmental Protection Agency, or by writing to:

In the U.S.A.: Regional office of
Environmental Protection Agency, or
401 M. Street S.W., Ste. #200
North East Mall
Washington, D.C. 20460 (202) 475-9605

In Canada: Ask for Radiation Protection Services at your provincial Health Ministry.

For information on water treatment to remove radon write to:
Professor Lowry, Dept. of Civil Engineering
451 Aubert Hall
University of Maine at Orono
Orono, ME 04669 (207) 581-1220

Formaldehyde

Testing for formaldehyde is somewhat more costly and less conclusive than for radon. (Each formaldehyde test costs about $30, including analysis.) While radon levels have been directly linked to lung cancer risk, the formaldehyde levels commonly found in houses will have widely varied effects, depending on individual susceptibility. Most people can smell formaldehyde when it reaches levels commonly considered to be irritating (.1 ppm), but they may not recognize the odor or may have become accustomed to it. Others who are sensitive may react to levels below .1ppm which cannot be detected by odor.

Test for formaldehyde if you have any of the following conditions in your home:

• If anyone in your home suffers from chronic respiratory illness, such as acute asthma or emphysema.

• If anyone in your home is suffering from environmental sensitivity.

• If you have moved into a home built or renovated in the last 10 years and not had control over the choice of building materials, paints, floor coverings, cabinets, and insulation.

• If you live in a mobile home built in the last 10 years.

• If your home was built to current energy efficient standards.

• If you know or suspect that your home has had U.F.F.I. installed in it at any time (even if it has been removed).

FORMALDEHYDE TEST DEVICES

Formaldehyde air test devices are small cannisters or badges filled with liquids or chemicals which absorb formaldehyde from the air. They are then sent to a laboratory for analysis.

These devices should be placed 6 to 8 feet above the floor in living areas for the period recommended by the supplier. Do not place these tests inside cabinets or on furniture which may be producing formaldehyde. Areas to test are the kitchen, bedrooms, and living room. To establish the "worst case" condition, it is best to test during the heating or cooling season, when the home is closed up and ventilation is minimum.

INTERPRETING RESULTS

The results from the laboratory analysis will be expressed in *ppm* (parts per million).

• If levels are below .05 ppm (total aldehydes), you home is in the range of the least contaminated conventional homes measured. However, chemically sensitive individuals may still react at this level. Improved ventilation or specific air purification can be considered in this case. (See the Home Ventilation chapter).

• If levels are .05ppm to .1ppm (total aldehydes), your home is considered "safe" by government agencies. However, many people can detect formaldehyde odors at this level, and some will react with respiratory or other symptoms. Consider improved ventilation and removing the formaldehyde bearing materials, such as particle board floor underlayment. (See the Materials and Selection chapter.) Sealing edges and surfaces of particleboard that cannot be easily removed (eg., on kitchen cabinets) will also help to reduce contamination.

• If levels are .1ppm to .5ppm (total aldehydes) these exceed all maximum standards, and serious reactions and sensitization will occur for many people. In this case, use improved ventilation, major removal of formaldehyde bearing materials (see the Materials and Selection chapter), and possibly specific air purification for removing formaldehyde. (See the Home Ventilation chapter.)

• If levels are greater than .5 ppm (total aldehydes), relocate immediately in a safe home until renovations can be done. These are very alarming levels and a professional investigator should be called.

PROFESSIONAL TESTING

Environmental testing services can perform these and other tests for you, or bring equipment to your home for rapid or even immediate results. These services usually cost $100 and up for a home visit. (For a list of approved agencies, contact your local health department or branch of the E.P.A. (Addresses are listed at the end of this chapter.)

FABRIC AND MATERIAL TESTING

There are simple home formaldehyde test kits for fabric and other materials. They are available from suppliers specializing in products for the chemically sensitive. (See the section ENVIRONMENTAL ILLNESS AND YOU.) *These tests are not very sensitive and will definitely not test for formaldehyde in air.* They can be useful, however, for testing fabric and upholstery which may contain unacceptable mildew, moth, or crease resistant treatments.

RESOURCES

Formaldehyde air test suppliers:

Air Quality Research Inc.
901 Grayson St.
Berkeley, Ca. 94710 (415) 644-2097

PRO-TEK
DuPont Fabric & Finish Department
Applied Technology Division
Barley Mill Plaza
Marshall Mill Building
Wilmington, DE 19898

(Approx. $235/10, plus $20–$35 each for lab analysis.)

Further information on formaldehyde and a list of suppliers and services contact your regional Environmental Protection Agency Office (see the end of this chapter for addresses).

U.S. Department of Housing and Urban Development, 451 7th St. S.W.
Washington, D.C. 20024 (202) 755-6270

If you live in Washington state, Oregon, Idaho, or Montana, you can get further information from your district office of the Bonneville Power Administration.

Other Volatile Organic Compounds

(Xylene, toluene, benzene, ethanes, ethers, ethylenes, naphthalenes.) Testing for other volatile organic compounds is generally very complex and must be done by professional investigators. (They require taking air or water samples to a laboratory, or bringing complicated equipment to the home.)

Water borne volatile organics are a serious problem in some areas where groundwater drinking supplies have been contaminated by industry. Where this is the case, send tap water samples to a testing service for specific analysis for organic compounds. Before going to a private testing lab, inquire if your public health authority has testing services.

Test your air or water for these compounds if any of the following conditions apply to your home.

• If a physician has found unusual levels of organic compounds in blood or hair samples that cannot be explained by exposure at work or other causes.

• If your home is located near chemical dump sites or where soil or water are known to be contaminated by industry.

Testing should be undertaken with the help of a consulting physician or public health authority. (For help finding a specialist physician see the section ENVIRONMENTAL ILLNESS AND YOU.)

Pesticides, Herbicides, Other Organochlorines, Toxic Metals

Tests for these materials are all very complex and will require professional advice.

Tests the air, water, and soil from your yard if any of the following conditions apply.

• If any occupant has been diagnosed with environmental illness.

• If a physician has found unusual levels of pesticides or other compounds in blood or hair samples that cannot be explained by exposure at work or other causes.

• If your home is located near chemical dump sites, intensive agriculture using chemicals, or where soil, air, or water are known to be contaminated by industry.

• If your home has received repeated or unusual extermination treatments in the past.

WATER TESTING

It will be necessary to test your water if you wish to treat it, because treatment systems *must* be specially selected for the type of contamination present. (See the chapter, Water Treatment.)

Test your water if:

• You receive water untreated from a shallow well, spring, river, or lake.

• You live in an area with known or suspected industrial pollution of the groundwater or surface water.

• You receive your water from *any* source other than an approved municipal water system.

• Anyone in your household has a recognized sensitivity to chlorine products.

• You find the taste, odor, or appearance of your water unacceptable for any reason.

HOW TO TEST

If you receive water from a municipal supply, your water authority can supply some water test results. However, these results may *not* accurately describe the water in your home. Generally, the further you are from the chlorination plant the lower the chlorine levels will be. At the same, time other contaminants such as carcinogenic vinyl chloride from plastic water mains (if they are in use in your area) and sediments, are likely to be higher. Water authority test results can only be used as a rough measure if they were not done in your home.

If you do not receive water from a city system, but from a well or shared local service such as a stream, lake, or spring, check with local health authorities for instructions on water testing. If you must pay for a private lab test, consider sharing the cost with a neighbor who is on the same water supply. A basic lab test usually costs about $25, and will give you bacteria counts and levels of dissolved minerals (hardness). If you need information on chlorine, or chlorine compounds, or other compounds, the cost may be greater. (See the chapter, Water Treatment.)

Follow test instructions closely for accurate results. You must use a sterile glass sample jar with a tight fitting metal top. Lab instructions usually require that you first sterilize your cold water tap by holding a butane lighter or torch flame briefly under the opening. The water is then run rapidly for 5 minutes, and then turned down to a steady trickle for 1 minute before taking the sample. The jar should be closed immediately, and taken to the lab as soon as possible.

INTERPRETING TEST RESULTS

Full interpretation of water test results is a very complex matter. Your local health department can advise you regarding bacteriological contamination and can help interpret water hardness. However, if other chemicals are present in your water sample, you will need the advice of an environmental health specialist, such as a clinical ecologist, to interpret the data.

PROFESSIONAL TESTING

Testing should be undertaken with the help of a consulting physician or public health authority. (For help finding a specialist physician, see the section ENVIRONMENTAL ILLNESS AND YOU.)

Asbestos

Visual inspection of your home can determine if it contains hazardous asbestos products. Check ceiling tile, insulation, fireproofing, furnace ducts, plaster, and wallboard. (See Resources, below). Due to regulations introduced in the 1970's controlling the use of asbestos products, these are most common in older homes. *If* they are in stable condition and *not* part of an air handling system (such as heating duct liners or joints), small amounts of asbestos are probably best left undisturbed. They should be isolated from living spaces wherever possible, as by enclosing them with new wallboard. However, if the materials are visibly crumbling, or part of air ducts, or if renovations will disturb them, hire a competent professional service to remove them. Everyone in the house should be prepared to relocate to a safe home while cleanup is under way. (See Protecting Yourself, in the chapter Construction Trades and Services.)

Combustion Gases

Chimneys may work in reverse due to house de-pressurization, spilling dangerous gases, such as carbon monoxide, into the home. You may have this problem if you live in a weathersealed house with conventional gas or oil heating. (Using fireplaces and large exhaust fans in a tightly closed house is a frequent cause.)

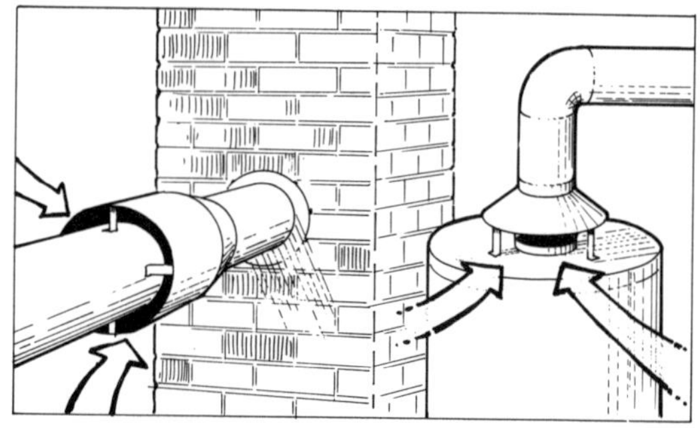

Fig.27-1 Draft regulators

HOW TO TEST

Close the house up tightly and operate all exhaust devices. Include kitchen and bathroom fans, clothes dryers, and outside vented vacuums. Locate the draft regulator on the chimney pipe of your furnace or water heater. (Draft regulators are loose fitting collars or fittings directly above the unit.) Start the furnace or water heater and hold a smoking taper (eg. a twisted paper) near the draft regulator and observe the smoke; it should be drawn into the pipe. *If the smoke is rejected you have a dangerous situation.* Repeat this test with the fireplace in use.

If your chimney is reversing you need a larger outdoor air source to prevent house de-pressurization. Consult a heating or ventilation specialist.

FOR FURTHER INFORMATION ON TESTING AND RELATED SERVICES

IN THE U.S.A.:
Contact your regional **EPA** Office:

Room 2203
JFK Federal Building
Boston, MA 02203
(617) 223-4845

26 Federal Plaza
New York, NY 10278
(212) 264-2515

841 Chestnut Street
Philadelphia, PA 19107
(215) 597-8320

345 Courtland Street, NE.
Atlanta, GA 30365
(404) 881-3776

Suite 1300
One Denver Place
999 18th Street
Denver, CO 80202
(303) 283-1710

1201 Elm Street
Dallas, TX 75270
(214) 767-2630

726 Minnesota Avenue
Kansas City, KS 66101
(913) 236-2803

230 South Dearborn St
Chicago, IL 60604
(312) 353-2205

215 Fremont Street
San Francisco,
CA 94105
(415) 974-8076

1200 Sixth Avenue
Seattle, WA 98101
(206) 442-7660

IN CANADA:
Contact your Provincial Environment Ministry, or local Public Health Office.

28 CONSTRUCTION TRADES AND SERVICES

Building or renovating a home in a health conscious manner is not easy, and will require the cooperation of all concerned and complete control by *YOU*.

Contractors, trades people, and architects have very little experience with the health concerns discussed in this book. Though most will now be aware of radon and formaldehyde, and may have some information on how to control them, few will be aware of other hazards, alternative materials, ventilation and air purification systems, and health conscious construction techniques.

If you intend to build or renovate to the strictest hypoallergenic standards for the environmentally sensitive, your task will be even more demanding. Of course, if you are a builder, or will be doing your own work, or at least directly supervising it, your task will be easier, because the rigid control required for every step will be in your hands.

Preparing Yourself

The need to make as many decisions beforehand about design, materials, and methods cannot be overemphasized. Selecting a single material, or a device, such as an air or water purification system, can require a great deal of research, adding hours or even days to your preparation time. Making these decisions under duress when construction is under way is difficult even for conventional construction; it is far more difficult in health conscious construction.

RESEARCH

Read everything you can find on the subject. (See Further Reading, in the GETTING HELP section.) If you are learning to live with environmental sensitivity, or only want to take the best health precautions, the experience of others and shared resources can be tremendously valuable. Consider joining a chapter of H.E.A.L. (Human Ecology Action League), or another health and environmental action group (see the ENVIRONMENTAL ILLNESS AND YOU section), use their resources, and get involved.

• Try to find contractors, designers, or trades who might have special experience with health conscious work. Check with your local health action group or allergy association.

• Check their references and talk with their previous customers.

• Ask them detailed questions about methods and materials.

• Make it clear that you expect to have total control over every choice of material and method, and final approval before the final payment.

• Consider adding a clause to any contractual agreement, to state your special needs and require your final approval.

• If possible, bring together all those who will be working on your job to go over the details of the project. Good cooperation starts with good coordination.

• Expect to pay a little more for the extra time and dedication required to deliver a good, health conscious job.

If you suffer from environmental sensitivity, seek the help of a health professional, such as a clinical ecologist or a building consultant for the environmentally sensitive, when planning your project. Your special needs will influence the decisions that you must make. (See the section, ENVIRONMENTAL ILLNESS AND YOU.)

If you have difficulty finding a suitable contractor or trade, consider specialists in energy efficient construction. They have experience with exacting details and methods far beyond those of conventional projects. *However, energy efficiency experts must be carefully briefed on the need to select materials with extreme caution.* Many are accustomed to using a wide range of high performance sealants, plastic products, and other materials which are unacceptable to the health conscious.

SUPERVISION

It is absolutely essential that you become involved in the construction, approving choices and checking the work. This will stretch the limits of the most harmonious and patient working relationships, so be prepared for some strain. Remember that your contractor or trades people can be your best allies. Once they become aware of what you are trying to do, you may get a good deal of support and some helpful ideas. Many builders and contractors are becoming aware of the risks to their own health in working under contaminating conditions and may welcome the opportunity to work on your project.

PROTECTING YOURSELF DURING CONSTRUCTION

A high quality respirator mask is absolutely essential for many aspects of demolition and construction. *Masks are available* (see below) *with special filters which will remove some gases and vapors, as well as airborne particles.*

Always use a mask during:

Demolition Debris can contain any number of hazards, including asbestos, lead, pesticides, and allergenic dusts.

Cleanup Sweeping or vacuuming raises large amounts of dust. (Moistening surfaces will help to reduce dust.)

Sanding, mixing, sawing (Or any activity which produces dust.)

Painting (Or using adhesives, cleaners, and waxes which produce volatile vapors.)

When it is necessary to use paints, adhesives, etc., which produce dangerous vapors, do the work outdoors, if possible, and use brush techniques instead of spraying. If you must use them indoors, place a large fan in a window or door opening to bring in outside air, and open windows on the opposite side to generate cross ventilation. Make sure that everyone in the area is wearing a proper respirator mask.

Safety supply companies are the best places to go for a respirator. Those available from your local hardware store are not likely to be adequate. Expect to pay about $50 for a good permanent unit, and from $1 to $8 for replacement filters of various types.

Look for a N.I.O.S.H. (National Institute of

Occupational Safety and Health) rating on the mask, and be sure that it fits your face and has secure straps. Always follow the manufacturer's instructions. Consult the table of recommended filters for each type of hazard that is included with the mask. Some suppliers and manufacturers also have toll-free telephone services and will provide advice on protection.

A good industrial respirator mask is more than a dust mask, and will protect your health if used properly. It will absorb or neutralize most vapors from paints, adhesives, welding, cleaners, plastics, etc., with specific filters.

Whenever possible, isolate the area where the work is taking place by covering doorways and openings with a tarp. Tape it to walls, floors, and ceilings to reduce dust. *Do not leave on a forced air heating or cooling system connected to an area in which renovations are taking place.* Dust and fumes will enter the system, be carried throughout the house, and will contaminate the ducts, filters, fan, and heating or cooling unit.

Gloves, long sleeved shirts, and hats are also important protection when handling paints, adhesives, or dusty projects. You can absorb significant amounts of dangerous materials through skin contact. (These articles of clothing should be laundered carefully and separately from other clothing.)

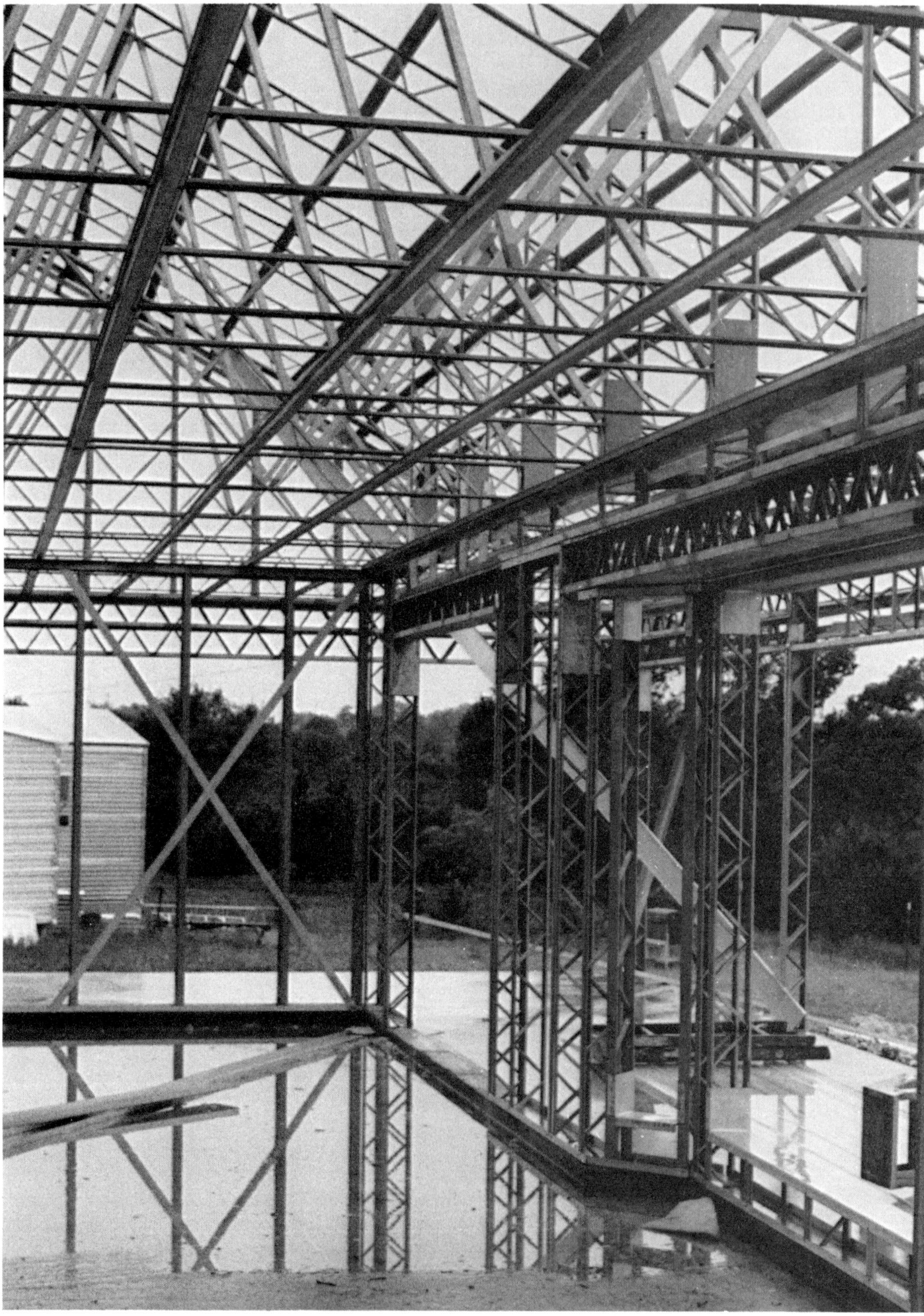

Metal framing for a health conscious home. Photo: Dona Shrier

29 CONSTRUCTION NOTES

Introduction

The construction methods for health conscious building are different in some important ways from those in common use today, particularly those in mass produced housing. Some of the techniques are new to housing, such as the use of lightweight steel framing systems for walls and floors, or aluminum foil air/vapor barriers in place of polyethylene plastic. However, most methods are traditional, such as the use of interior plaster mixed on site.

Many of these methods simply combine good design with conscientious construction practice—a commodity all too rare in current buildings. Others are simply safe and reliable alternatives to the use of hazardous chemicals, such as cement mortar for setting ceramic tile instead of adhesives, metal shields for preventing termite entry instead of residual pesticides, or screw fasteners in place of construction adhesives.

The traditional methods are labor intensive, but allow better control over the contents of building materials and the way they are applied. Though the labor cost will be higher, this will be offset in the long term by the limited use of costly "convenience" materials, and the durability, quality, and value of the finished home.

Planning for Light

Exposure to sunlight and daylight is one of the many important considerations in home planning. Careful orientation of rooms and openings for light will mean benefits in winter, well being, and comfort, with improved interior appearance, function, and energy efficiency.

Northerly exposures are preferred for activities requiring constant light such as studios, and cooler temperatures, such as storage rooms. In hot climates, bedrooms are also often located on the north side.

Easterly exposures are preferred where morning sun can be an advantage, such as in kitchens and breakfast rooms.

Southerly exposures are preferred where midday sun is an advantage, such as for sunrooms, greenhouses, and playrooms.

Westerly windows are usually avoided due to problems with afternoon overheating.

Bedrooms may be oriented north, east, or south, depending on preference for morning light and daytime sun. West exposures are almost universally undesirable, due to summer overheating lasting well into the evening.

The effects of light and heat on the home can be altered dramatically by trees and outside shading devices. A living room, for example, can be oriented toward a westerly view, if shade is provided to reduce overheating and glare.

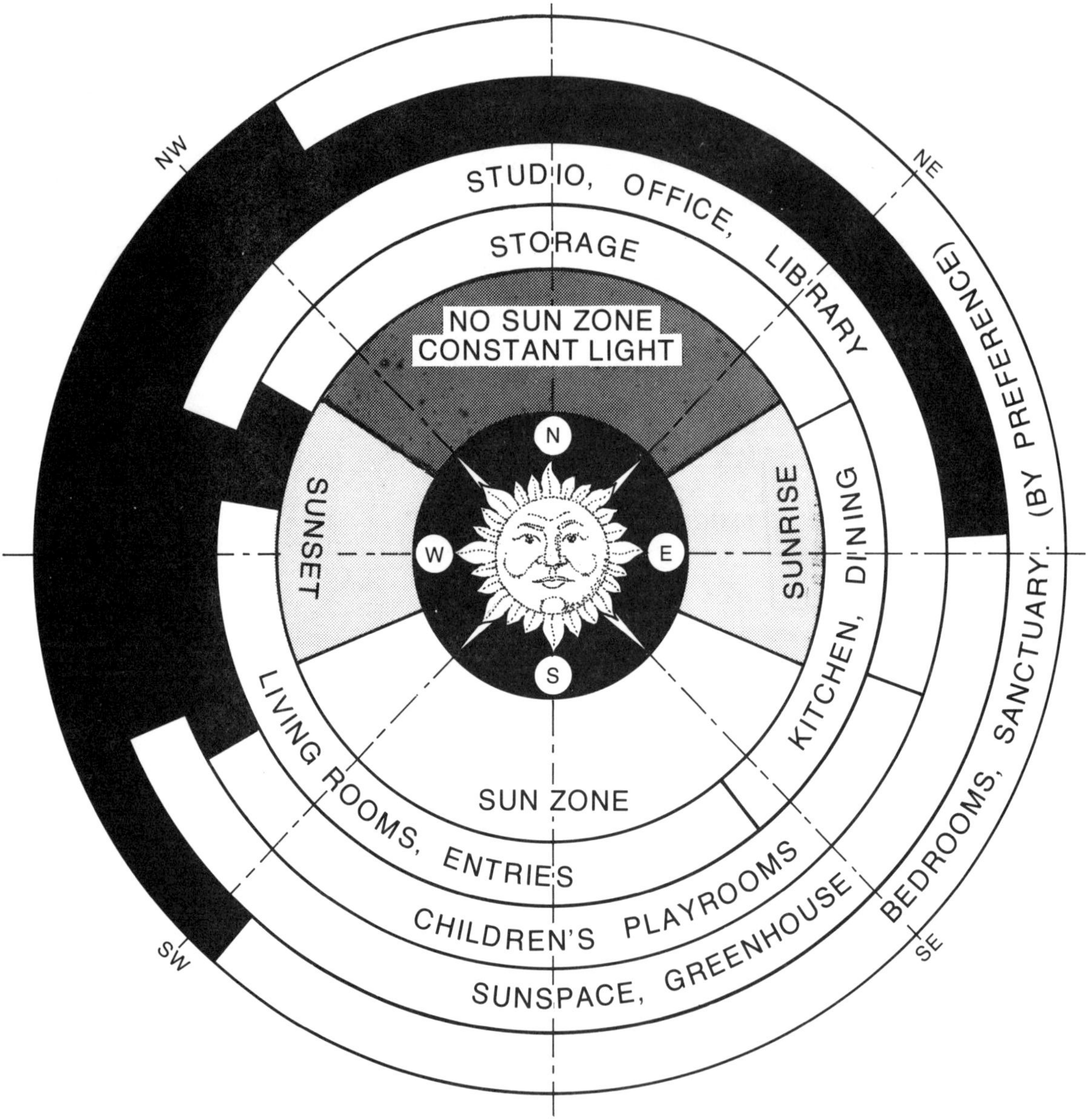

Fig. 29-1 Natural Light Exposure For Rooms

Use this diagram when planning a home to choose the most desirable room and window locations for your situation.

Foundations

Moisture control, prevention of cracking, prevention of radon entry, and termite protection, are the major concerns with foundations.

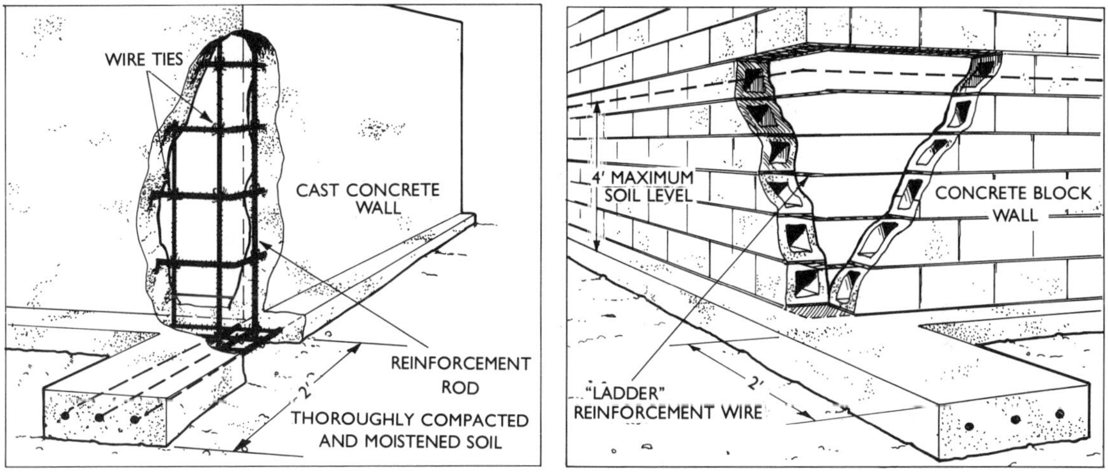

Fig. 29-2 Foundation Footings and Reinforcement. *For a cast concrete wall, thoroughly moisten and compact soil before placing a gravel base and concrete forms. Extend wall footings 2 feet beyond corners to minimize settling and cracking of walls. Place a minimum of three pieces of 1/2" reinforcing steel in footings, and use* Reinforcement Rod *vertically and horizontally at corners in poured concrete walls. For concrete block walls use* Ladder Reinforcement Wire *in horizontal joints below grade. Do not attempt to use concrete block instead of poured foundations where more than 4 feet of earth burial is required.*

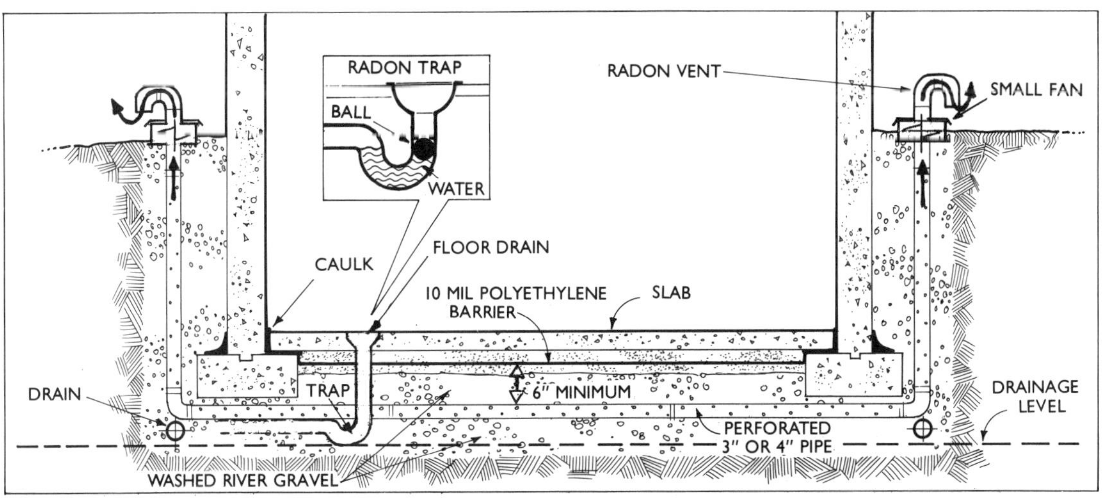

Fig. 29-3 Basement Foundation Venting For High Radon Areas. *In high radon areas install* Perforated Vent Pipes *in* Washed River Gravel *above the final level of* Perforated Drains. *Use a* 10 Mil Polyethylene Barrier *in sand under slab.* Caulk *the barrier to walls and footings. More effective: Add a* Small Fan. *Fit all* Floor Drains *with* Radon Traps.

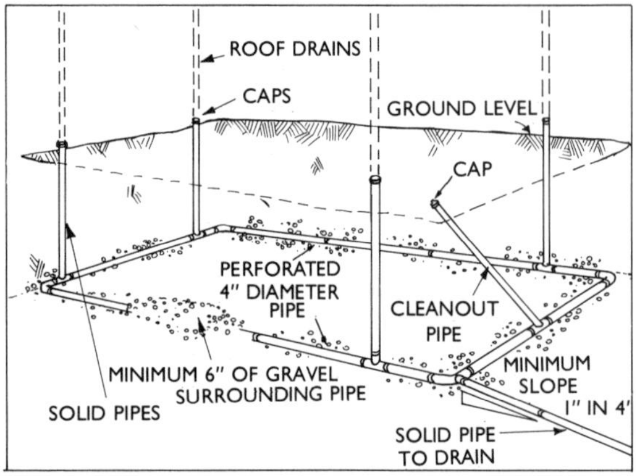

Fig. 29-4 A Typical Foundation Drainage System. *Place* Perforated Pipe *with the perforations facing down on a 6" bed of washed gravel. Rigid plastic, clay, or cement pipe are best. The pipe is placed level, and located just below the wall footings. Use* Solid Pipes *to connect the* Roof Drains *to the system, and a* Solid Pipe Drain *placed at a minimum slope of 1" per 4 feet to connect to a disposal point.*

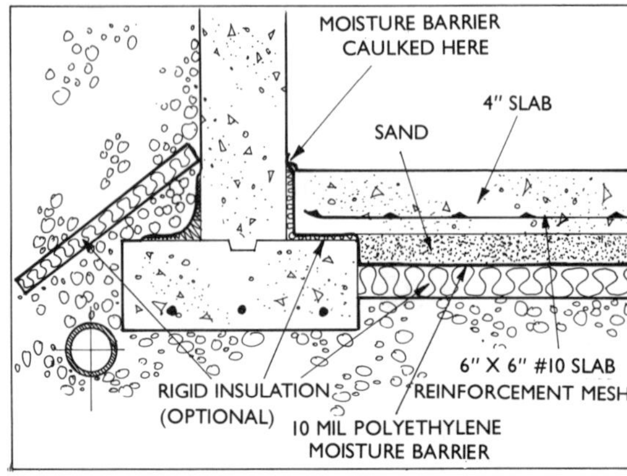

Fig. 29-5 Slab Drainage and Sealing. Place *the* Slab *on a* 10 Mil Polyethylene Moisture Barrier, *which is set in 2' of moistened sand and caulked to the wall. The slab is reinforced with* 6" X 6" #10 Slab Reinforcement Mesh *placed in the lower 1/3 of slab.* Rigid Insulation Board *is optional under slab and at perimeter. Use only insulation types rated for under slab use.*

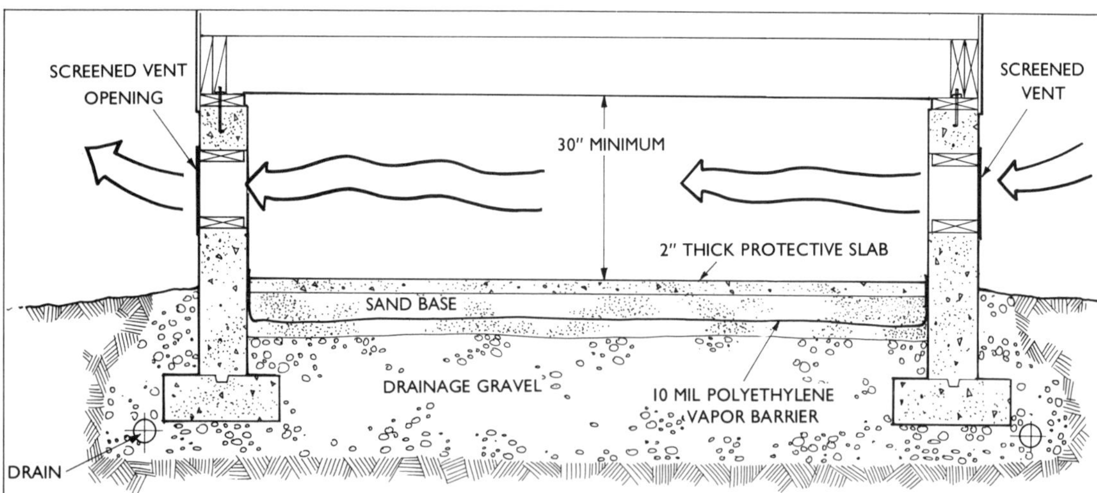

Fig. 29-6 Crawl Space Sealing and Venting. *Place a* 2" Protective Slab *over the* 10 Mil Polyethylene Moisture Barrier, *which is set in 2"of moistened sand. This slab will protect the moisture barrier and keep the crawl space clean. It must be handled carefully during construction, to prevent cracking.* Place screened Vent Openings *on opposite sides of the crawlspace, allowing at least one square foot of area for each 150 square feet of ground area.*

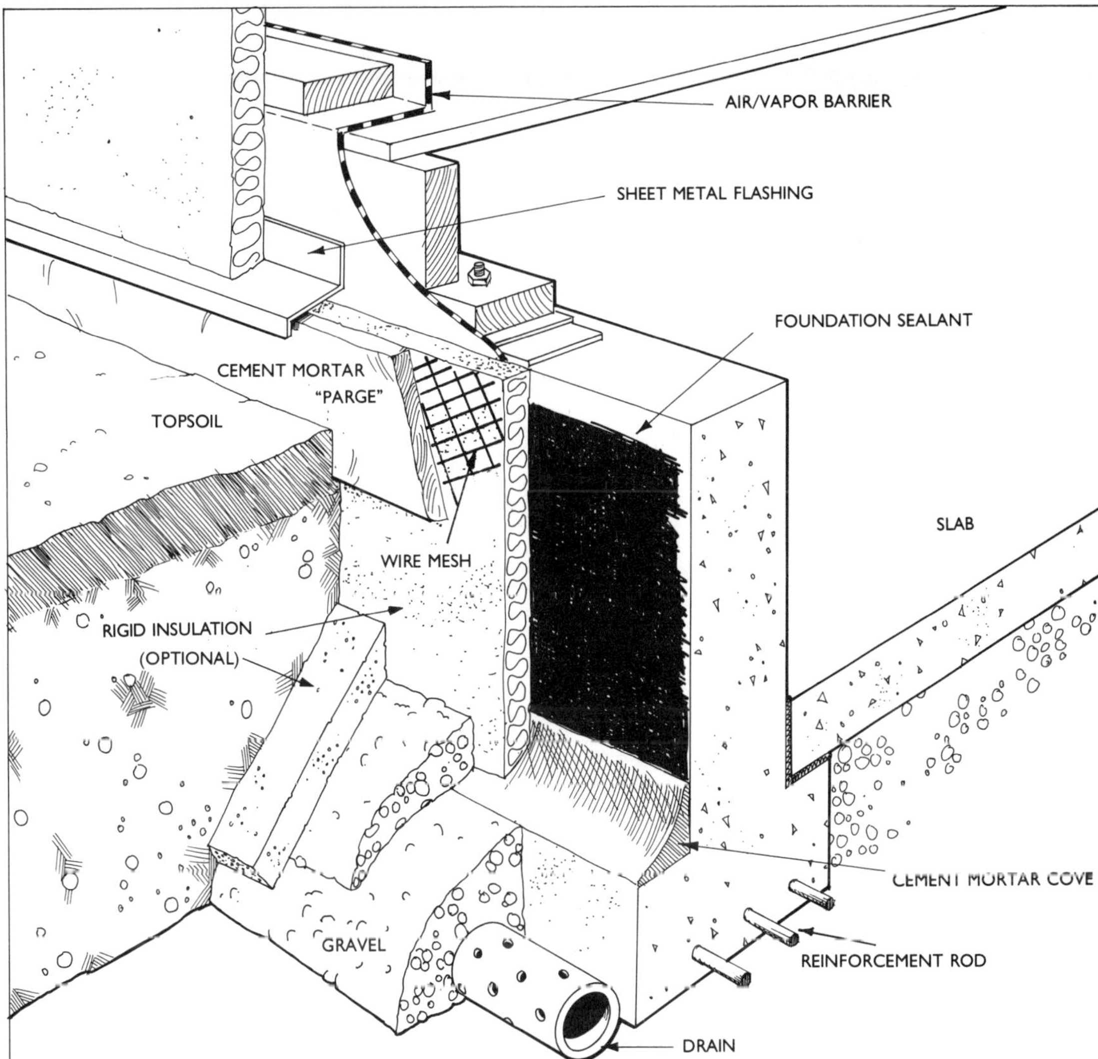

Fig. 29-7 Foundation and Footing Drainage and Sealing. *Form a* Cement Mortar Cove *with a trowel between the wall and footing. Apply* Foundation Sealant *to the wall, then* Rigid Insulation *(if desired) and washed gravel up to the surface.* Topsoil *is placed over the gravel (if desired) and sloped away from the building.* Rigid Insulation *will require a* Cement Mortar ("Parge") *coating for protection. Apply wire stucco mesh or wire lath to the insulation first.*

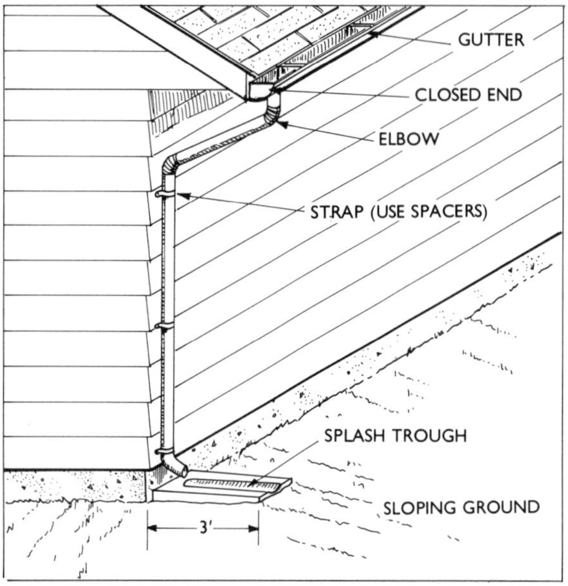

Fig. 29-8 Preventing Water Damage to Old Foundations. *Existing buildings without proper foundation drainage can be protected from excess moisture by installing gutters and downpipes leading to a splash trough. This trough carries water away from the foundations.*

TERMITE CONTROL

Termites can only survive in damp soil near a ready supply of woodfiber for food. They can build tubes above the ground to a height of about 12″ to reach a food source. Careful construction methods are an effective and safe alternative to the use of chemical treatments for termite control. Sheet metal shields which project at least 2″ from foundations will protect wood parts from termite entry. Sheet metal strips, cast into concrete foundations at joints, will also prevent termite entry through cracks after settling. Use only corrosion resistant metals, such as copper or galvanized steel.

To eliminate a potential food source for termites, always remove all stumps and roots from soil during land clearing and excavation, remove all wood formwork from cement foundations before backfilling, and clean up wood construction scraps regularly to prevent their burial.

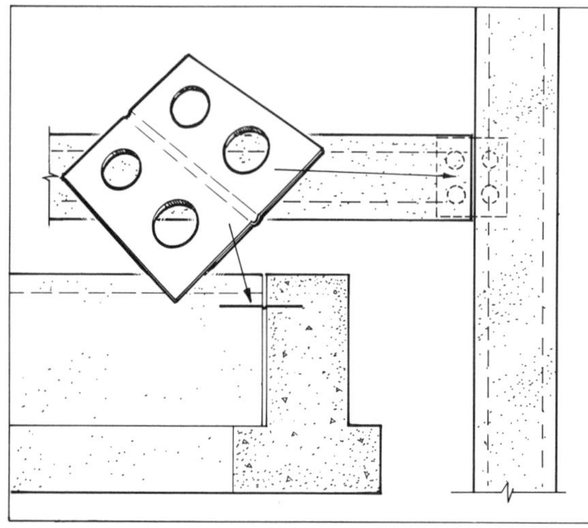

Fig. 29-9 Termite Shields at Wall and Floor Junctions

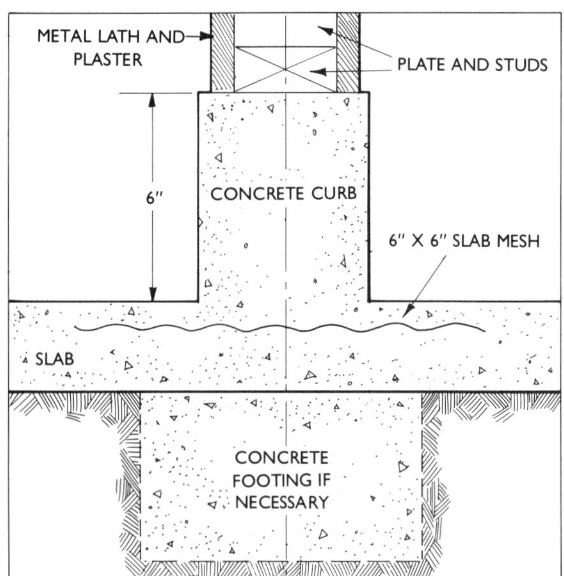

Fig. 29-10 Basement Floor Construction at Partition. *Raise wood construction at least 6″ above concrete floors. Reinforce slab under partitions to reduce cracking, and provide a footing for load bearing walls.*

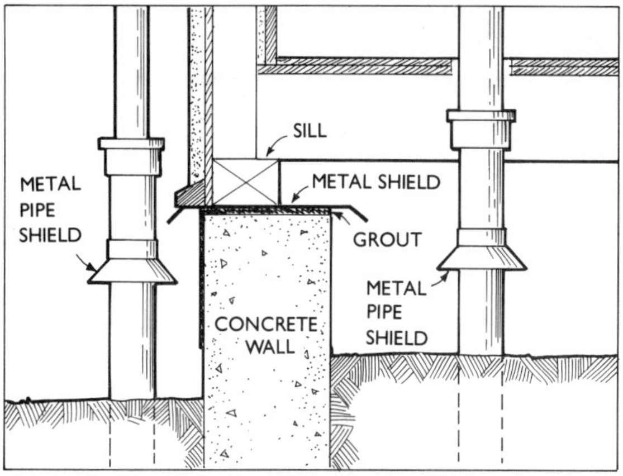

Fig. 29-11 Termite Shields for Basements or Crawl Space Foundations. *The concrete wall must project at least 12" above soil level. Grout a* Metal Shield *to the wall before placing the wood* Sill *plate. Also install circular* Metal Pipe Shields *on drain pipes leading to the building, either inside or out.*

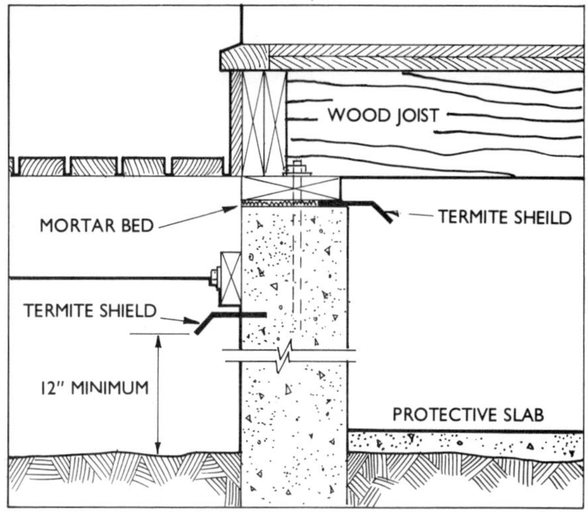

Fig. 29-14 Shield For Entrance With Wood Steps and Floor

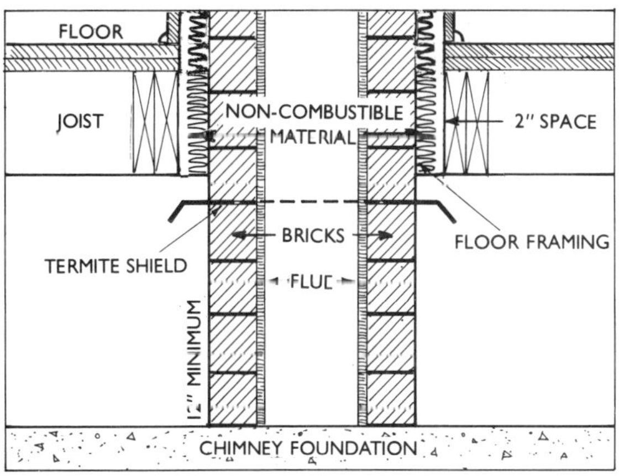

Fig. 29-12 Termite Shield at Chimney Foundation

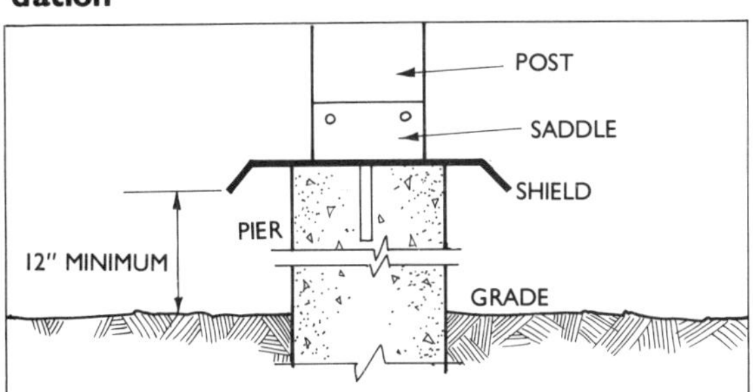

Fig. 29-13 Shield On Concrete Pier With Saddle and Wood Post

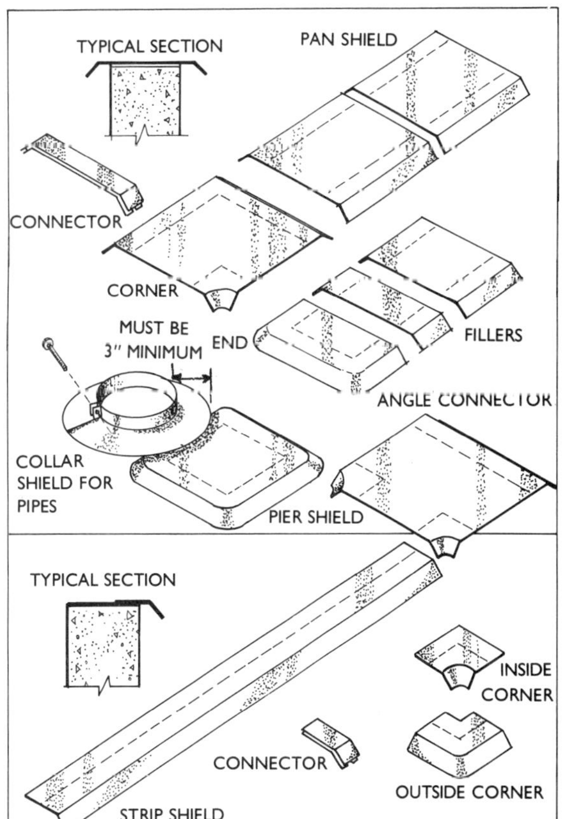

Fig. 29-15 Types Of Termite Shields

Framing Systems

Steel framing systems for both structural walls and floors, and for lightweight non-load-bearing partitions, are in common use in commercial construction. They can be readily adapted to home construction. Steel systems are especially appropriate for those sensitive persons who cannot tolerate the plant terpenes contained in softwood lumber, or the hazardous glue or fungicide treatments which many wood framing members contain.

WALL SYSTEMS

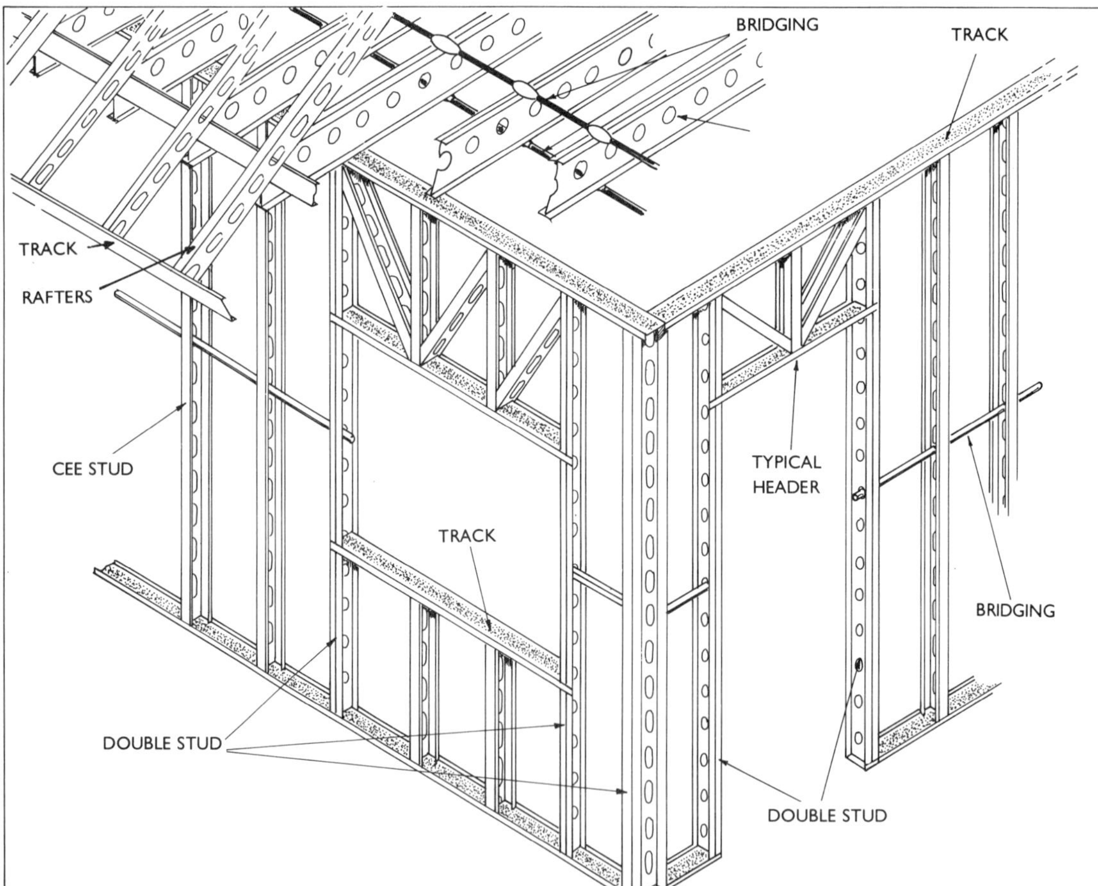

Fig. 29-16 Light Steel Structural Framing. *Most fastening can be done with screws and bolts, with a minimum of drilling. Lighter members can be cut with heavy snips. A special electric chop saw, or other metal saw, is required for heavier pieces.*

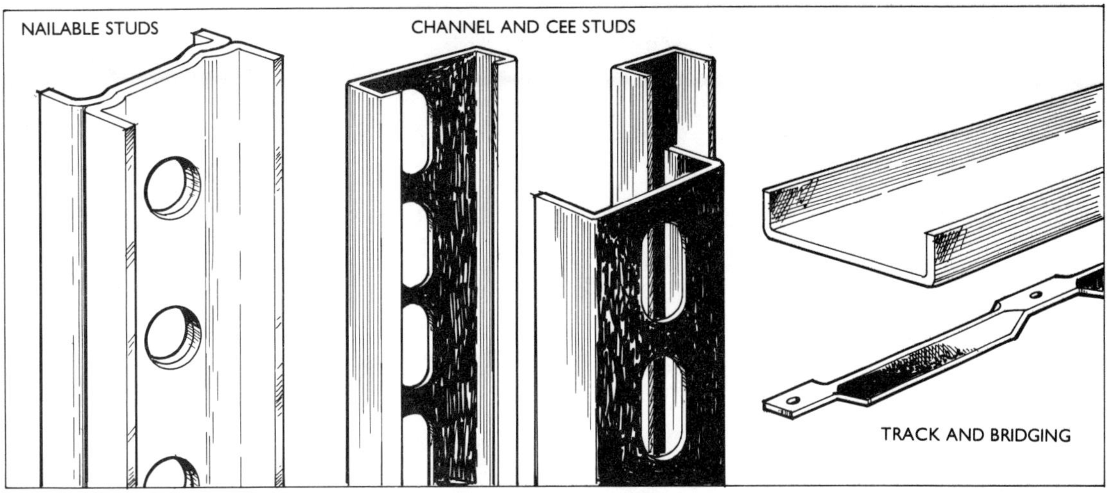

Fig. 29-17 Metal Stud Types

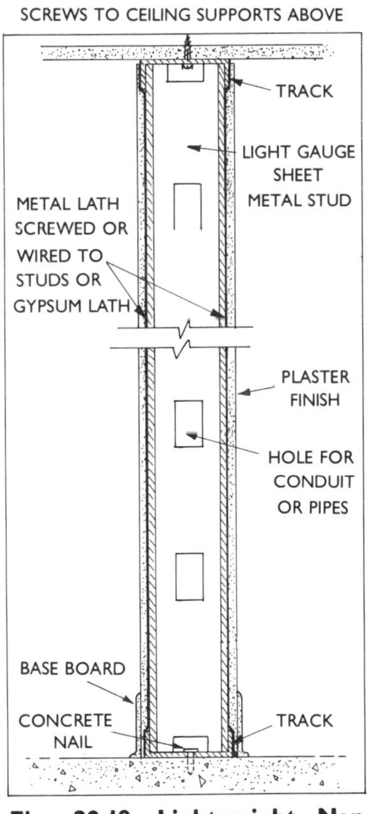

Fig. 29-18 Lightweight Non Load-Bearing Metal Partition Framing. *These light sheet metal studs and tracks, available from commercial drywall systems suppliers, are inexpensive and easy to handle.*

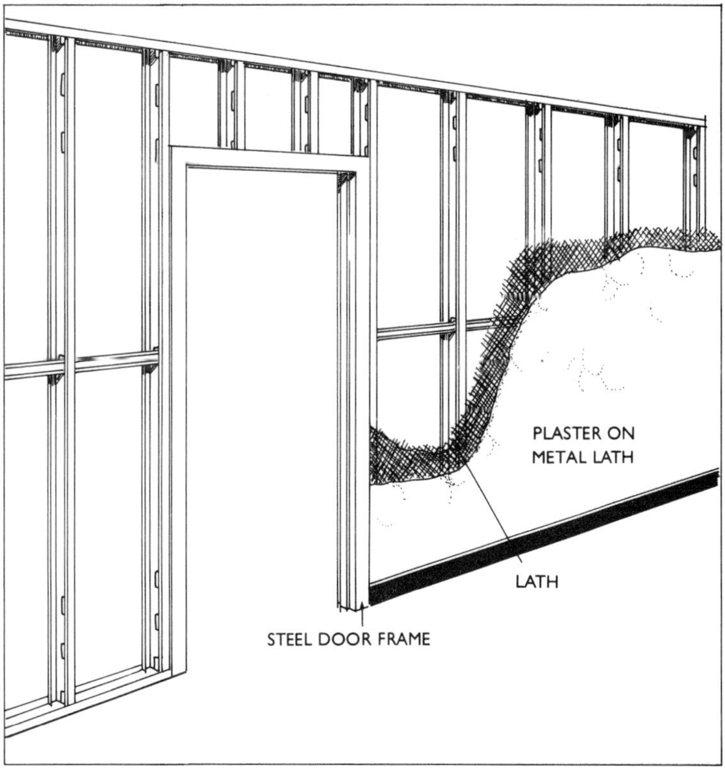

Fig. 29-19 Plaster On Metal Lath Wall System

MASONRY/STEEL OR CONCRETE/ STEEL HYBRID WALL SYSTEMS

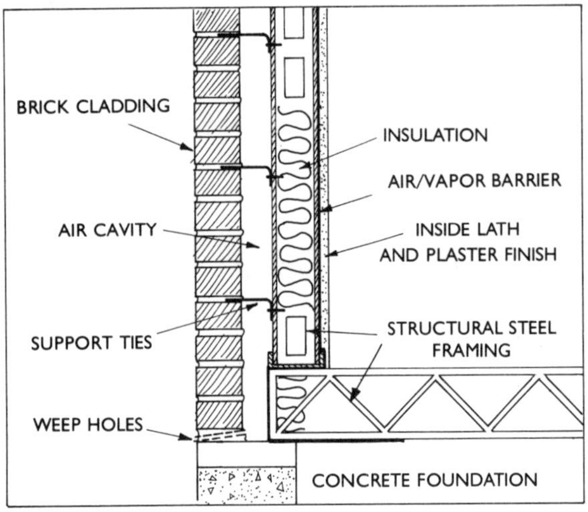

Fig. 29-20 Exterior Structural Steel Wall with Brick Cladding. *An air cavity must be provided with weep holes to drain moisture.*

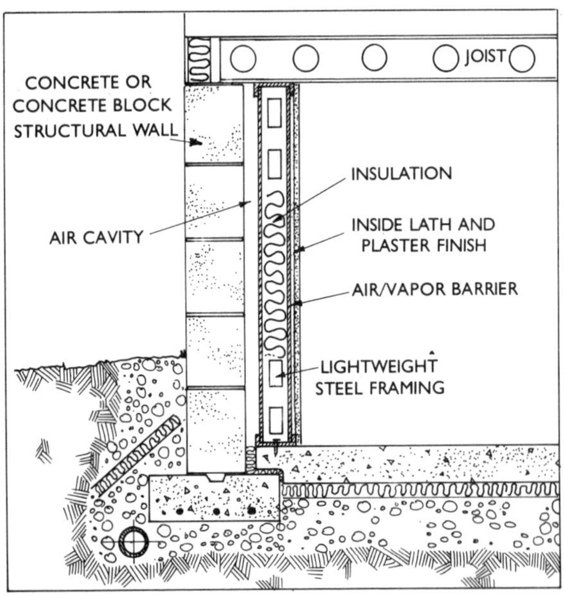

Fig. 29-21 Non-structural Steel Frame Wall on Concrete or Block. *Note: Allow 2 to 6 weeks for concrete to cure before installing wall, in order to reduce moisture content.*

FLOOR SYSTEMS

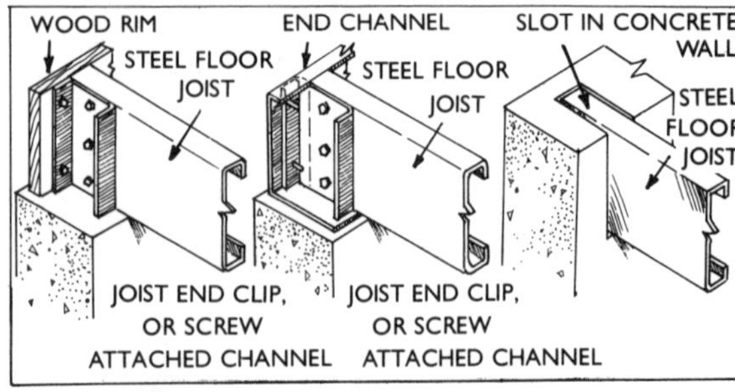

Fig. 29-22 Steel Channel Floor Joists for Light Construction. *Lightweight steel joists are available in sizes comparable to wood joists, for short spans. Fasten with an all steel Clip and Screw system. Or combine steel joists with wood or concrete systems.*

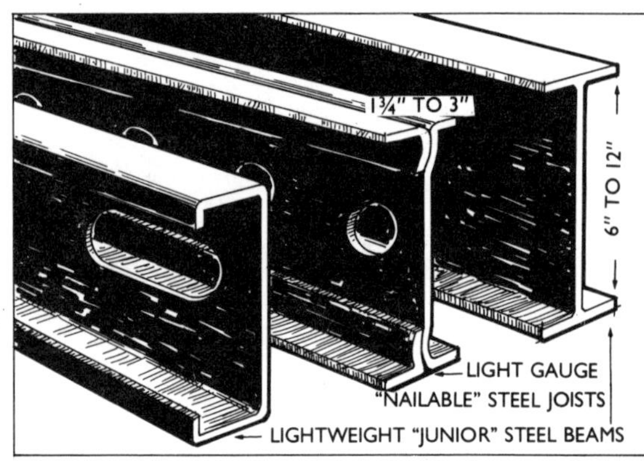

Fig. 29-23 Lightweight Steel Floor Joists (Available for spans up to 22'.)

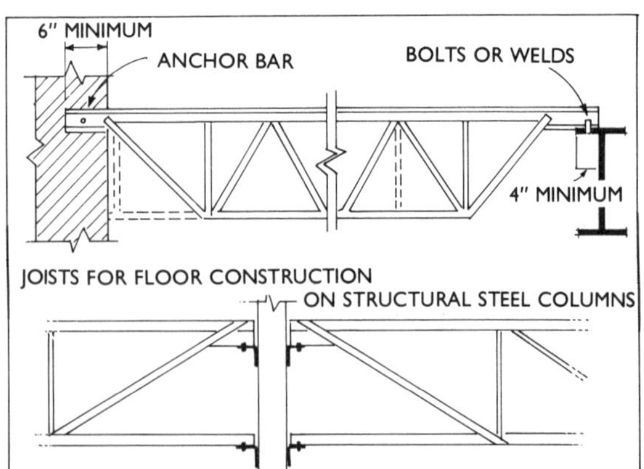

Fig. 29-24 Long Span Steel Joists for Floor or Roof Systems. (Available for spans up to 90'.)

COMPOSITE CONCRETE/STEEL FLOOR SYSTEMS

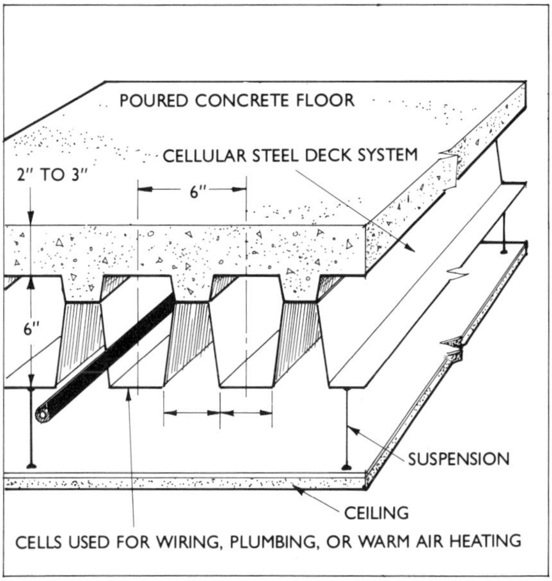

Fig. 29-25 Cellular Steel Deck System (Available in 20′ lengths.)

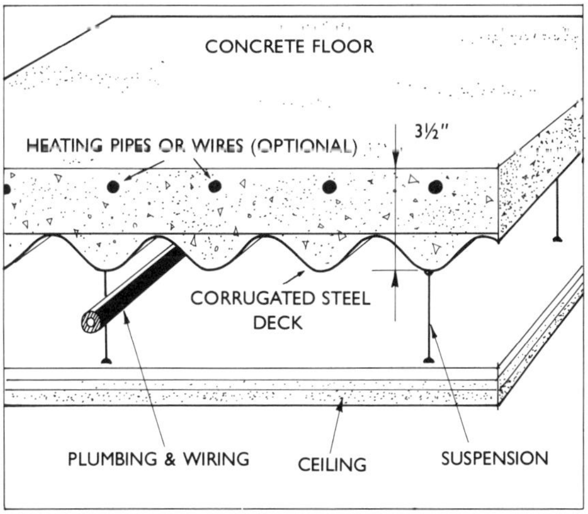

Fig. 29-26 Heavy Gauge Corrugated Steel Deck with Concrete Floor. *The steel deck acts as both a form for concrete, and a permanent reinforcement* (Available in 20′ lengths.)

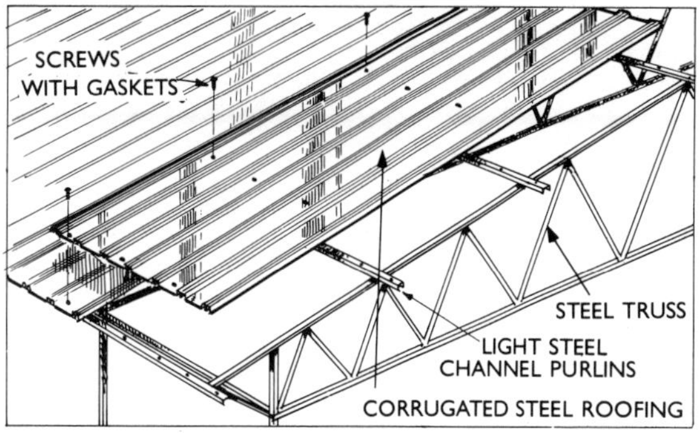

Fig. 29-27 Steel Corrugated Roof Screwed to Steel Purlins on Steel Roof Truss. (Roofing available in lengths to 20′.)

ROOF VENTILATION METHODS

To prevent moisture damage it is essential to ventilate the roof space above the insulation. Extra ventilation with an attic fan will improve summer comfort and reduce cooling costs.

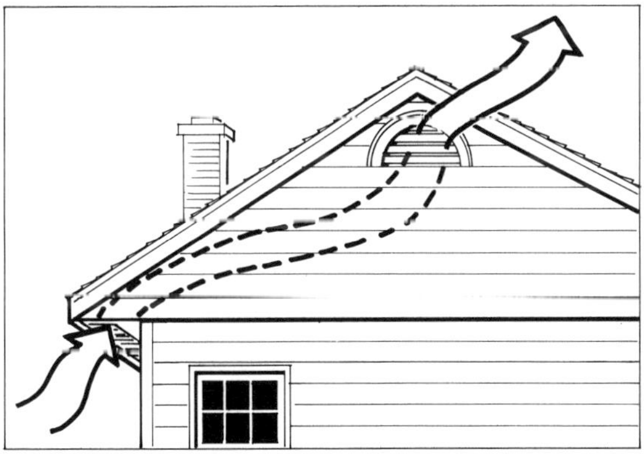

Fig. 29-28 Typical Soffit and Gable Roof Vent

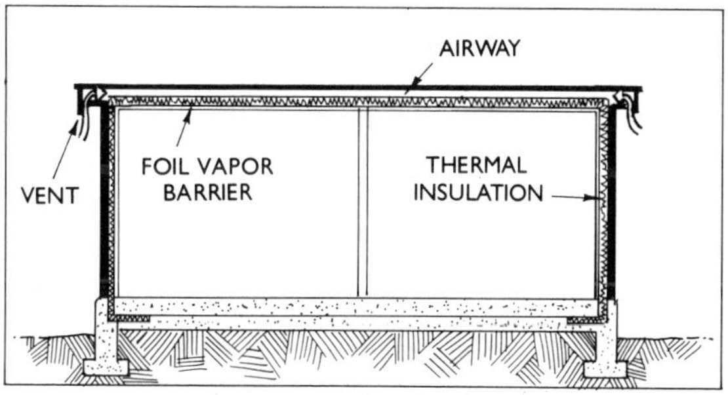

Fig. 29-29 Flat Roof Ventilation

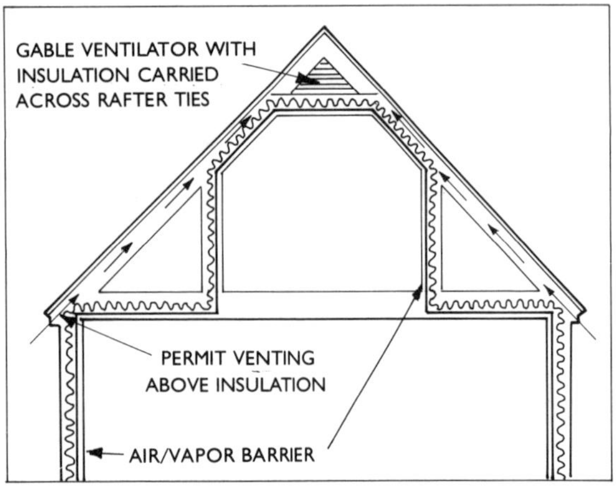

Fig. 29-30 Gable Ventilator with Insulated Attic

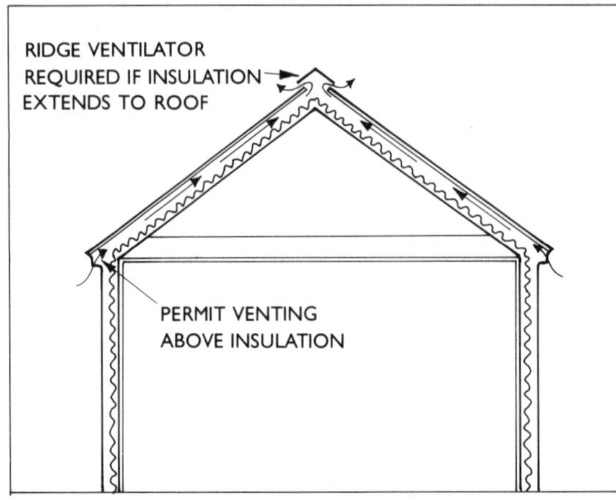

Fig. 29-31 Ridge Ventilation with Open Ceiling

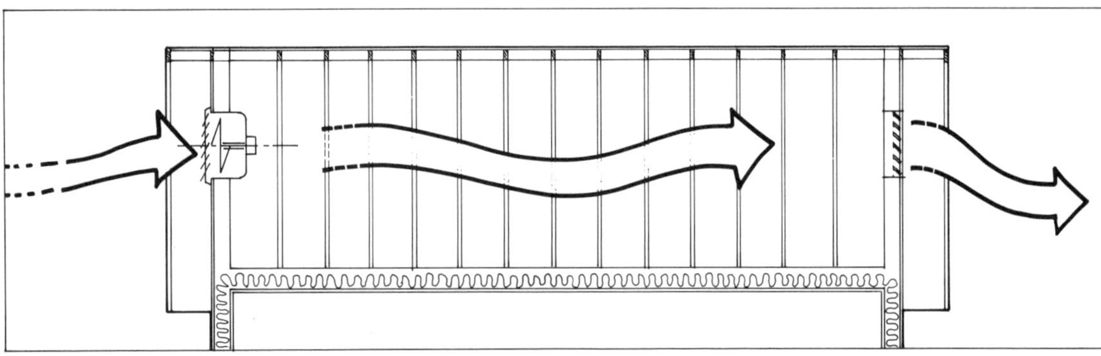

Fig. 29-32 Fan Ventilation of Attic Space

Insulation

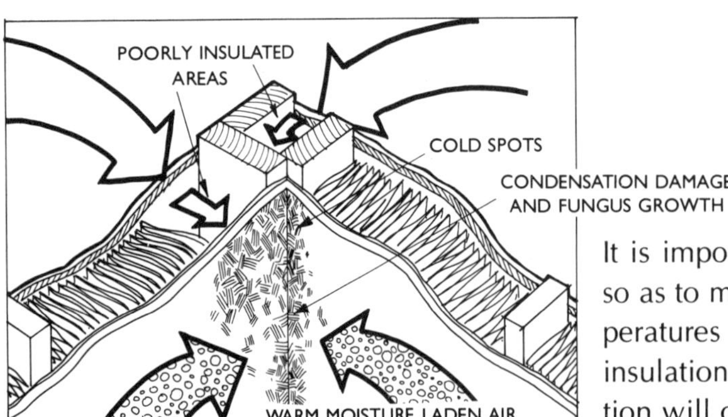

Fig. 29-33 Insulation Gaps

It is important to apply insulation carefully, so as to maintain even wall and ceiling temperatures inside the home in winter. Gaps in insulation due to settling or careless installation will cause cold spots, which encourage condensation and fungus growth.

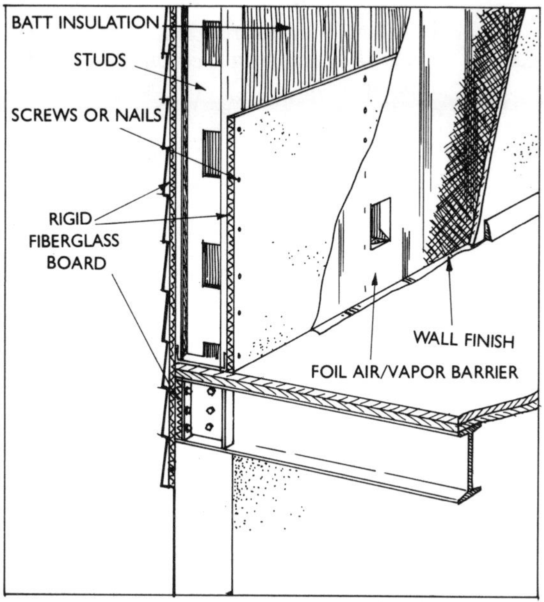

Fig. 29-34 An Insulated Wall. *Fasten* Rigid Fiberglass Board *to the exterior before applying exterior finish. Carefully fit* Batt Insulation *to the cavity spaces, cutting it around electrical boxes and taking care not to compress it. Lightly fasten* Rigid Fiberglass Board *to the interior with* Screws. *Apply* Foil Air/Vapor Barrier *and lightly fasten it with staples along seams. Then tape the seams with foil tape, and apply the wall finish.*

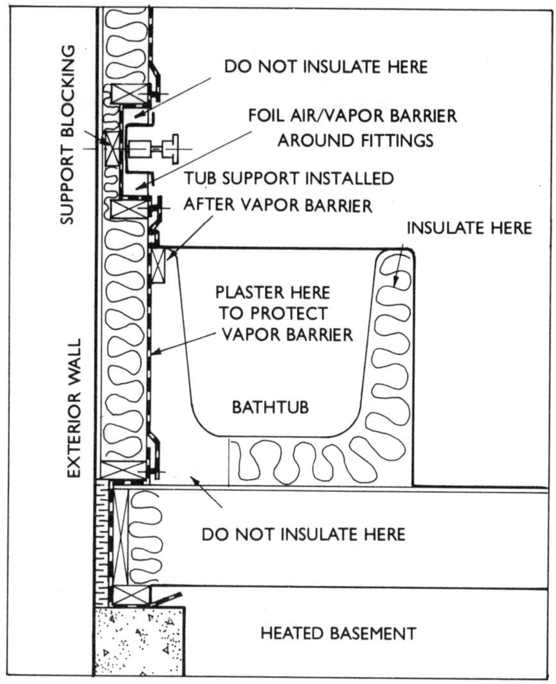

Fig. 29-36 Tub Enclosure Insulation Over Heated Basement. *Wall insulation and wall covering is continuous behind tub. Place no insulation between tub and cold wall due to trapped moisture hazard.*

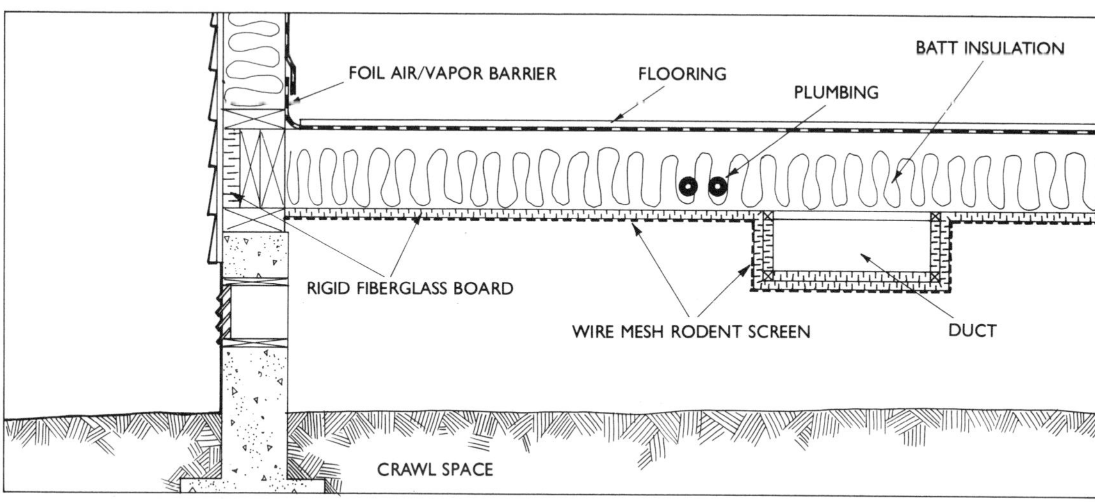

Fig. 29-35 Floor Insulation Over Unheated Crawl Space

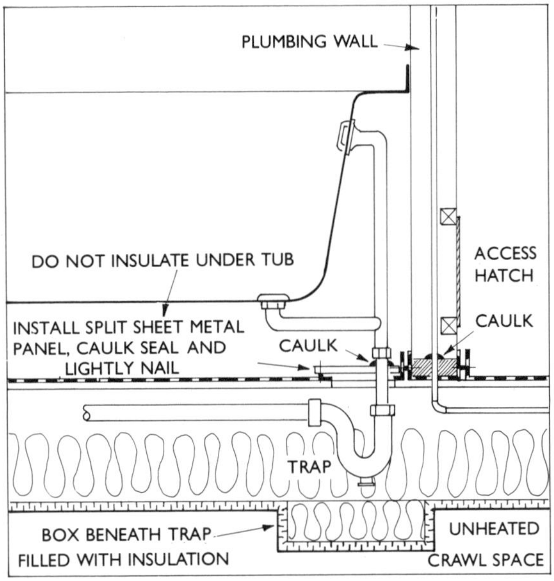

Fig. 29-37 Tub Enclosure Insulation Over Crawl Space. *Floor insulation is continuous under tub and drain trap. No insulation is placed between tub and cold floor due to trapped moisture hazard.*

The Air/Vapor Barrier

The air/vapor barrier is one of the most critical features of health conscious building. The barrier must: prevent the leakage of warm, moisture laden indoor air into building cavities, where it will cause condensation damage and fungus growth; prevent the diffusion of water vapor contained in room air through the building shell; and prevent the leakage of outgassed fumes from insulation and building materials back into room air.

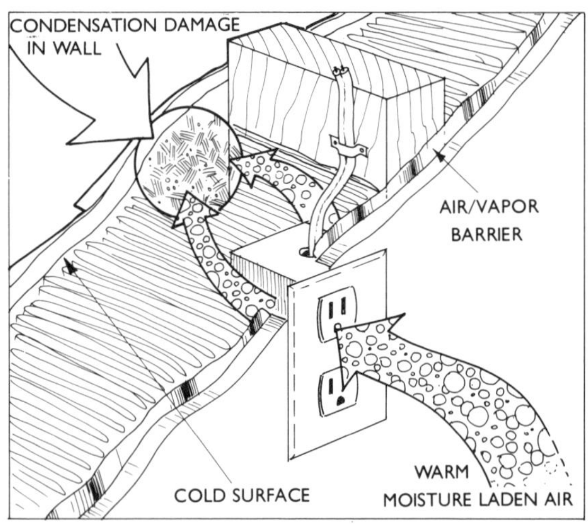

Fig. 29-38 Condensation Damage Due to Poor Air Seal. *During the cold season, warm room air leaking out through openings in the air/vapor barrier passes through the insulation until it reaches a cold surface. Here part of its moisture content condenses, forming a moist spot which will then support mold growth and cause building damage.*

By far the most important of these three functions is the air barrier function. The air leaking through a typical poorly sealed electrical outlet will carry more moisture with it into building cavities than what can pass by diffusion through 1,000 square feet of typical plaster or drywall. For this reason a great deal of effort must be devoted to ensuring a good air seal when installing the air/vapor barrier.

The air/vapor barrier material represented in the accompanying diagrams is a plain aluminum foil type sealed with a foil tape. This material is a hypo-allergenic substitute for the usual polyethylene plastic sheet. It is available from suppliers of specialty building products and from some builders supply stores.

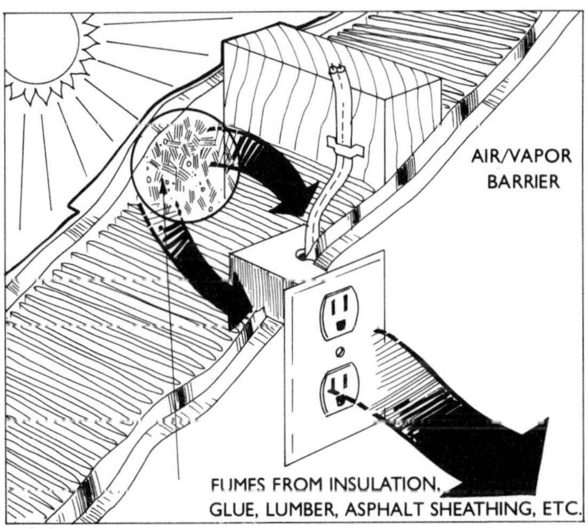

Fig. 29-39 Leakage of Wall Cavity Air Into Home Due to Poor Air Seal. *An imperfect air/vapor barrier allows contaminated air from the building cavities to leak back into the home when the outdoor temperature is high, or when wind pressure forces drive it in. This air contains gases from glue, insulation, plastics, and wood building materials.*

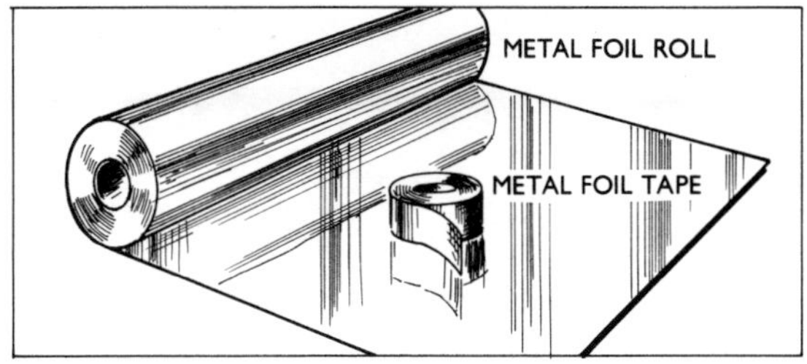

Fig. 29-40 Air/Vapor Barrier Material

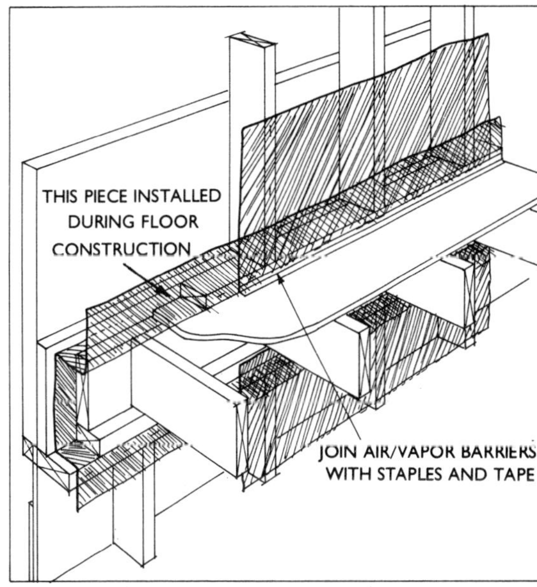

Fig. 29-41 Continuous Air/Vapor Barrier Around Floor Framing

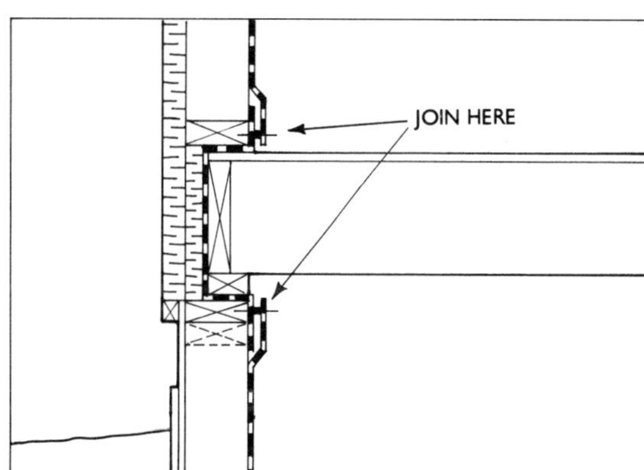

Fig. 29-42 Section of Air/Vapor Barrier (Fig. 29-41)

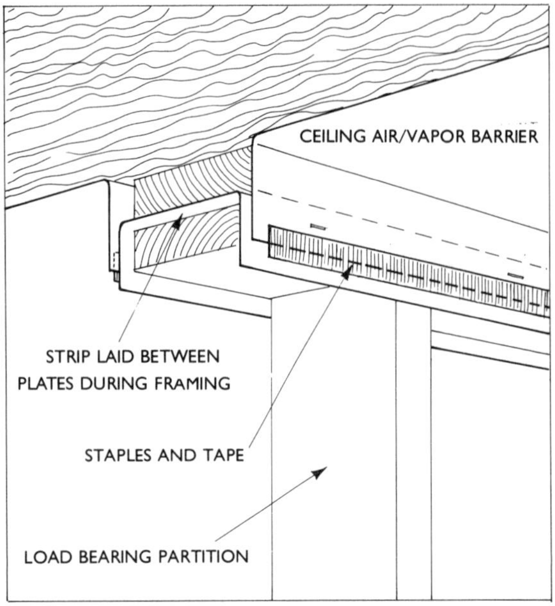

Fig. 29-43 Sealing Air/Vapor Barrier to Interior Partitions at Ceiling

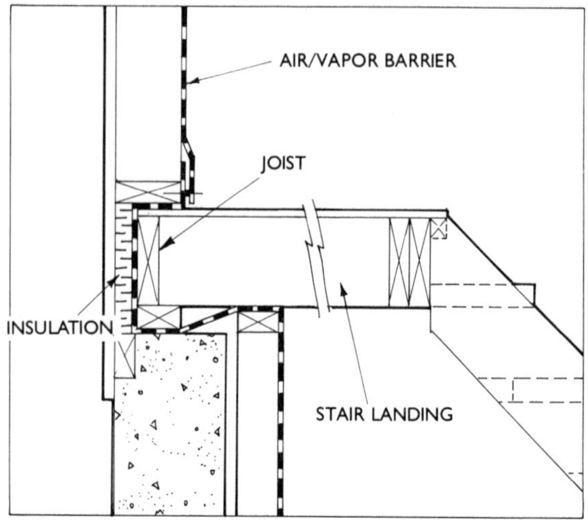

Fig. 29-45 Air/Vapor Barrier Detail at Stair Landing

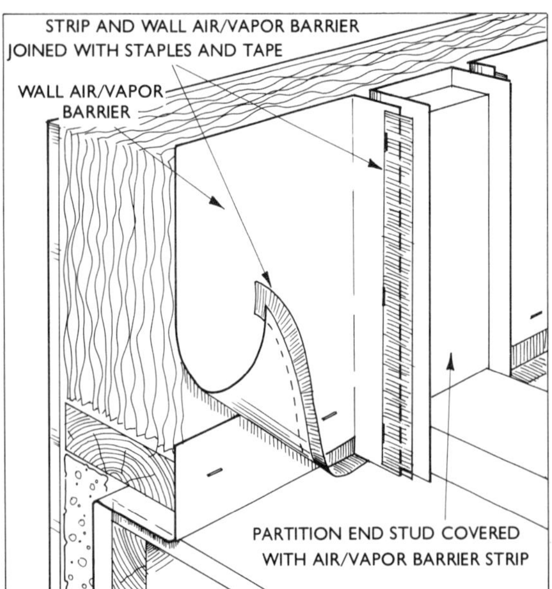

Fig. 29-44 Sealing Air/Vapor Barrier to Partition at Exterior Wall

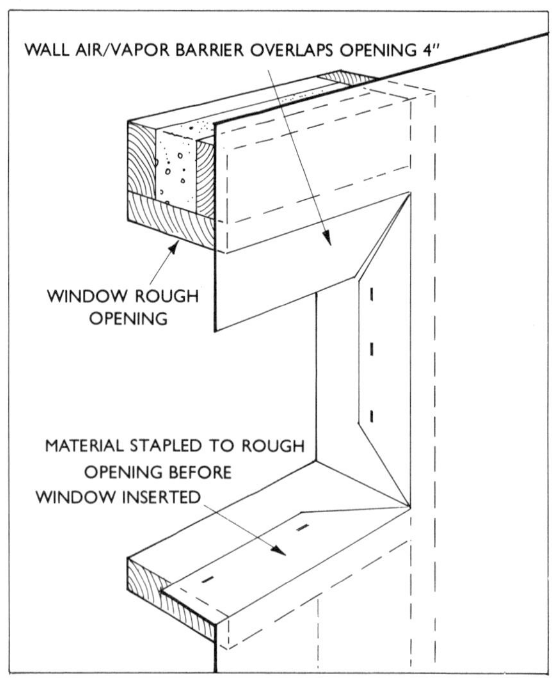

Fig. 29-46 Preparing Window Opening

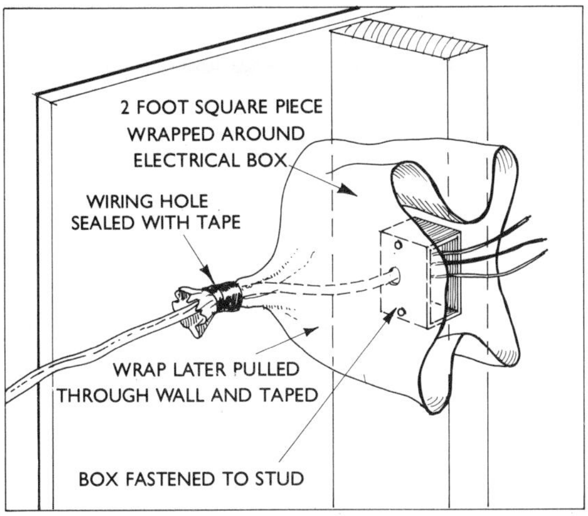

Fig. 29-47 Simple Method For Preparing Electrical Box for Sealing to Wall Air/Vapor Barrier

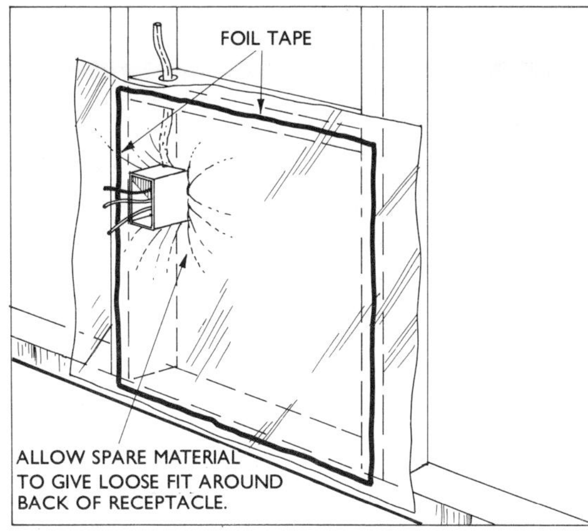

Fig. 29-49 Alternative Method For Sealing Electrical Boxes

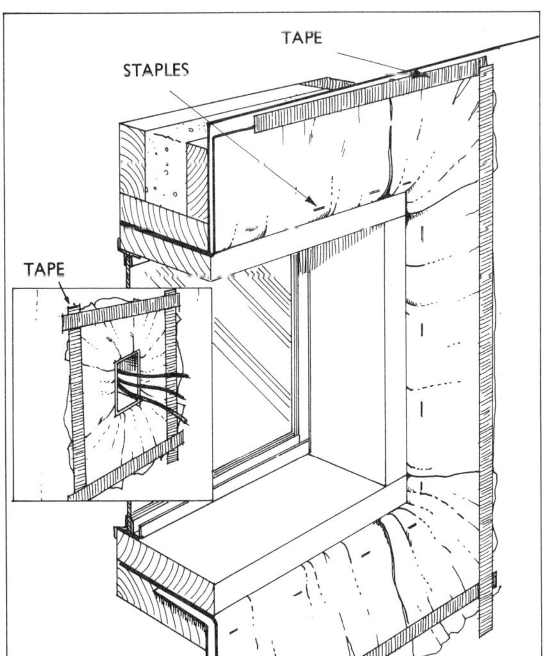

Fig. 29-48 Joining Window Frame and Electrical Outlet Pieces to Wall

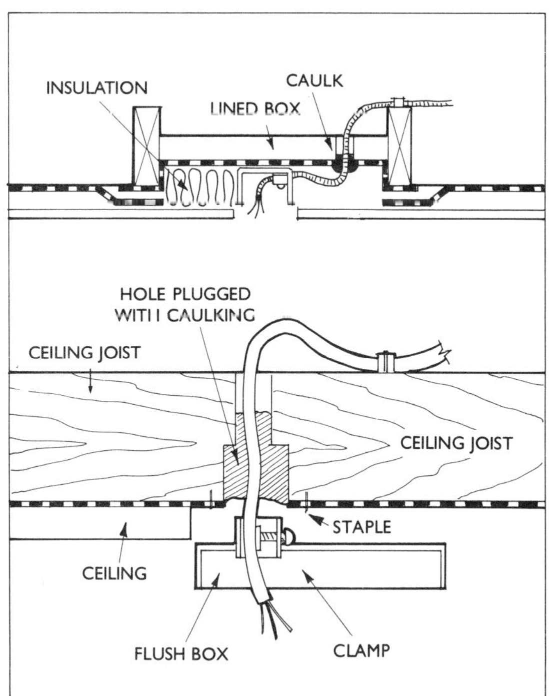

Fig. 29-50 Alternative Sealing Methods For Ceiling Fixtures

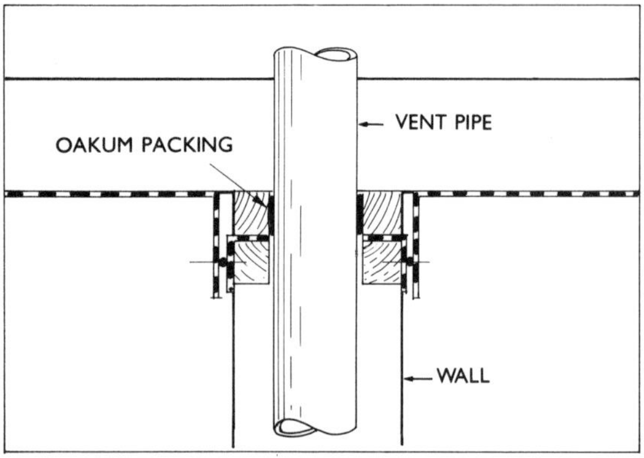

Fig. 29-51 Pipe Sealing Method

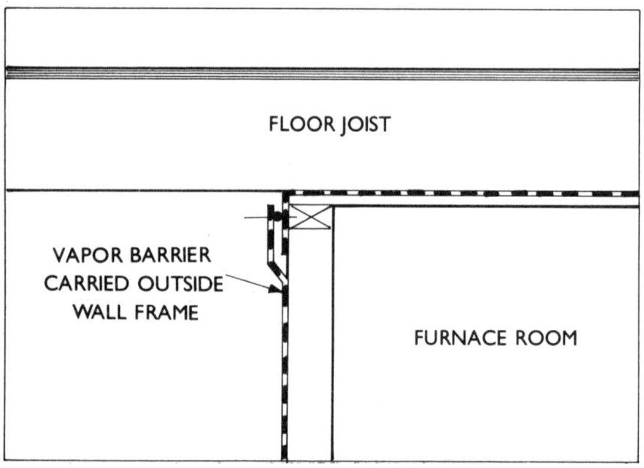

Fig. 29-52 Furnace Room Air/Vapor Barrier

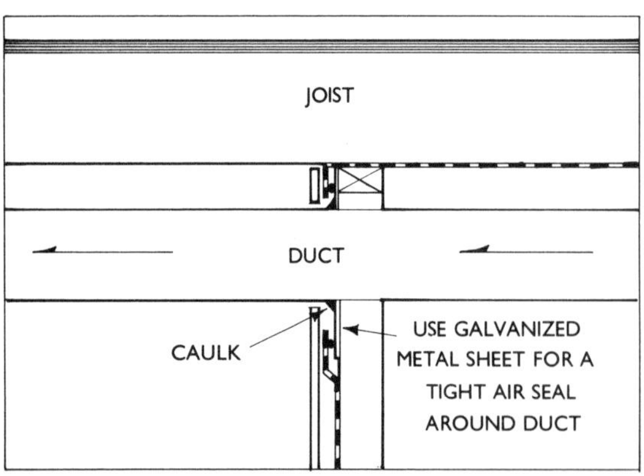

Fig. 29-53 Sealing Air Ducts Passing Through Walls. *Note: Keep warm air ducts clear of combustible material. Consult local fire codes.*

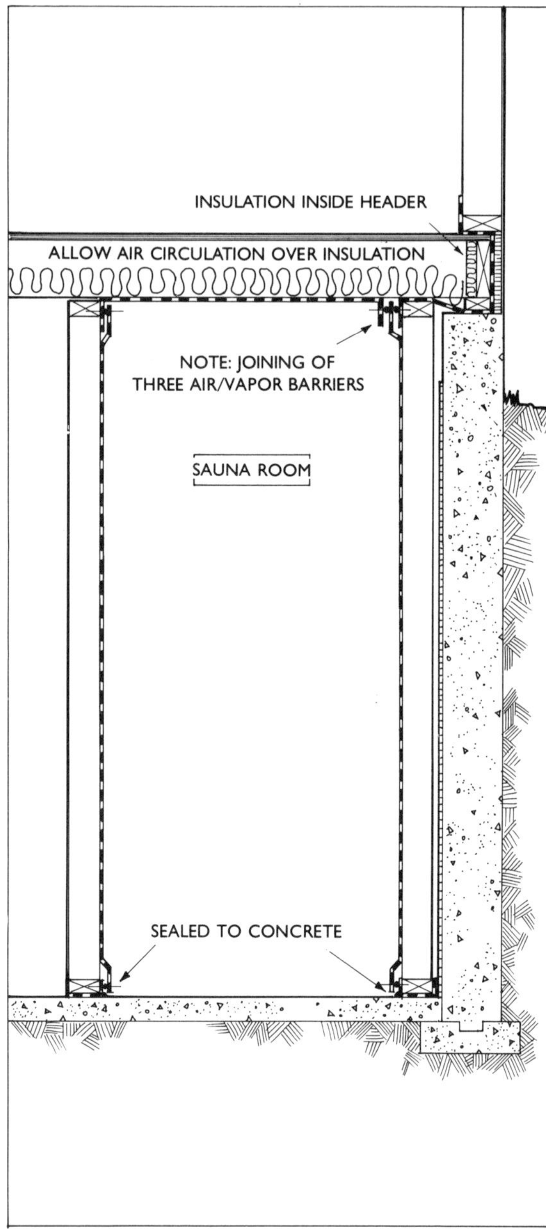

Fig. 29-54 Air/Vapor Barrier Sealing of a Sauna Room. *Sauna rooms must be totally isolated from surrounding walls, floors, and ceilings by a tight* Air/Vapor Barrier. *Use metal foil securely taped and stapled on all inside surfaces.*

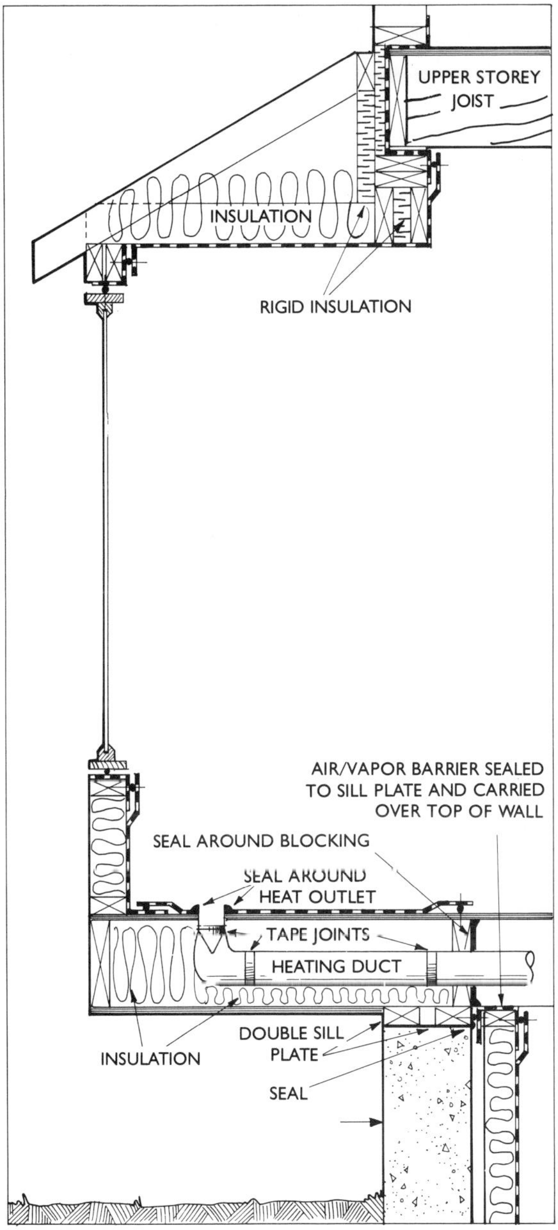

Fig. 29-55 Air/Vapor Barrier For Bay Window

Floor Coverings

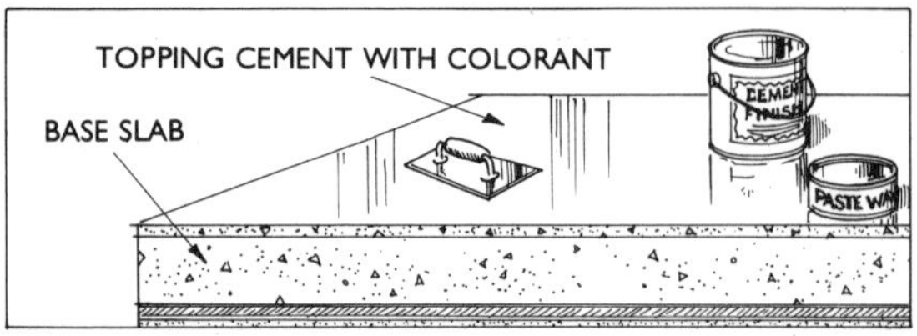

Fig. 29-56 Concrete Colorant and Paste Wax Finish. *A topping cement layer is applied to a concrete slab (new or existing), with a colorant and finish additive. The smooth troweled surface is allowed to cure, and then waxed periodically with a paste wax.*

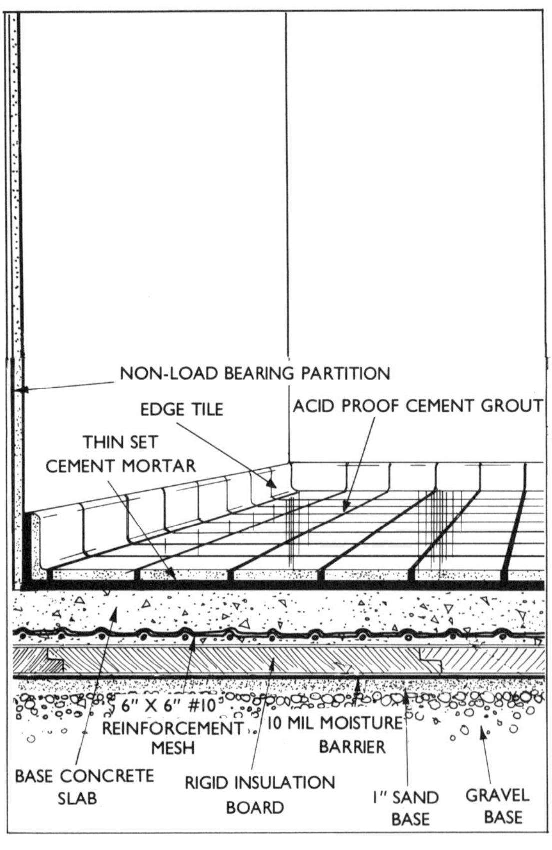

Fig. 29-57 Ceramic Tile Setting on Insulated Concrete Slab

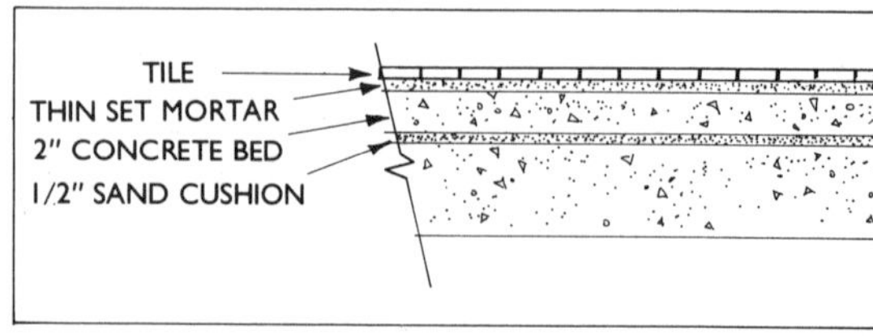

Fig. 29-58 Alternative Ceramic Tile Setting Method

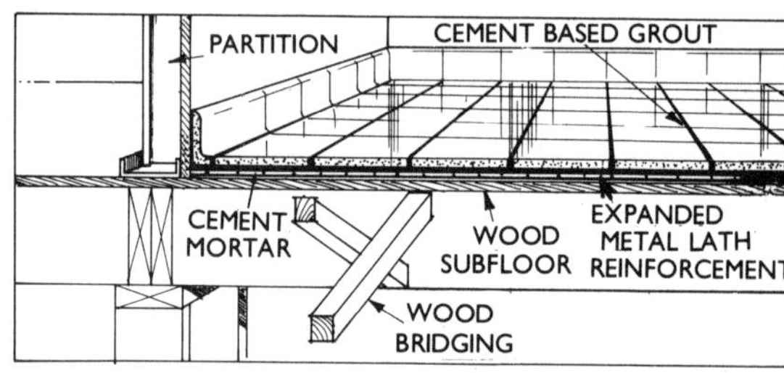

Fig. 29-59 Ceramic Tile on Reinforced Wood Floor. *Note: Floor system must be adequate to support load. For old construction, restrict tile settings in mortar to 10' floor spans, or 100 sq.ft. maximum. Floors over 100 sq. ft. can be reinforced with posts, added joists, or bridging.*

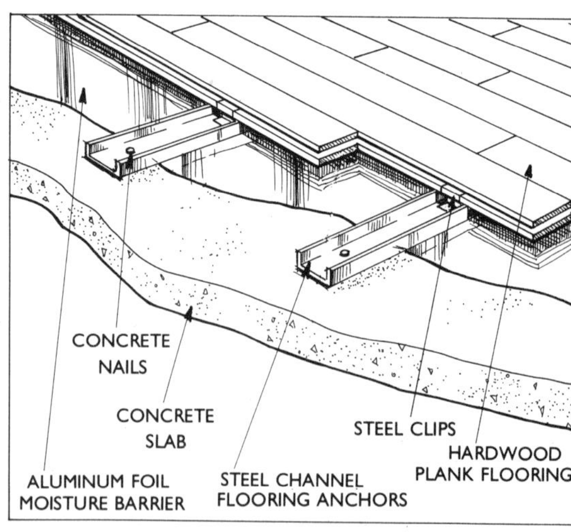

Fig. 29-60 Hardwood Floor on Concrete Slab. *A hardwood floor can be applied to a concrete slab using an all steel channel system. But, if there is heating in the slab, the heat transfer will be reduced.*

Wall And Ceiling Coverings

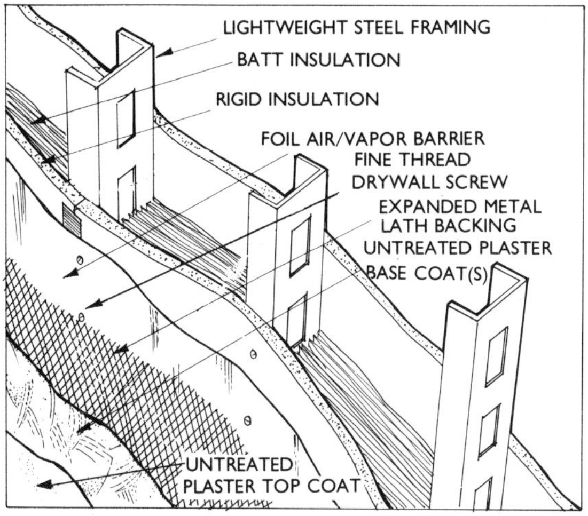

Fig. 29-61 Untreated Plaster Wall or Ceiling Covering on Metal Framing. *Note: Untreated plaster formulations contain only cement, lime or lime putty, sand, and gypsum.*

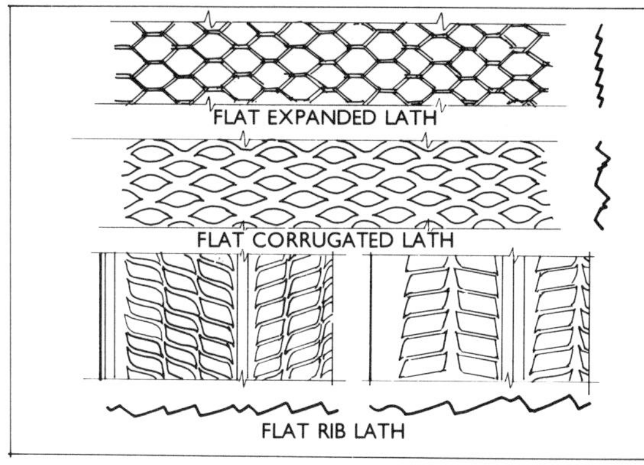

Fig. 29-63 Types of Metal Lath

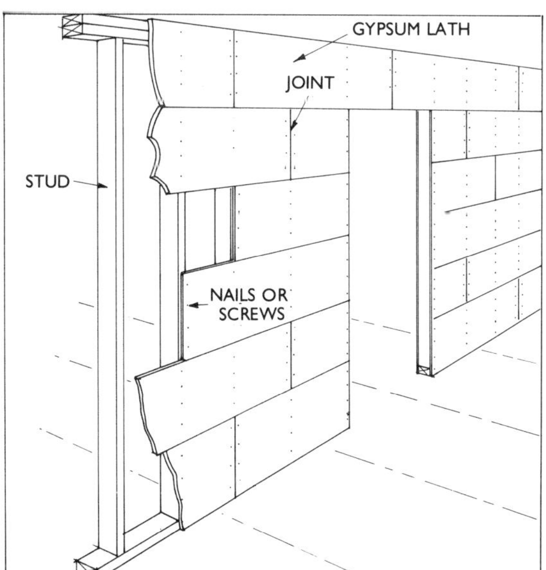

Fig. 29-62 Gypsum Lath Base For Plaster Finish. *Gypsum lath, similar to drywall, may be used in place of metal lath, if individually acceptable.*

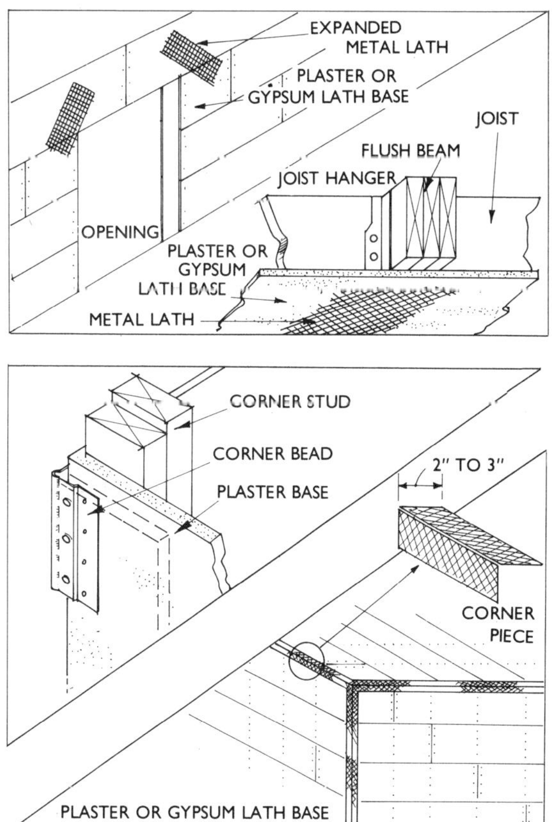

Fig. 29-64 Uses of Metal Lath

Fig. 29-65 Tub Enclosure Detail. *Cement board (available at builders suppliers), or metal lath and plaster, may be used as a base for tile in the tub enclosure. Do not use drywall or gypsum lath in the tub or shower enclosure, because it will absorb moisture and deteriorate.*

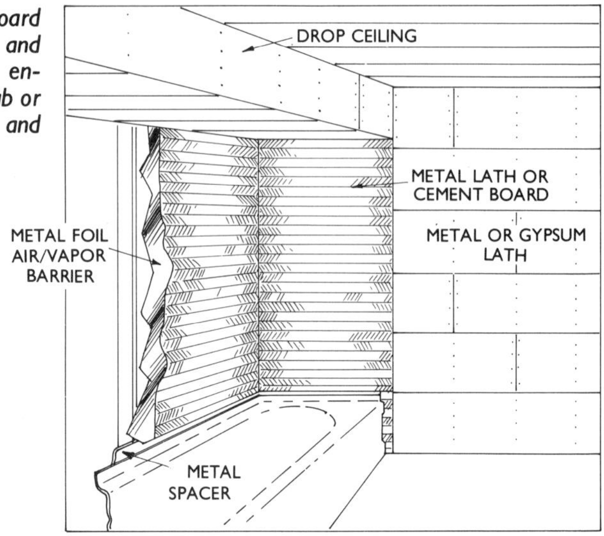

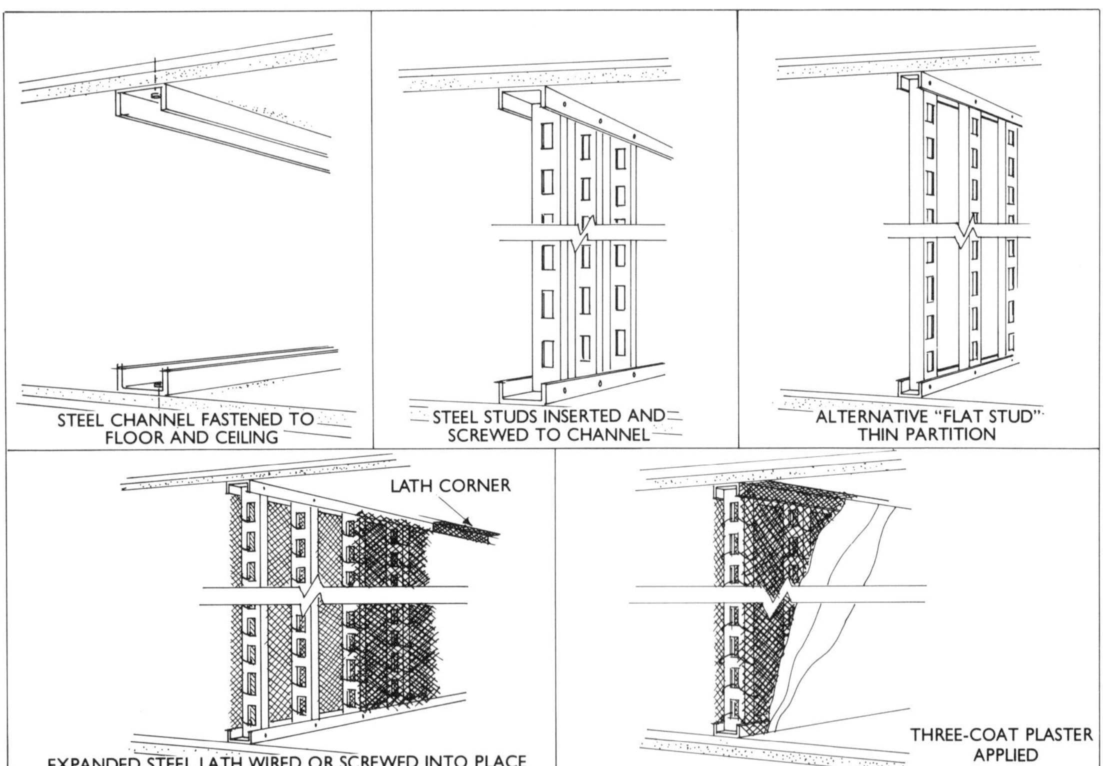

Fig. 29-66 Solid Plaster and Steel Partition System. *This system is for simple non load-bearing partitions. Standard sheet metal channel framing is shown, but special thin track and channel systems are available for this use in some areas.*

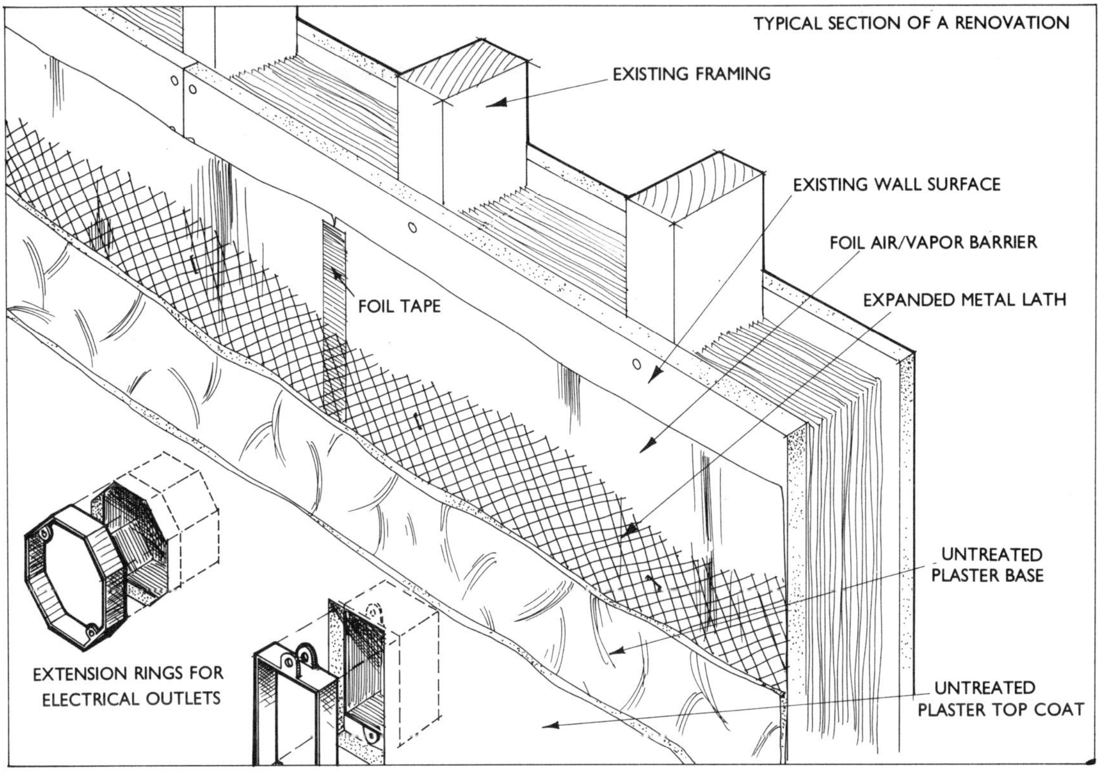

Fig. 29-67 Adding An Untreated Plaster Finish to An Existing Wall or Ceiling. *An existing room can be refinished to cover and seal old construction. Electrical outlets can be extended using steel* Extension Rings *available at electrical suppliers. Be sure to carefully seal* Air/Vapor Barrier *to all openings with tape or caulking.*

Sound Control

Careful planning when building is the first strategy for sound control in the home. A major cause of objectionable noise in most locations is windows and doors facing streets or close neighbors. A further problem is sound transmitted through outside walls and shared walls. Careful location of openings and soundproof wall construction can reduce these problems.

The control of sound generated inside the home is largely accomplished by soundproof wall and ceiling construction, as well as by sealing cracks and openings between rooms. If this is done, the only remaining means of sound transmission is by flanking paths of sound where sound can leak past barriers.

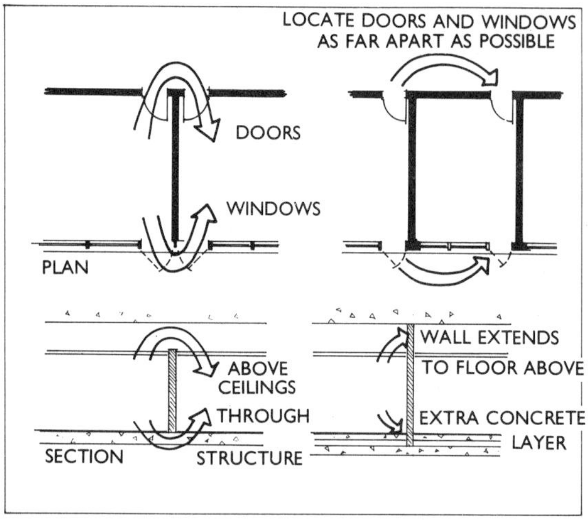

Fig. 29-68 Flanking Sound Paths. *Sound can travel around, above, or below soundproof walls, if there are paths open to it.*

LIGHTWEIGHT SOUND ISOLATION SYSTEMS

These sound isolation systems are particularly effective for reducing the transmission of impact sound, such as the sound of footsteps on the floor above.

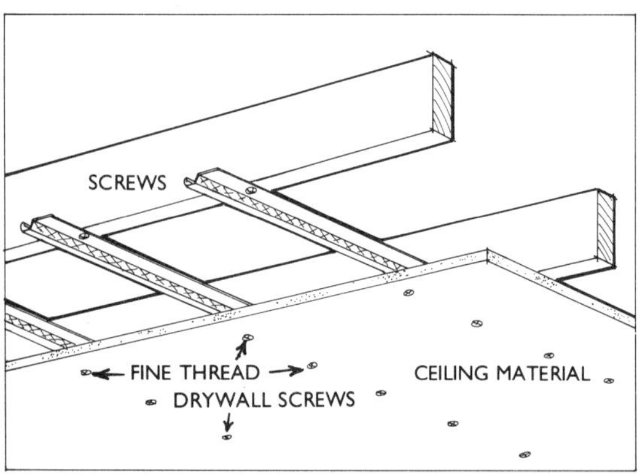

Fig. 29-69 Ceiling System. *Fasten steel resilient suspension bar to the floor frame with screws or nails. Then screw the ceiling material to the suspension portion of the bar. Careful sealing of all seams and openings in the ceiling is crucial to the performance of these systems. Steel resilient bar is available from drywall system suppliers and builders suppliers.*

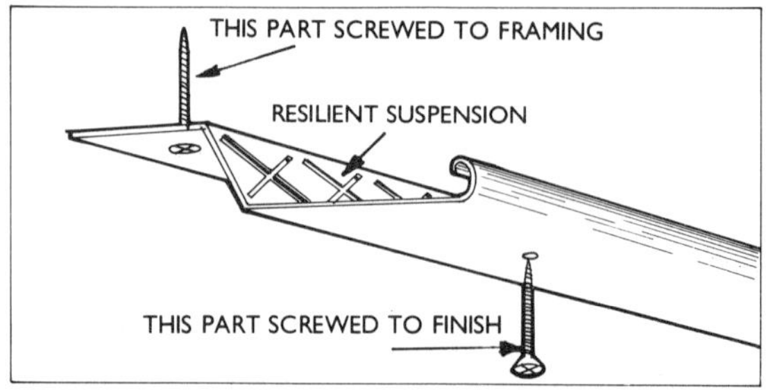

Fig. 29-70 Detail of Steel Resilient Bar

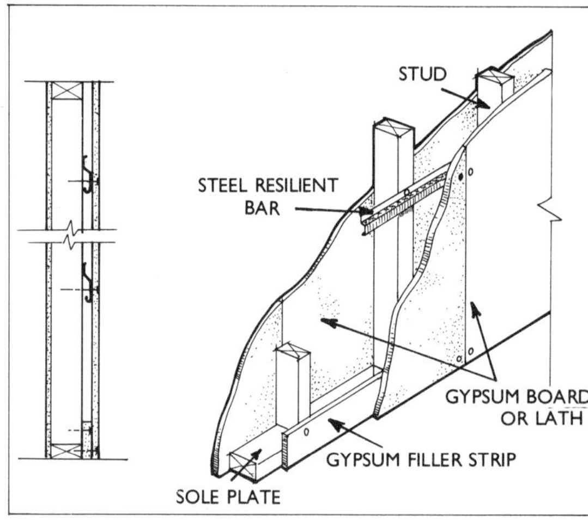

Fig. 29-71 Wall System. *Resilient suspension can be used horizontally for walls. It can be used on one or both surfaces.*

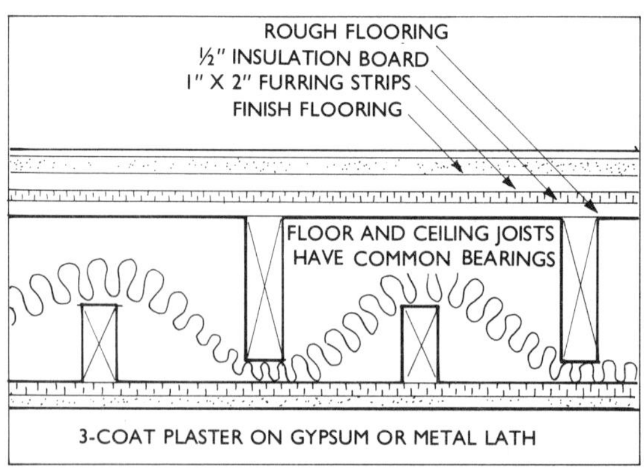

Fig. 29-72 Alternative Soundproofing System for Floors. *Conventional framing is built independently for floors and ceilings, to reduce sound transmission.*

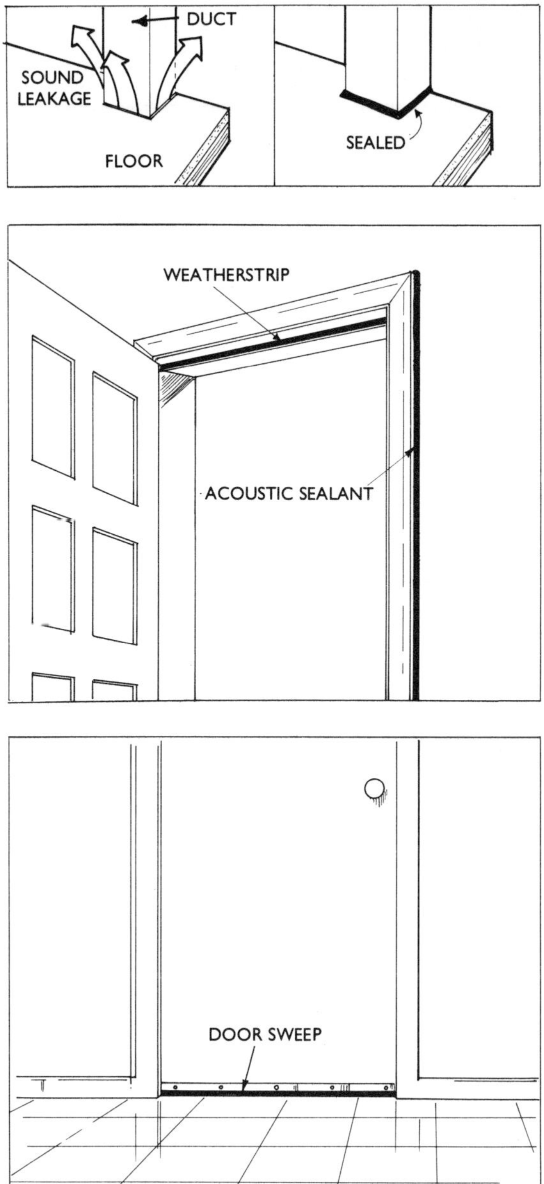

Fig. 29-74 Sealing Sound Leakage Paths. *Blocking all gaps and cracks around doors, windows, trims, and ducts, will reduce the flanking paths available to sound.*

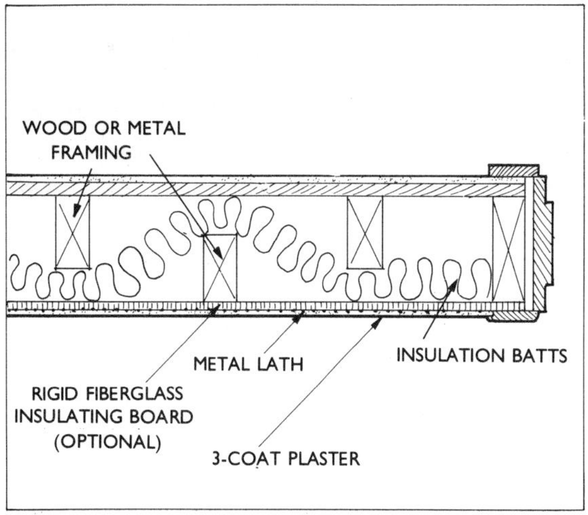

Fig. 29-73 Alternative Soundproofing System for Walls. *Conventional framing is built independently for the two sides of the wall.*

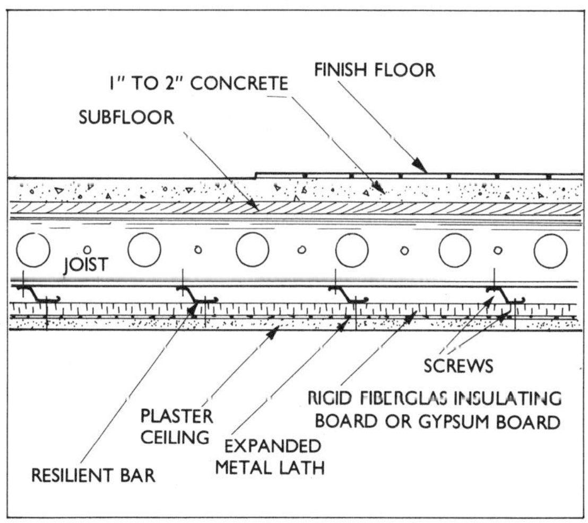

Fig. 29-75 Massive Sound Reduction System For Floors. *The addition of a 1" to 2" layer of concrete to the subfloor before the application of the finish floor is very effective for reducing airborne sound transmission, such as conversation and music. A resilient bar ceiling suspension below will further improve sound isolation.*

Wiring And Lighting

Installing electrical wiring in thinwall steel conduit will reduce exposure to plastic and oil based wiring materials, as well as to the electrical fields associated with home wiring. This commercial type of wiring is more costly than conventional cable wiring, but is readily available through electricians and electrical suppliers.

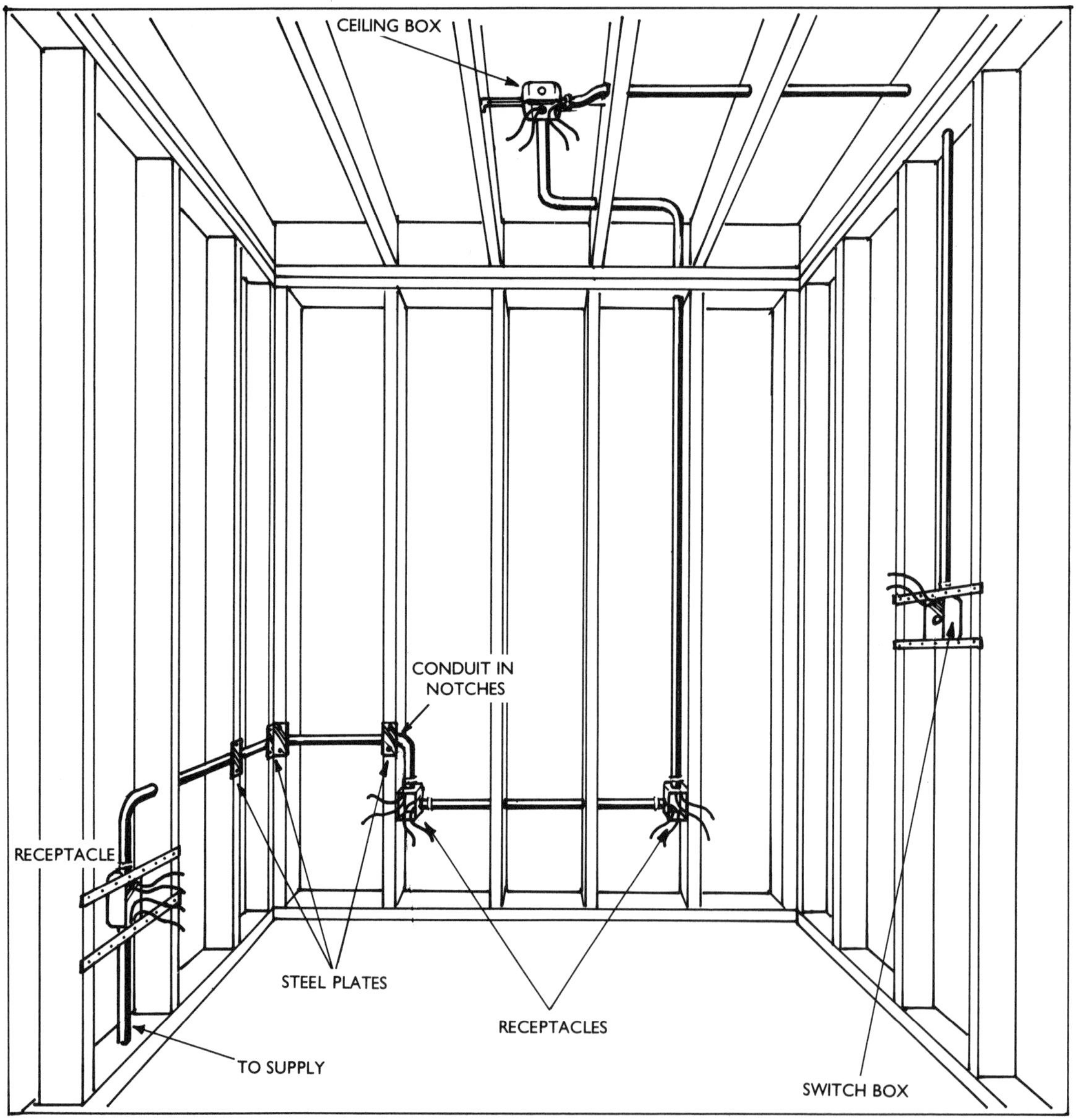

Fig. 29-76 Typical Conduit Wiring.

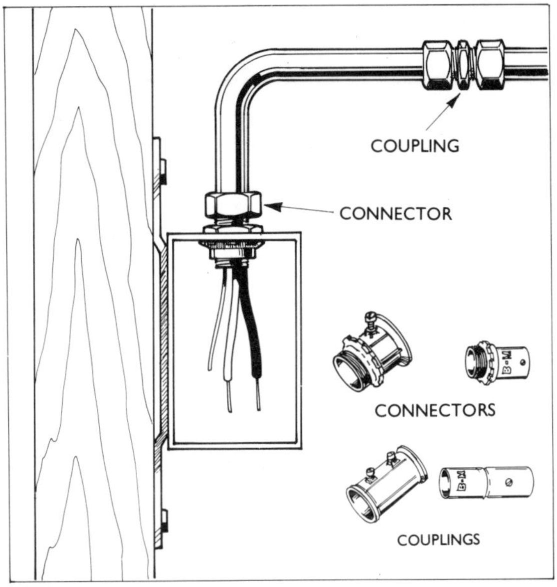

Fig. 29-77 Typical Steel Box and Conduit Connection.

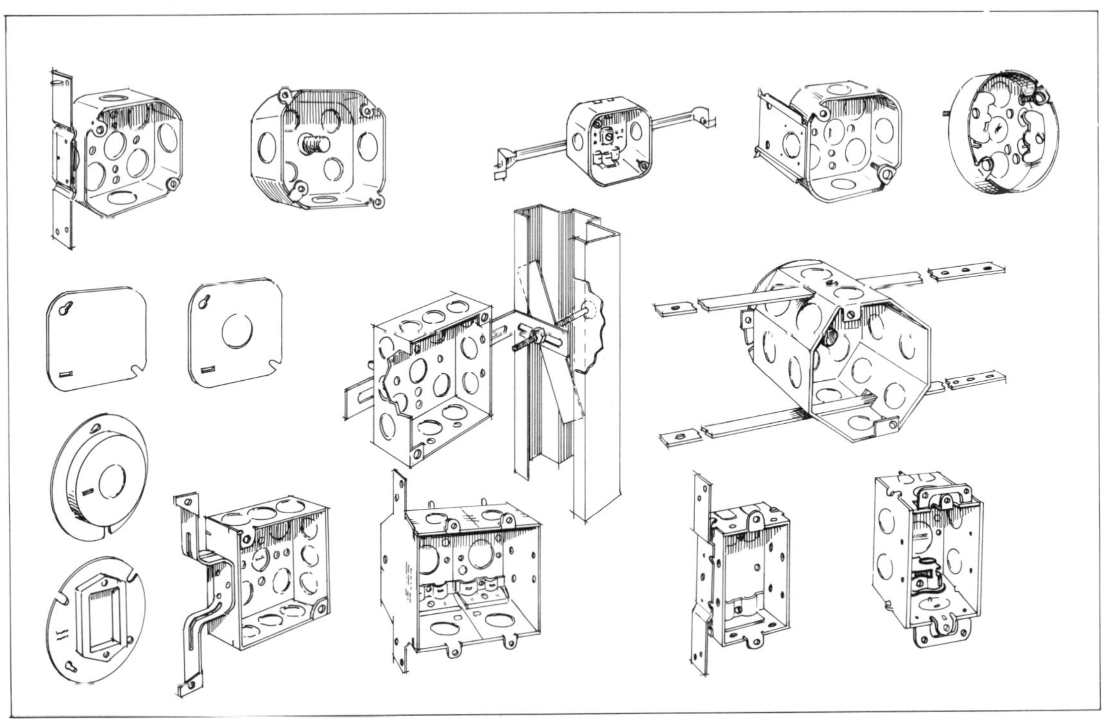

Fig. 29-78 Steel Electrical Boxes. *All wiring should be done with metal boxes and covers. Plastic boxes produce contaminating fumes when heated, and they do not shield electrical fields.*

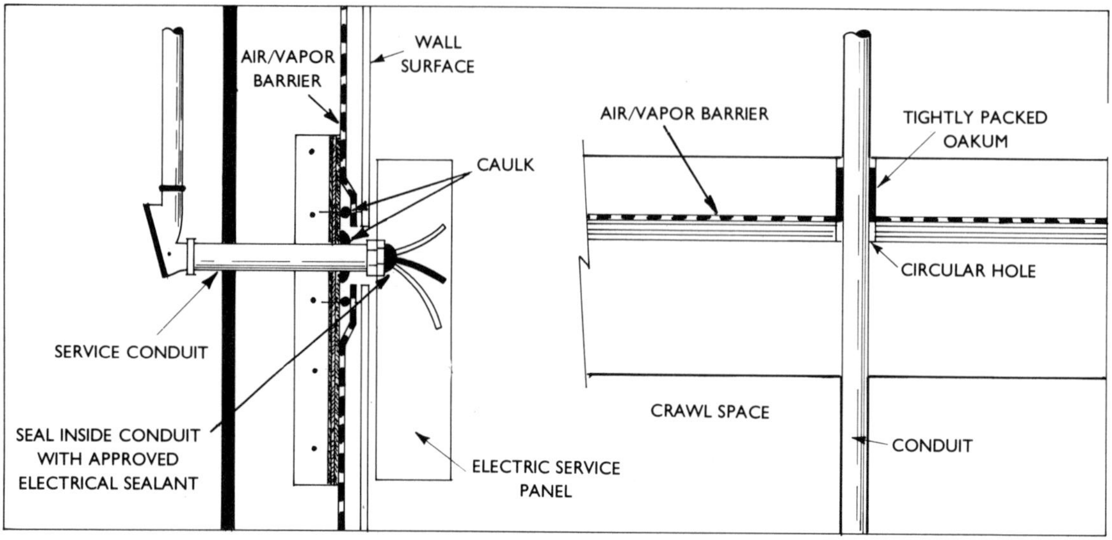

Fig. 29-79 Sealing Conduits

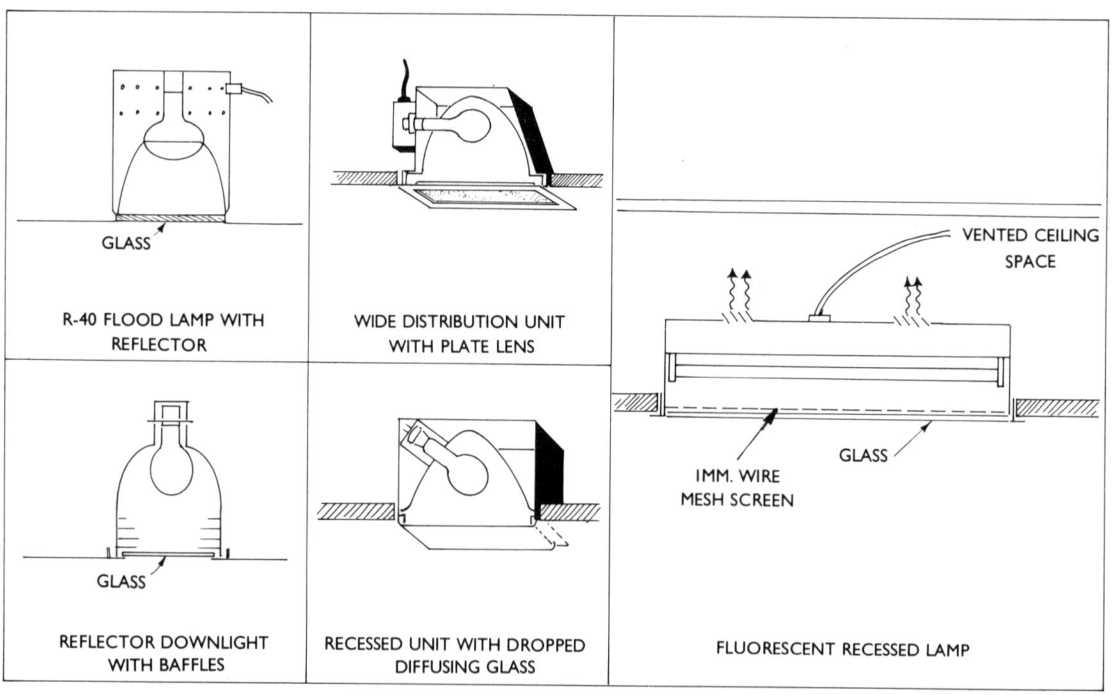

Fig. 29-80 Ceiling Lighting Vented to Ceiling Space. *Light fixtures with glass covers which are vented to the ceiling space will not release dust or fumes to the room. Note: Wire reinforced glass or wire mesh screen on glass may be used to reduce electrical fields.*

OTHER BUILT-IN LIGHTING SYSTEMS

Note: All installations must comply with local electrical and fire safety codes. Only fluorescent lamps are usually permitted in recessed applications.

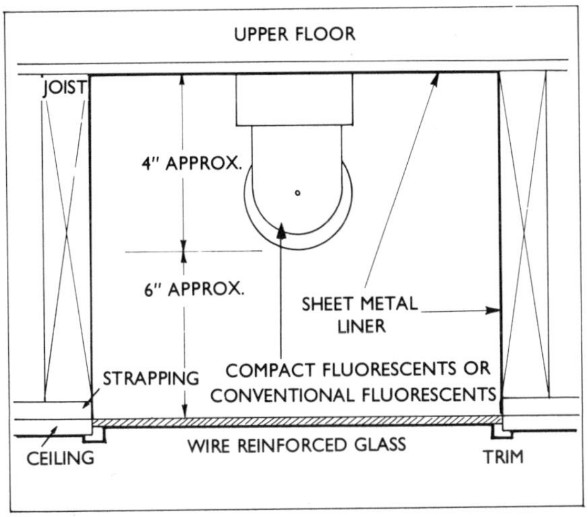

Fig. 29-81 Recessed Ceiling Panel Lighting

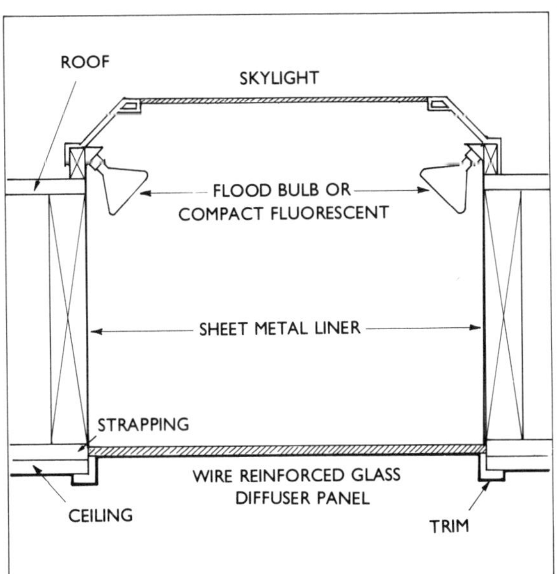

Fig. 29-82 Flood Lighting Added to Skylight

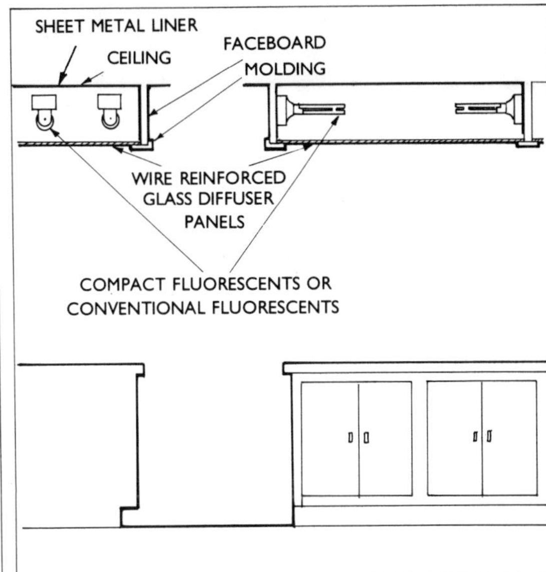

Fig. 29-83 Soffit Lighting

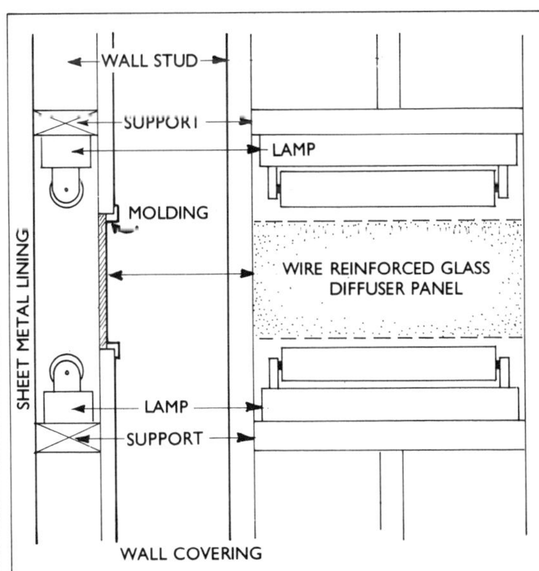

Fig. 29-84 Wall Panel Lighting

Plumbing

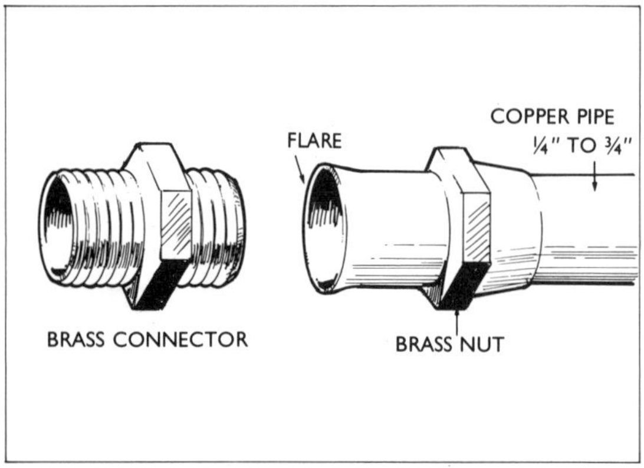

Fig. 29-85 Solder-Free Flared Water Pipe Fittings *(Copper pipe measures are inside diameters.)*

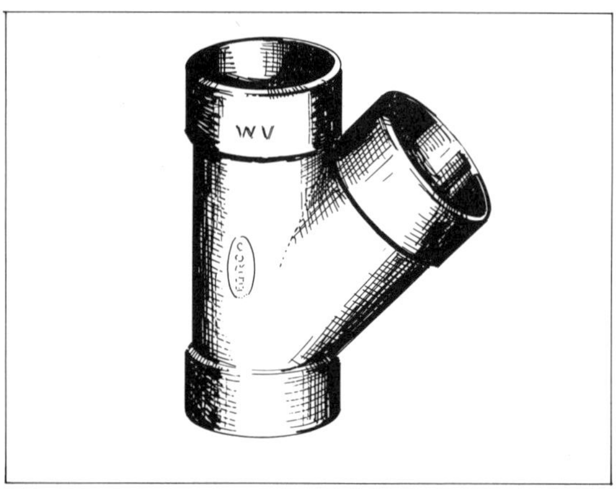

Fig. 29-86 Brass "DWV" Type Drain Fittings. *An alternative to plastic, soldered connections.*

BRASS AND CAST IRON DRAIN PIPE SYSTEMS

All metal drain pipe systems are more costly than plastic systems, but do not produce fumes in the home.

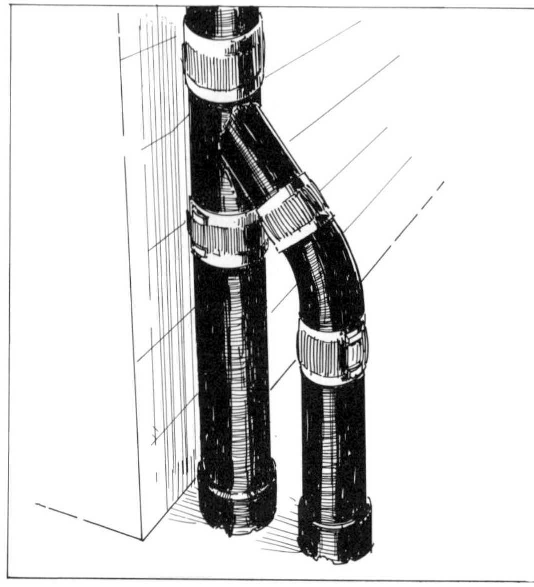

Fig. 29-87 Cast Iron "No Hub" Type Drain Fittings. *Stainless steel band and rubber connections.*

PLASTIC DRAIN SYSTEMS

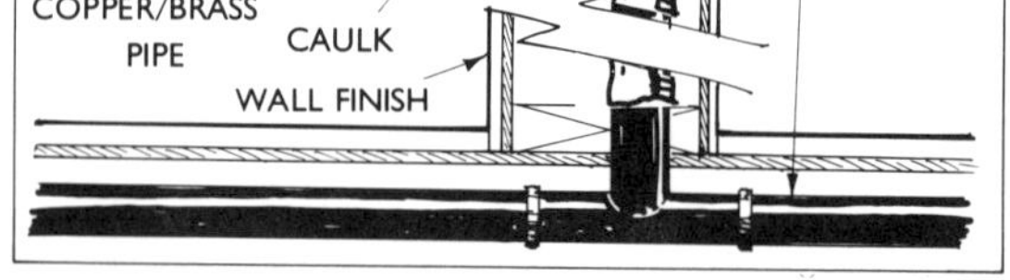

Fig. 29-88 Sealing Plastic Drain Pipes with Metal Foil. *Where plastic drain pipes must be used indoors, they can be tightly wrapped with metal foil and taped with foil tape to reduce outgassing of plastics. All pipe inside the room, such as drains under sinks, should be all-metal.*

Heating

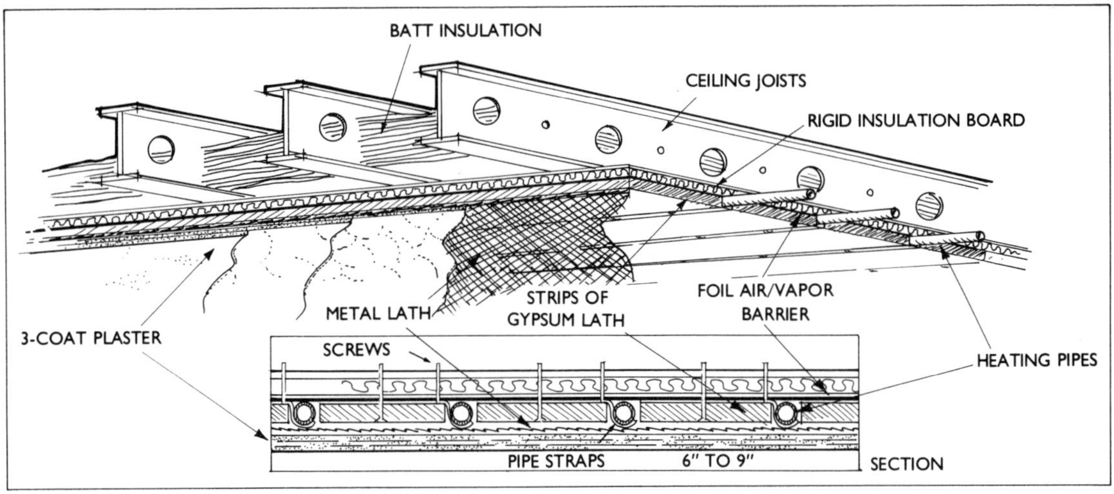

Fig. 29-89 Ceiling Heating With Heated Liquid. *Strap* Heating Pipes *spaced from 6" to 9" apart to the ceiling, which has been prepared with* Rigid Insulation Board *covered with metal* Foil Air/Vapor Barrier. *Then fasten filler strips of* Gypsum Lath *between the pipes and apply a* Metal Lath *and* Plaster *finish.*

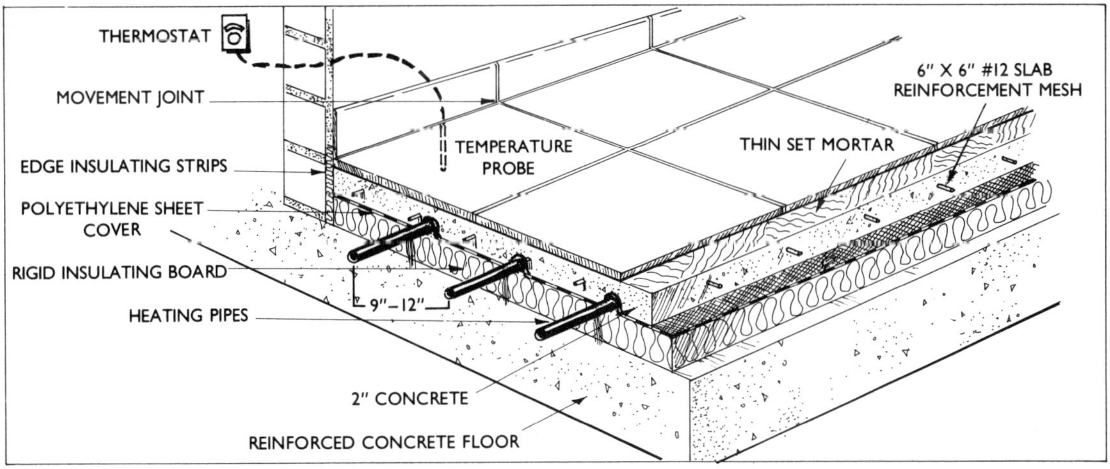

Fig. 29-90 Floor Heating With Heated Liquid. *Place* Heating Pipes *spaced 9" to 12" apart on* Rigid Insulation Board *on top of a* Reinforced Concrete Floor. *The pipes are covered with polyethylene sheet or other suitable protection from the concrete, and a* 2" Concrete Topping *with* 6" X 6" #12 Slab Reinforcement Mesh *is poured on top. A* Finish Floor *of ceramic tile or stone is then installed on top with cement mortar. An* Edge Insulating Strip *is installed on the perimeter, and a* Movement Joint *provided at the baseboard to allow for expansion. A* Temperature Probe *should be installed in the concrete or on the surface, to maintain floor temperature below 85°F.*

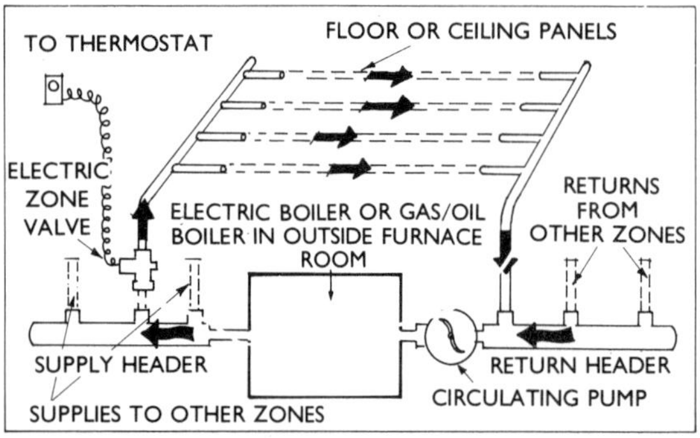

Fig. 29-91 Heating Panels And A Typical Boiler System

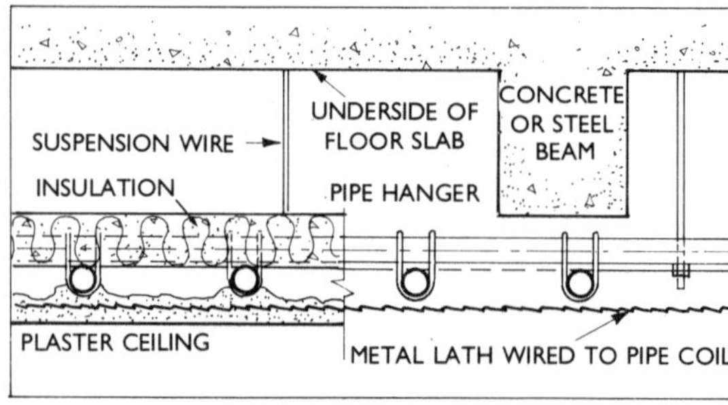

Fig. 29-93 Suspended Ceiling Heating Panel
This system can be hung from any type of floor construction, whether wood or concrete.

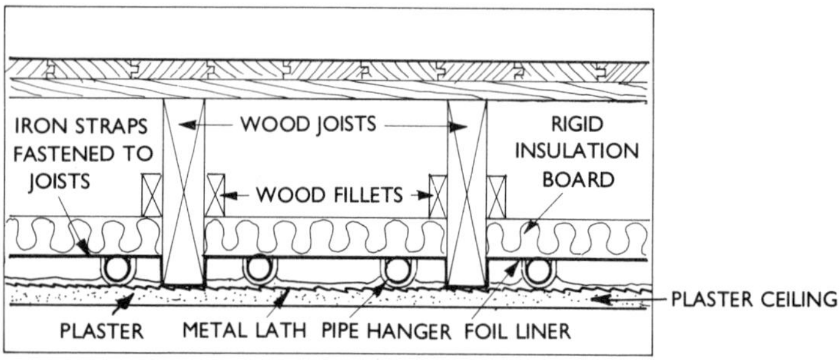

Fig. 29-92 Ceiling Heat Over Existing Wood Construction

Built-In Vacuum System

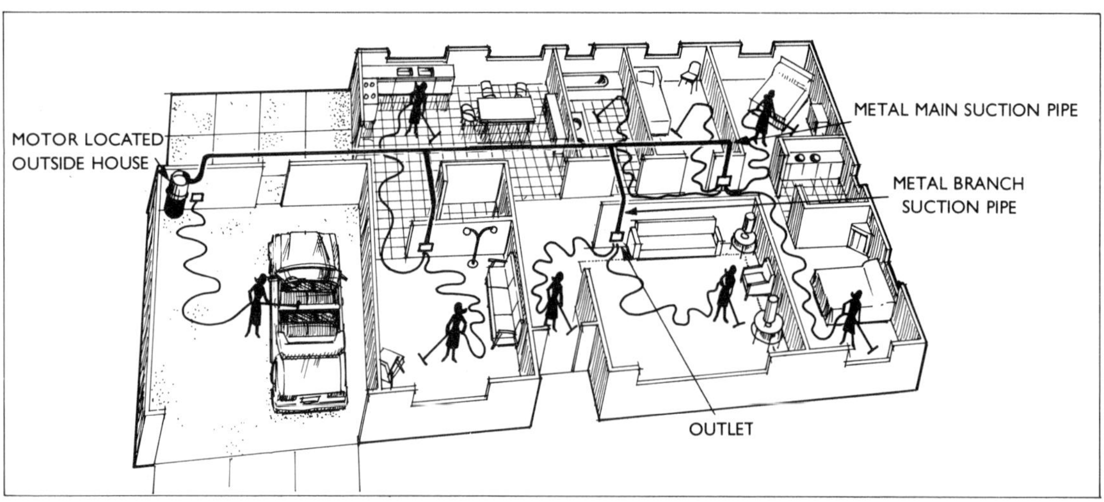

Fig. 29-94 Built In Vacuum System

Construction Details

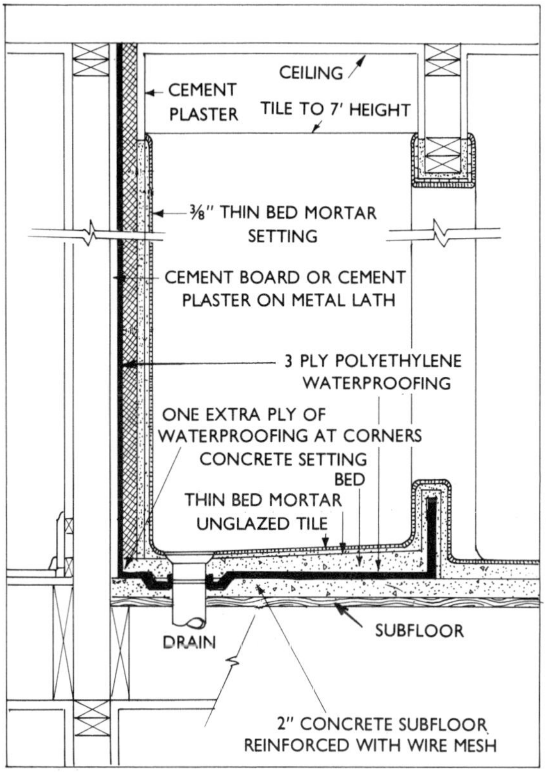

Fig. 29-95 Tile Shower Construction

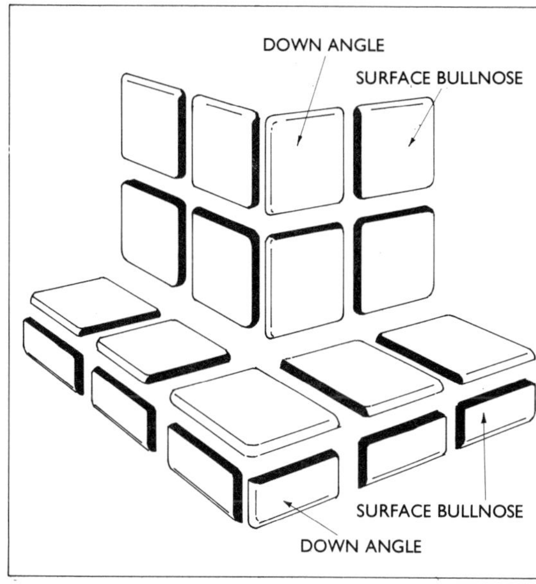

Fig. 29-97 Available Bullnose Tile Shapes

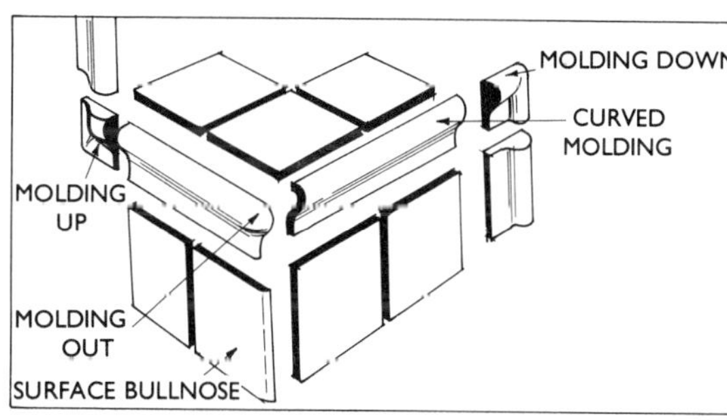

Fig. 29-98 Tile Molding Shapes

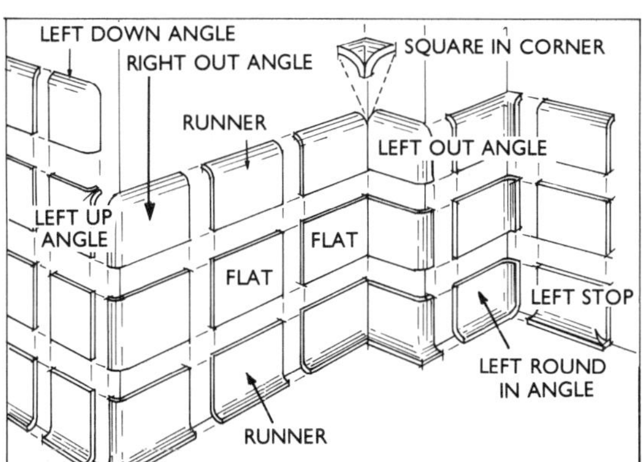

Fig. 29-96 Standard Tile Shapes and Trims

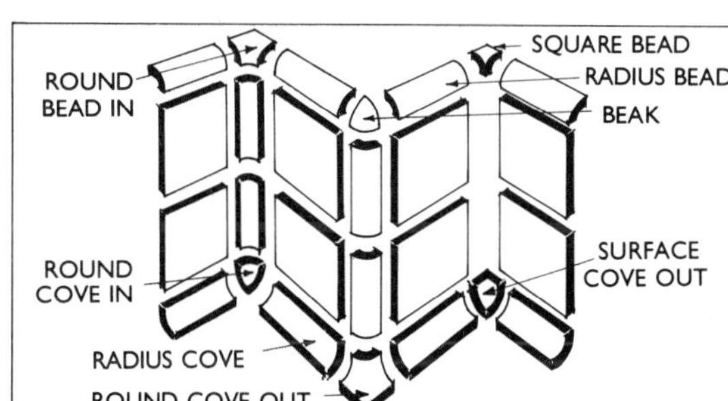

Fig. 29-99 Tile Molding Shapes

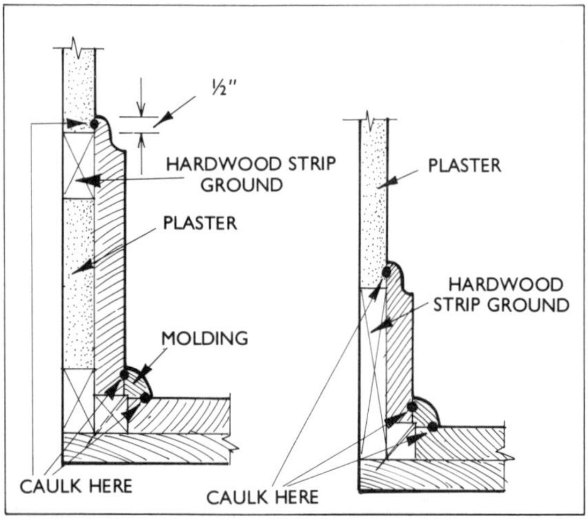

Fig. 29-100 Plaster Grounds For Baseboards. *Grounds are wood fillers set into plaster for fastening trims.*

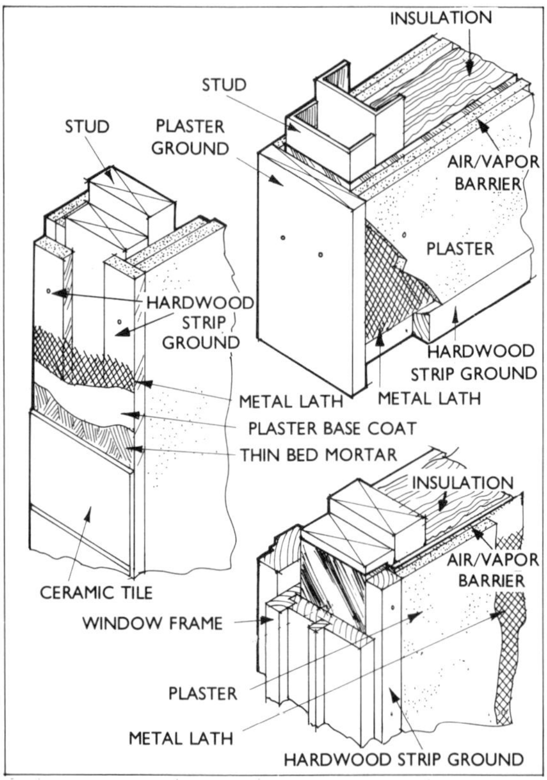

Fig. 29-101 Plaster Details For Doors and Windows. *Tile is a durable way to finish door and window openings.*

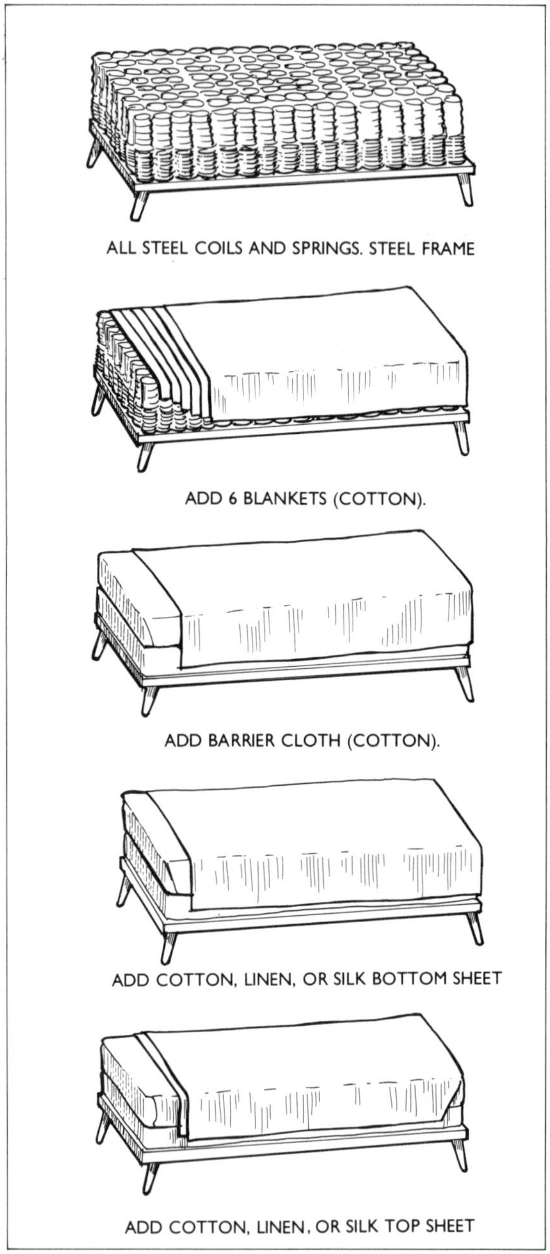

Fig. 29-102 A Simple Washable Bed. *A simple, well ventilated bed can be made from entirely washable components. This bed is dust free, mold free, and free of chemical fireproofing and mold treatments. (Courtesy of the Human Ecology Foundation of the Southwest, Dallas, Texas.)*

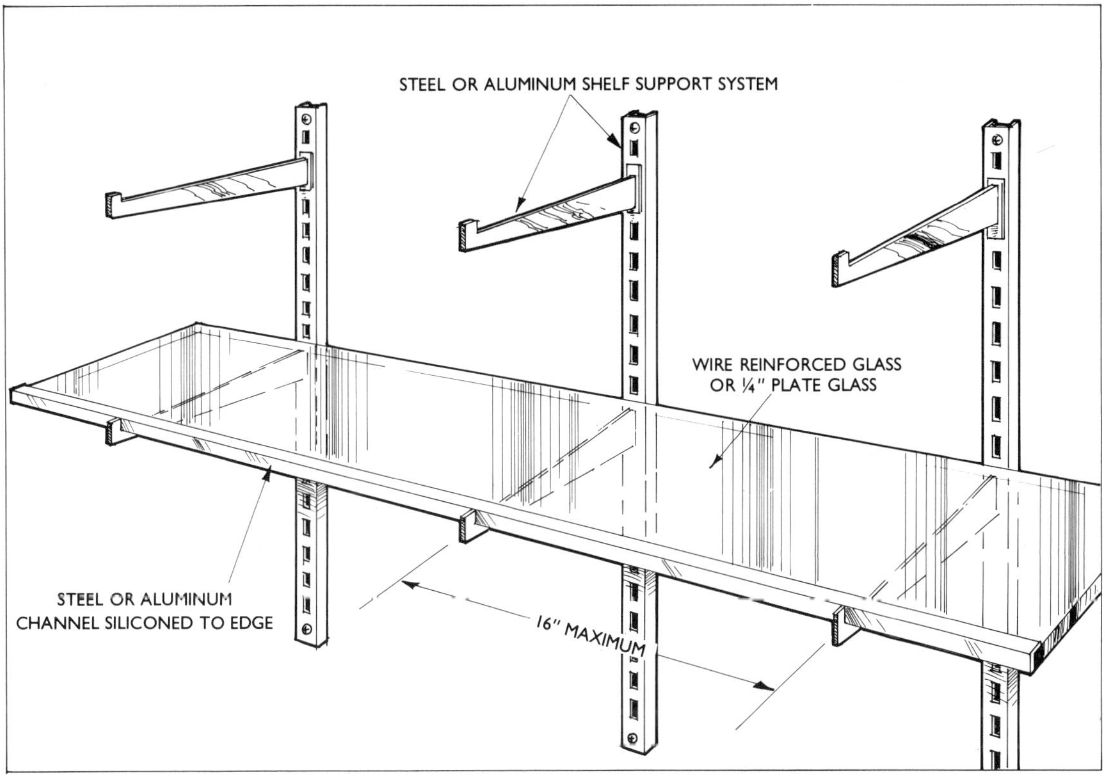

Fig. 29-103 A Simple Glass and Metal Shelving System. *Such a system is free of wood, plastics, glue and paint.*

SELECTED FURTHER READING

General

Healing Environments, Carol Venolia. Celestial Arts, Berkeley, CA., 1988

A holistic approach to the healthy home.

Air Quality (Indoor)

Indoor Air Pollution and Housing Technology, Bruce M. Small. Canada Mortgage and Housing Corp., Ottawa, Canada, 1983

A lengthy, detailed study of indoor pollution including housing for the environmentally sensitive. Available from: Canadian Housing Information Centre, 682 Montreal Rd., Ottawa, Ontario. K1A 0P7.

Indoor Air Quality and Human Health, I. Turiel. Stanford University Press, Stanford, Ca., 1985.

A reference text.

Indoor Air and Human Health, Richard Gammage and Stephen Kay. Lewis Publishers, Chelsea, Mich., 1985.

A reference text.

Indoor Air Quality, Beat Meyer. Addison Wesley, Reading, Mass., 1983.

A reference text.

Asbestos

Asbestos in the Home, U.S. Consumer Product Safety Commission. Available for sale from: U.S. Government Printing Office, Washington, D.C. 20402. (202) 783-3238

A guide for asbestos identification and removal in the home.

The Asbestos Hazard, Paul Brodeur. New York Academy of Sciences, N.Y., 1980.

A readable description of the uses and health hazards of asbestos, including a history of industrial uses with case studies.

Chemical Hazards in the Home

The Poisons Around Us, H. A. Schroeder. Indiana University Press, 1974.

A guidebook to environmental hazards in accessible language.

Controversial Chemicals, Kruus and Valeriote. Multiscience Publishers, Montreal, Canada, 1979.

An excellent description of common environmental hazards.

Handbook of Toxic and Hazardous Chemicals, M. Sittig. Noyes Publishers, Park Ridge, N.J., 1981.

A technical reference book on 600 chemical hazards, including health risks and safe handling methods.

The Non-Toxic Home, Debra Lynn Dadd. Jeremy P. Tarcher Inc., Los Angeles, Ca., 1986.

A readable popular work on common household chemical hazards and safer alternatives.

Electromagnetic Pollution

The Zapping of America, Paul Brodeur. Norton Publishing, N.Y., 1977.

The story of the hazards of microwave emissions, written in simple language, with anecdotes.

Biological Effects of Environmental Electromagnetism, Herbert L. Konig. Springer Verlag, N.Y., 1981.

A scientific review of current knowledge on the topic.

Environmental Illness

See Further Reading in this book in the chapter, Resources for the Environmentally Ill.

Environmental Pollution

Well Body, Well Earth, Mike Samuels and Hal Zina Bennett. Sierra Club Books, San Francisco, 1983.

An excellent sourcebook filled with information on health and the environment.

Healthy Living in An Unhealthy World, Edward Calabrese and Michael Dorsey. Simon and Schuster, N.Y., 1984.

An excellent technical acount of the links between toxic environmental exposure, nutrition, and disease.

Formaldehyde

Formaldehyde, Everything You Wanted To Know, Consumer's Federation of America, 1424 16th St., N.W., Washington, D.C., 20036.

A free pamphlet. Send a stamped, self addressed envelope.

The Susceptibility Report, Bruce M. Small. Sunnyhill Research Foundation, RR #1, Goodwood, Ontario, Canada, L0C 1A0. (Available from the author).

A report on urea formaldehyde foam in the home, and remedies.

Home Heating

The Household Environment and Chronic Illness, Pfeiffer and Nikel. Thomas Publishers, Springfield, Ill., 1980.

A collection of articles including heating and health topics.

Home Maintenance

The Natural Formula Book For Home and Yard, Dan Wallace (ed.), Rodale Press, Emmaus, Pa., 1982.

An excellent reference book on inexpensive and safe alternatives to many home maintenance products.

Strategies for Healthful Residential Environments, Karl Raab. Canada Mortgage and Housing Corporation, Ottawa, Canada, 1984.

An excellent monograph on safe home maintenance. Available from: Canadian Housing Information Centre, 682 Montreal Rd., Ottawa, Ontario, K1A 0P7.

Household Appliances and Products

Consumer Reports, Consumer's Union of the United States.

See specific issues for consumer items.

Canadian Consumer, Consumer's Association of Canada.

See specific issues for consumer items.

Light and Color

Human Factors in Lighting, P. R. Boyce. Applied Science Publishers, London, 1981.

An excellent theoretical text on lighting.

Lighting Design and Applications, Journal of the Illuminating Engineering Society.

A practical professional guide to lighting.

"Indoor Pollution, Lighting, Energy and Health," H. Levin and L. Duhl, in *Architectural Research,* James Snyder (ed.). Van Nostrand Reinhold, N.Y., 1984.

An excellent article drawing on a wide range of environmental health issues.

Color and Value, Joseph Gatto. Davis Publishers, Worcester, Mass., 1974.

A good text on color use and color mixing.

Natural Pest Control

Encyclopedia of Natural Insect and Disease Control, Roger Yepsen. Rodale Press, Emmaus, Pa., 1984.

An excellent reference book on safe methods for controlling garden and house pests.

Radon

Radon Reduction Techniques, U.S. Environmental Protection Agency. Available free from: Center for Environmental Research Information, 26 W. St. Clair St., Cincinatti, Ohio 45268. (513) 569-7941

A good practical manual for builders.

Radon, The Invisible Hazard, Michael LaFavore. Rodale Press, Emmaus, Pa., 1987.

An excellent and up to date book on all aspects of radon, presented in simple language.

Sound

Noise, Buildings and People, Derek Croome. Pergamon Press, Oxford, England, 1977.

A very thorough text on environmental engineering and noise control design in buildings.

Ventilation and Air Purification

The Sandia Report, Indoor Air Quality Handbook For Designers, Builders, and Users. U.S. Department of Energy, Sandia Labs.

Available from U.S. Government Publications Office, Washington D.C., 20402

Consumer Reports, "Air Filters." Jan 85.

Canadian Consumer, "Air Filters." Apr 86.

Water

Consumer Reports, "The Selling of Water." Sept 80.

Consumer Reports, "Water Filters." Feb 83.

Domestic Water Treatment, J. Lehr, T. Gass, et al. McGraw Hill, N.Y., 1980.

A technical guide to local water supply and treatment for home and farm.

INDEX